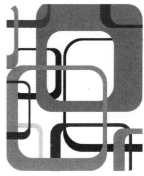

A Contemporary Approach to Substance Abuse and Addiction Counseling

A Counselor's Guide to Application and Understanding

Ford Brooks and Bill McHenry

AMERICAN COUNSELING ASSOCIATION
5999 Stevenson Avenue
Alexandria, VA 22304
www.counseling.org

A Contemporary Approach to Substance Abuse and Addiction Counseling

A Counselor's Guide to Application and Understanding

American Counseling Association
5999 Stevenson Avenue
Alexandria, VA 22304

Director of Publications
Carolyn C. Baker

Production Manager
Bonny E. Gaston

Editorial Assistant
Catherine A. Brumley

Copy Editor
Susan B. Klender

Cover and text design by Bonny E. Gaston.

Library of Congress Cataloging-in-Publication Data

Brooks, Ford.
A contemporary approach to substance abuse and addiction counseling : a counselor's guide to application and understanding/Ford Brooks and Bill McHenry.
    p. cm.
Includes bibliographical references and index.
ISBN 978-1-55620-282-7 (alk. paper)
1. Drug abuse counseling.   2. Alcoholism counseling.   3. Addicts—Counseling of.
4. Substance abuse.   5. Health counseling.   I. McHenry, Bill, 1971–   II. Title.

RC564.B74 2009
362.29'186—dc22   2008053753

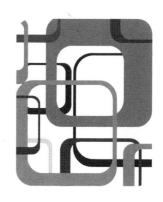

Table of Contents

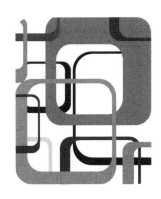

About the Authors

Ford Brooks, EdD, LPC, NCC, CAC, is an associate professor in the Department of Counseling and College Student Personnel at Shippensburg University of Pennsylvania. He coordinates the Clinical Mental Health Program as well as Practicum and Field Internships for the Counseling Department. Ford provides counseling, supervision, and training services to clients, supervisees, and agencies/schools in the South Central Region of Pennsylvania.

He received his doctorate in counseling from The College of William and Mary, his master of science degree in rehabilitation from Virginia Commonwealth University (with specialization in alcohol and drug counseling), and a bachelor of arts degree from the University of Richmond in psychology. Ford has been a professional counselor for over 23 years, working primarily with clients who suffer from addiction and co-occurring mental disorders. He has worked in hospital, inpatient and outpatient clinics, private practice, and university student affairs settings. Much of Ford's clinical work and writing has focused on relapse prevention and spirituality issues in addiction.

Bill McHenry, PhD, LPC, NCC, is an assistant professor of Counseling and College Student Personnel at Shippensburg University of Pennsylvania. He is the director of *Growing Edges*, which is the Shippensburg University Community Clinic. His doctorate is in counselor education from the University of South Dakota. He has been a professional counselor for 14 years. His professional experiences include working with clients (individuals, groups, couples, and families) with substance abuse/addiction issues in schools, universities, rehabilitation programs, mental health agencies, and college counseling centers.

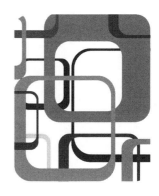

Acknowledgments

I (Ford) would like to thank Carolyn Baker for her work with this project and belief in our mission: to educate counselors on alcohol and drug issues. Her editorial comments were significant and useful in our revisions. Additionally, I would like to thank Susan Klender for her copy edits, Catherine Brumley for her editorial assistance, and Bonny Gaston for production and cover design. I would also like to thank our reviewers for the time and energy they gave to provide us constructive feedback. To my friend and colleague, Bill McHenry, I am eternally grateful for your help in getting this project off the ground and co-constructing a meaningful text. Without you this project would not have happened. Heartfelt thanks go to Dr. Jill Schultz for her feedback on preliminary chapters. Her encouragement and compassion were invaluable to the spirit of this book. Many thanks to brother Andrew Brooks for allowing me the space to write initial drafts of the text in his Forest City, Maine, abode; Marty and Linda Kurdt for their continual support with this project; and last but not least, to my wife Kathryn for her patience and endless sacrifice. Bill and I want to thank our graduate assistants Tomomi Kikkawa, Becky Eby, and Isaiah Varisano for their help in preparing the revised manuscript.

I've had the pleasure of working with many counselors and teachers over the years who have, in their own ways, contributed to this book and deserve recognition: Mary Moyer, Jay Douglas, Jay Maynard, Dennis Holman, Robert Johnson, Bill McDowell, Donnie Conner, Michael Weldon, Kathy Benham, Ron Forbes, M.D., Marcia Lawton, Charles Matthews, Father Martin, Bill Maher, Peter Coleman, M.D., Jim Leffler, Dan Evans, Shirley Near, Carolyn Carver, and Perry Campanella. Last, but certainly not least, I would like to thank the students, supervisees, and clients who have been so willing to share their journeys with me. It is for you this book was written.

I (Bill) would like to thank our editorial team, especially Carolyn Baker for believing in this project, supporting our work, and making the process smooth and professional through every turn. To the reviewers of our work, thank you for your insightful suggestions, clear direction, and respectful frames. You made our book better in many ways.

Thank you to my family for your support, guidance, and the peace you continue to provide in my life. Finally, I want to thank Ford for the opportunity to create this meaningful and important book. Throughout the process I was in constant awe of your patience, skill, knowledge, and respect for both our readers and the clients we serve.

Drug and Alcohol Counseling:
An Introduction

To the Fish and the Owl
The Alpha and the Omega
Synchronicity at the Time of Death
Brought Forth Life and Spirit
—Ford Brooks

A client presents during his intake evaluation that he is using three grams of cocaine four times a week and is about to lose his job, his marriage, and all of his life's savings because of his use. He is coming to you for help, yet is resistant to inpatient drug and alcohol treatment.

A 16-year-old female student is referred to you for "behavioral problems" in the classroom and was just suspended for smoking cigarettes in the bathroom. During the session you suspect she is under the influence of drugs.

A 60-year-old male comes in for issues of depression, yet during the session you detect the faint smell of alcohol.

In each of these cases, what would you do and how might you proceed? Working with clients who suffer from substance abuse and addiction problems is very challenging and at the same time can be very rewarding. As clinicians who have worked with this client population and counselor educators who teach this subject, we wish to convey information, suggestions, and strategies to best work with this clinical issue and population.

Our Stories

When I (Ford) started as a counselor in the drug and alcohol field, I struggled because I was a novice with only basic understanding of the requirements to work with drug and alcohol addicted clients. Despite being anointed a master's-level alcohol and drug rehabilitation counselor, I toiled and labored to understand the use of "self" in effecting positive change, especially with clients experiencing significant emotional and physical pain. I could not fully envision the power of compassion; nor could I fully grasp the negative presence *my* frustration could have on clients. I struggled to grasp how spontaneity and hope could possibly be as important as confrontation, urine screens, and alcohol and drug education.

When I (Bill) started working with clients who had drug and alcohol issues, I struggled. My previous counseling experiences were with *other* types of clients exhibiting *other* types of problems. I labored to effectively connect and make meaning of the stories of drug and alcohol clients. As I saw clients relapse, I saw failure; as I saw clients using again, I framed it as wrong. My dichotomous thinking regarding alcohol and drug clients retarded my general nature of believing in and valuing the *journey*.

The Counseling Relationship

One of the main reasons we wrote this text was to encourage readers to more fully engage in the helping process with drug and alcohol addicted clients. In essence, we hope to help you avoid our mistakes and to provide you with informative and creative approaches to working with this unique population of clients. We consider genuine compassion and deep understanding to be the core values manifested by effective counselors. We cannot stress this enough. Although such values are appreciated by many types of clients, we suggest that they are crucial in counseling clients who use drugs and alcohol.

The amount of shame, guilt, embarrassment, and terror that drug abusing and addicted clients feel can be beyond description. Therefore, clients need a sense of safety, understanding, and compassionate care in the counseling relationship in order to change and grow. My (Ford's) first supervisor described it as "loving your clients to wellness." I took her wisdom and found how clients responded and grew when I did just that, therapeutically loved them.

We want counselors reading this text to own this fact: *Your way of being in the therapeutic relationship impacts client growth*. Counselors bring to the therapeutic relationship a "self" (e.g., compassion, genuineness, spontaneity, and creativity), which is used as an instrument of change in the counseling relationship.

Carl Rogers (1957) suggested that certain counselor characteristics were necessary in the therapeutic relationship in order for clients to feel supported and begin the change process. He believed the counselor's ability to be genuine, express accurate empathy, and provide unconditional positive regard were significant in the foundation of counseling relationships. We agree with Rogers. Clients are well-served when counselors are authentic, accurately empathize and understand their clients' worldviews, and have compassion for their clients.

What helps maintain the helping attitude is for counselors to frame client anger, blame, and dishonesty as a function of survival in a chaotic, chemically induced world. By so doing, counselors can understand their clients' drug and alcohol use as an important *relationship* they will protect with whatever means possible. A genuine, truthful, and in-the-moment relationship allows clients to know, without question, that they are understood and cared for during their emotional pain and time of crisis. The connection that is forged between counselors and clients following a drug and alcohol crisis can be profound. In an effort to help empathize with drug and alcohol addicted clients, Gideon (1975) encouraged counselors to frame clients as disconnected, isolated (from self and others), and afraid. He emphasized the value of understanding clients' experiences and creating an environment of trust and safety.

One way such a relationship can transcend technique is as follows: Clients, who for years have been isolated in addiction and reveal for the first time how sad and depressed they have felt, can immediately begin to experience a sense of relief and connection after sharing their torment with an understanding human being. Genuine and authentic counselors increase the likelihood of engaging with their clients in a trusting, therapeutic relationship, which can result in clients attempting change with new behaviors (W. R. Miller & Rollnick, 2002).

Counselors who are *truly with* clients during these low points (perhaps to depths that many people will never approach) are privileged to hear such astonishing stories. Therefore, we suggest counselors need to both realize and appreciate the courage it takes to share such pain after *so* much isolation. Please pause for a moment and consider the previous message. We encourage you to reflect on the strength, bravery, and perhaps enormous pain clients go through as they share their stories. Recognize this: You are uniquely quali-fied to provide *your* distinct gifts, talents, and compassion for the human spirit.

Mistaken Images of Drug and Alcohol Addicted Clients

We suggest counselors assess for and then address those biases they might have with clients who use, abuse, and are addicted to alcohol and drugs. For some counselors, terms of *substance abuser*, *alcoholic*, or *addict* may conjure strong negative images of individuals nursing inexpensive bottles of liquor wrapped in a brown paper bag, or gaunt, unkempt folks with needle marks and bloody clothing, or maybe young students struggling in school because of their marijuana use. It should be noted, however, that the majority of drug and alcohol ad-dicted individuals hide their use, are indistinguishable from nonusers most of the time, and function in society, albeit at times under the influence.

For many counselors, the field of drug and alcohol counseling harbors a challenging and perplexing population. Such a frame on the part of a counselor can mitigate the de-velopment of both a helping attitude and an open, compassionate heart. Remaining open and compassionate can be particularly difficult when clients become angry, minimize their alcohol and drug use, or seemingly lack motivation in treatment–goal follow-through. Without counselors developing a well-thought helping attitude, clients are many times blamed and labeled as *resistant*. Paradoxically, such reactions by counselors typically yield an increased defensiveness from the client, where the resistance is in response to both the counselor and the counseling approach (here we suggest to the reader that this is similar to a self-fulfilling prophecy by the *counselor)*. What counselors want to create is a helping attitude, which includes the following seemingly paradoxical attitudes: to be supportive yet questioning, to be unconditionally present yet at times direct, and to possess an overall attitude of realistic optimism.

Establishing a Genuine Helping Relationship

A starting point may be for counselors to foster a helping attitude when working with cli-ents who use and are addicted to alcohol and drugs. This is evident when the counselor's personal exploration of bias has entered the therapeutic process. One example is a counsel-or who is angry and disgusted by a heroin-using client. This counselor, with all the desire to be helpful and effective, will have substantial difficulty in developing a helping attitude. However, if this same counselor comes to understand and respect the nature of abuse and addiction, and can empathize with the client's emotional suffering, a helping attitude is possible. Counselors need to maintain this respectful and helpful attitude. One way to do this is to continue to develop knowledge and understanding in the area of use of drugs and alcohol. For example, as counselors realize the powerful effects of narcotics coupled with an understanding of the client's life in relation to heroin, empathy and ongoing support on behalf of the counselor is possible (through both the good times and bad moments).

Another effective procedure is to unlearn previous lessons, notions, and knowledge. Start fresh with *Zen Mind, Beginner's Mind* (Suzuki, 2006). This approach views each cli-ent interaction as new and interesting. For counselors to see with fresh eyes each day, the mental approach of the beginner's mind can also be effective in maintaining a helping attitude and demonstrating empathy. How many times are counselors handed a case file three inches thick only to be told sarcastically by the staff, "Good luck"? Counselors want to approach clients as if it were their first time in counseling, otherwise counselor bias and prejudice ensure this assuming failure. The beginner's mind is curious and open to all client messages and pieces of the story yet to be told. This curiosity and open-minded attitude staves off counselor apathy or fatigue, while facilitating the development of new strategies to increase therapeutic effectiveness.

First, we hope you find our writing style comfortable and that you benefit from the book's construction. We've approached writing this text the way in which we work with clients: as genuine and as clear as possible. We've found that counselors-in-training and counselors tend to be intimidated and fearful of working with clients who abuse and are addicted to alcohol and drugs. Counselors-in-training sometimes discount their own skills and assets in effecting change when they are not recovering themselves. This is very unfortunate. In response to such concerns, we believe we've created a body of information that will increase awareness and knowledge while reducing the amount of apprehension in working with this population.

Significant Aspects of This Book

Relapse prevention, developmental issues, spirituality, and ecological aspects of life are significant aspects of this book. Because addiction is relapse prone, we have devoted an entire chapter to relapse prevention. Included are methods of working with developmental "stuck points" during the clients' process of getting sober and clean. For example, approaching clients who have relapsed for the third time is clinically different from working with clients who have entered treatment for the first time. The work of Terence Gorski (1989) has significantly contributed to relapse prevention treatment with addicted clients. In addition to his model, our text also takes into consideration co-occurring disorders (both emotional and physical), environment (family and community), gender/cultural/diversity issues, and spiritual/faith/support issues. Relapse prevention focuses on connecting patterns of behavior that can lead to the use of drugs and alcohol after a period of abstinence. Identification of patterns helps clients examine their developmental deficits, which contribute to relapse.

Developmental life pattern analysis, a rarely identified and explored aspect to recovery work, can contribute significantly to therapeutic planning. Clients' life patterns originate from developmental deficits within the first years of life. From such origins, clients create methods of coping, which may include isolation and disconnection. In adult life, these same coping skills impede client success in the recovery process by blocking connection with others and maintaining the disconnection from feelings.

Also in this text is the intertwining of spirituality in the recovery process. Although there is some debate and disagreement by helping professionals on the issue of spirituality in the treatment of addiction, the majority of treatment centers in the United States continue to use the 12 steps of Alcoholics Anonymous (AA), a spiritually oriented program of recovery. The debate has led to the creation of various and varied support groups, which are highlighted in this text.

In addition to relapse prevention, developmental perspectives, and spirituality, we present a community counseling approach based on the ecological model of Bronfenbrenner (1976, 1988). His approach offers a multicultural and community perspective that can be blended with treatment and prevention planning. Whether those reading this text are working in schools, colleges, community/outpatient centers, companies, or hospital settings, the information available here can be applied and used in these settings. Because counselors work in a variety of clinical venues and with all age groups, we've provided information that is specific to each counseling genre.

For Whom This Book Is Written

- *For counselors-in-training.* For those new to the profession and still in the process of obtaining a degree, we cover alcohol and drug clients and options for treatment. We have provided the necessary information to effectively work in a variety of settings with clients who have addiction or substance abuse problems.

- *For counselors and counselors-in-training looking for employment in the addiction treatment continuum.* Many students, undergraduate and graduate alike, who want to work in the alcohol and drug treatment field are not necessarily clear where on the substance-abuse-helping continuum they would like to work. The continuum of substance abuse care includes detoxification, intensive outpatient treatment, inpatient care, as well as halfway house and long-term residential treatment. Students may also find themselves working in school-based assistance programs in which prevention, intervention, and education are vital components of client care. This book outlines and describes the variety of treatment modalities in existence today and explores the specific tasks and responsibilities of each modality.
- *For counselors currently working in drug and alcohol treatment.* Current drug and alcohol counselors will find the models of recovery, approaches to relapse prevention, and information on spirituality helpful in treating clients from a holistic perspective. Because group counseling is a primary modality of alcohol and drug treatment, group counseling and the therapeutic factors that occur in group are presented.
- *For counselors currently working in school, mental health, and college settings.* In some cases, clients may arrive for counseling services in these settings as the result of a precipitating event not necessarily labeled drug or alcohol related. In other cases, clients may seek help specifically to discuss their drug and alcohol use. The latter group may not necessarily be motivated in discontinuing their use, but rather, would like to cut back or control their consumption of drugs and alcohol. In either case, counselors need to understand both the assessment process and how to work effectively with clients who are ambivalent about their alcohol and drug usage. Referring alcohol and drug clients to structured treatment may not be appropriate, feasible, or possible. So what might counselors do?

In this text, we explore questions counselors need to be asking in such instances and provide information on drug terminology. Further, we present interviewing techniques to increase client motivation and change.

Overview of the Book

The remaining pages of this chapter outline the topics and information found in chapters 2–14. Brief in description, they provide counselors-in-training and counselors an understanding of each chapter and are constructed to be used as a quick reference.

Chapter 2: Diversity Issues in Substance Abuse Treatment

This chapter explores cultural and gender issues, including issues faced by gay, lesbian, bisexual, and transgendered (GLBT) clients as they relate to alcohol and drug treatment and relapse prevention. Historically, addiction treatment did not address issues of race/culture, gender, or diversity. Notably, AA was co-founded and develped by two White, European American males, which resulted in the use of the male pronoun in much of AA's initial writings. Because significantly high proportions of women entering alcohol and drug treatment have been sexually, emotionally, or physically abused, a section on women's issues is included in this chapter. These issues are reviewed, and options to facilitate effective planning with substance abusing and addicted women are addressed. Additionally, cultural awareness and race issues with alcohol and drug clients are explored. GLBT clients find difficulty in discussing their lives in alcohol and drug treatment as well as in support meetings, so methods and strategies on how to help these clients in treatment are addressed. In addition, clinical work with elderly clients and those clients with physical disabilities are explored in this chapter.

This chapter prepares counselors to understand the worldview of all clients in the counseling process. Throughout the text, multicultural, gender, and diversity vignettes with questions for discussion are presented.

Chapter 3: Types of Drugs and Their Effects

An overview of the varied drug classifications is provided in this chapter along with possible clinical interventions. Alcohol, stimulants and other amphetamines, marijuana, barbiturates, benzodiazepines, opiates, hallucinogens, inhalants, steroids, over-the-counter, and sedative-hypnotics are addressed. The signs and symptoms of intoxication and withdrawal risks and factors are also included. The concept of synergism (the impact of multiple drugs and how they potentiate each other), cross-addiction (addiction to drugs in different categories), and cross-tolerance (tolerance to drugs in the same category) are outlined. Included are descriptions of the psychotropic medications used in treating other mental disorders and the interplay with addiction treatment. Professional literature and information on each category is presented, with emphasis on application to the counseling setting. Counselors will be informed on the many classifications and the drugs in each category and the implications for treatment and referral.

Chapter 4: Assessment, Diagnosis, and Interview Techniques

This chapter presents information on various alcohol and drug assessment instruments that can be used during the substance abuse/dependency assessment. The use of motivational interviewing (MI) techniques, as developed by W. R. Miller and Rollnick (2002) are included to help counselors work with initial client resistance and ambivalence to counseling. Also in this chapter is a thorough description of the diagnostic criteria stated in the *Diagnostic and Statistical Manual of Mental Disorders* (American Psychiatric Association, 2000; *DSM–IV–TR*) and the differentiation between substance abuse and dependency.

Of significance is a description of how to effectively and accurately diagnose clients suffering from a co-occurring diagnosis, including suggestions for working with a variety of personality-disordered substance abusers. Because clients rarely have a single substance abuse/dependency diagnosis, a general understanding of the various mental disorders, along with knowledge of substance abuse/dependency criteria is necessary for accurate treatment planning. Depending on the counselor's work setting, accurate diagnosis can be a challenge. More specifically, the issue of how to develop an effective treatment team, even if the psychiatric resources are not in the counselor's setting, is discussed. The chapter explores issues such as when and where to refer, how to use drug testing and breathalyzers, and the use of external data and therapeutic leverage in the counseling process. After reading this chapter the counselor will be able to understand resistance, have a clear understanding of the diagnostic criteria in differentiating between abuse and dependency, and will be familiar with approaches to improving an accurate psychiatric diagnosis.

Chapter 5: Continuum of Nonuse to Addiction: A Biopsychosocial Understanding

This chapter reviews the biopsychosocial approach to addiction and helps readers understand more clearly the process of how clients move from nonuse to addiction. Additionally, information on genetics, as well as environmental/social and cultural perspectives, is explored and why some individuals appear more susceptible to addiction than others. Counselors will begin to understand the unique challenges that counselors face when working with this population. Building on the previous chapter, we apply MI techniques to case scenarios in order for the reader to understand the application of MI in the continuum.

Prevention models are described in terms of their application on or along the continuum of substance use or abuse (i.e., clients who have not yet used alcohol/drugs, clients who have used alcohol/drugs on occasion but are not yet dependent [at-risk], and those clients presenting multiple consequences and a history of alcohol/drug problems with or without symptoms of addiction). Significant to this chapter is information on how to appropriately match prevention strategies in helping clients at various points in the continuum. After reading this chapter the counselor should be able to understand the continuum of use to addiction and the appropriate application of prevention ideology. A graph is provided for readers to understand the continuum and how the stages of change (Prochaska & DiClemente, 1982; Prochaska, DiClemente, & Norcross, 1992), along with the work of Bronfenbrenner (1976, 1988), can be woven into a conceptual framework to work with clients.

Chapter 6: Treatment and Treatment Settings

Although many readers may not be alcohol and drug counselors specifically, this chapter helps counselors understand their role in the treatment process. A variety of work settings are discussed (e.g., secondary schools, college, and adult populations) as well as the implications for treatment and making the appropriate referral. An in-depth description of detoxification and inpatient treatment as well as outpatient and partial hospitalization programs are included. This understanding of the varied levels of treatment along the continuum (detoxification, outpatient, inpatient, partial hospitalization, halfway house) provides counselors with an in-depth view of what occurs in treatment. For many counselors, the alcohol and drug treatment process is misunderstood, and because of this a description of what occurs in treatment is presented. This understanding in turn will aid counselors in making accurate referrals and helping families and clients understand what to expect from treatment.

Additionally, this chapter focuses on how alcohol and drug treatment (external process) impacts the internal process of clients. A description of how counselors work with client defenses, denial and resistance, and how counselors help clients move from isolation to connection with others is provided. This chapter also provides counselors with an understanding of how they can help clients to verbalize their feelings, which is an important aspect of the healing process. After reading this chapter, counselors should understand what occurs in treatment, how treatment impacts clients, and what potentially unfolds internally for clients. From this chapter counselors may be able to create an approach unique to their settings and, at the same time, be aware of when to refer clients to a more intensive level of treatment depending on their needs.

Chapter 7: Developmental Approaches in Treating Addiction

Helping clients move from denial to awareness generally takes a great deal of facilitation and patience on the part of the counselor, as well as a tremendous amount of pain and suffering for the client. This chapter specifically addresses that internal client development from denial to awareness. The developmental model of recovery developed by Terence Gorski (1989) and Stephanie Brown's (1985) model of recovery are presented, along with William Gideon's (1975) approach from isolation to connectedness. The chapter identifies the stage goals in helping clients move, for instance, from the "drinking stage" to the "transition stage" in recovery. Counselors will understand the process for clients as they potentially move from use to nonuse and all the aspects of developmental surfacing that occur in recovery. Suggestions for counselors on how to help clients move from isolation to connectedness are also an aspect of the chapter.

Chapter 8: Family and Addiction

This chapter focuses on family development, the roles that are created in the family, the issues of family denial, and the systemic problems that arise from active addiction in the family. A connection between the cognitive framework of the addicted person and the denial of the family is made, as well as how to approach the family system. Suggestions are made on how to join with family members at their systemic level of development and how to appropriately address enabling behaviors. Counselors reading this chapter will be able to assess where clients may be in the recovery models presented and how to best approach and work with clients and their families.

Chapter 9: Grief and Loss in Addiction

This chapter describes the connection between clients' grief and loss issues and their use/abuse/addiction to substances. Models of grief and loss are reviewed, focusing on the direct and indirect mergers with substances. Special attention is paid to the synergistic relationship that feeds both the use patterns and reactions to loss for individuals. Potential proactive and therapeutic responses are provided to aid in working with the complications that grief and loss issues can have with clients abusing, addicted to, or in recovery.

Chapter 10: Group Counseling and Addiction

This chapter outlines and reviews numerous aspects of group work with alcohol and drug abusing and addicted clients. The appropriate use of confrontation and support and the importance of bringing the group into the here and now are explored. The use of process comments in a group and the integration of other skills are presented. Emphasis is placed on describing a variety of counseling group scenarios and how counselors can effectively intervene. Of particular note is the presentation of Yalom's (2005) therapeutic factors in a group. A discussion revisits a previous chapter concerning the various levels of care and how group approaches in these various settings can be different. As a result of reading this chapter, counselors should understand group development, process/content, the integration of 12-step recovery into groups, how to address denial, and the use of self as a counselor in the group counseling process.

Chapter 11: Relapse Prevention and Recovery

There is a significant difference between alcohol and drug treatment and relapse prevention treatment. Alcohol and drug treatment is structured for clients who have not previously entered a treatment program. Relapse prevention treatment, however, works with clients who have been through multiple alcohol and drug treatment experiences and who are admitting their addiction, yet are unable to stay sober/clean for any length of time without relapsing. This chapter reviews models of relapse prevention and the difficulties counselors face when treating this special population within a special population. This chapter introduces readers to the relapse dynamic and describes how to approach this population through mental, emotional, behavioral, and spiritual counseling techniques.

Cognitive therapeutic approaches are central in understanding the core beliefs of clients that contribute to relapse. Relapsing clients tend to be impulsive and compulsive and as a result need attention to daily decision-making skills. Time is spent in this chapter outlining effective ways clients can avoid making poor decisions, which ultimately lead to relapse. When clients relapse, the emotional issues that surface (e.g., depression, the shame of the relapse, self-hatred, and suicidal issues) need to be addressed.

In this chapter, counselors are informed on how to best help clients cope with a relapse. Also covered in this chapter is the importance of support meetings, identification of leisure activities, use of homework, and application of the 12 steps, as well as an overall examination of physical well-being.

Chapter 12: Spirituality and Support Groups in Recovery

This chapter explores spirituality and how it factors into recovery. The 12 steps of AA and the literature on spirituality are examined in order to help the clinician understand this aspect of recovery. This chapter brings together the 12-step philosophy of AA and the significant and vital impact that support groups factor into the recovery process. In addition to AA, other support groups such as Women for Sobriety and the Secular Organization for Sobriety are explored in order to provide counselors information when they have clients looking for alternatives to the 12-step program. Ideas on how to explore spirituality with clients as well as questions for counselors on this topic are brought forth for discussion. As a result, counselors reading this chapter will understand the integration of mind, emotion, behavior, and spirit into a comprehensive recovery plan.

Chapter 13: Addictions Training, Certification, and Ethics

In this chapter, various ethical codes, both from an association and certification viewpoint and the federal/state regulations regarding confidential records, are compared and contrasted. Also included are discussions concerning the recovering counselor and the issues of countertransference. Ethical issues concerning dual relationships, burnout prevention, and boundary setting are also explored. Ethical decision making with respect to appropriate treatment interventions is an important aspect for counselors to review and thus is an aspect of this chapter. The 2009 Council for Accreditation of Counseling and Related Educational Programs *Standards for Addiction Counseling* are found in Appendix 13.A at the end of the chapter. We've included this so students can identify the knowledge, skills, and abilities required for counseling clients and families with addiction problems. After most of the individual lines in the *Standards*, we've placed chapter numbers to aid readers in finding related material in our text.

Chapter 14: The Importance of Counselor Self-Care

Counselors working with this population truly need personal plans of self-care. Time is spent in this important chapter on the development and maintenance of counselor well-being through the use of personal counseling, supervision, and other suggested activities.

Summary

At the end of each chapter we've provided exploration questions that can be used in classes and suggested activities that can help the reader experientially understand the concepts presented in each chapter.

Exploration Questions From Chapter 1

1. What are the motivations for you to be a counselor?
2. What challenges, biases, or prejudices might you have when working with those addicted to drugs and alcohol?
3. What do you hope to gain by reading this text?
4. How might you implement ideas from this book?
5. Do you know of anyone personally who has struggled with addiction? What was it like for you?

Suggested Activities

1. Begin a journal to record your emotions as you read this text and attend your class on addiction studies. Record which emotions come up for you after attending class and completing reading assignments.
2. Attend at least two support meetings (e.g., AA, Narcotics Anonymous, Al-Anon, Nar-Anon, Secular Organization for Sobriety, Women for Sobriety) while reading this text and record your experiences and whether you would refer a client to any of the meetings you attended.

Diversity Issues in
Substance Abuse Treatment

I t is difficult for a single chapter to embrace, honor, celebrate, and inform students on multicultural, gender, and diversity issues pertaining to alcohol and drug counseling. We strongly suggest that multicultural counseling is deeply woven into every counseling relationship.

In this chapter you will be introduced to various worldviews, cultures, and experiences of alcohol- and drug-using clients and learn how these aspects of their identity significantly affect their therapeutic work with counselors. Presented here is a springboard of selected literature focused on infusing multiculturalism with addictions counseling. Throughout the text, gender-, cultural-, and diversity-related vignettes and questions for discussion are presented. Note, however, that *all counseling is multicultural.*

The spirit of this chapter continues further throughout the text. Our intent is to emphasize the value of connecting multicultural awareness to each and every aspect of counseling alcohol and drug addicted clients by intertwining vignettes that parallel current thought on multicultural and diversity training. Aspects of working with older persons and people with disabilities are explored later in the chapter.

The Role of Multicultural Awareness in Addiction Treatment

The addiction treatment field has learned over time that one treatment approach does not work with all clients, particularly in the area of relapse prevention. *One size does not fit all.* We want to pass this important lesson on to you. Unfortunately, most clients who abuse substances enter treatment, and regardless of their ethnic group, tend to receive the same treatment approach (Straussner, 2002). As such, the attention to worldview, culture, and diversity of clients has, until recently, been lacking. The imposition of treatment approaches, some of which may actually dishonor client culture, onto clients without understanding their ecological frame of reference ultimately can create resistance and disconnection from counselors and the overall treatment process (Sue & Sue, 2008).

Historically, alcohol and drug treatment providers used traditional approaches to substance abuse, which were developed by and for European American males (L. Schmidt, 1996). Terence Gorski, a nationally known relapse prevention specialist, concluded that 80–90% of his African American clients were discontinuing attendance in aftercare groups. He also recognized that a majority of the treatment programs around the area where he worked were structured and based on the assumption of clients being middle-class males

("Clinicians Add Cultural Element," 1998). This fact continues to support the current data that ethnic minorities may be more likely to drop out of treatment prematurely (King & Canada, 2004).

In addition to typical complications of treatment (e.g., self-pay vs. insurance, mandated vs. self-referred, outpatient vs. inpatient, relapse vs. first time in treatment), research suggests that many minority clients discontinue counseling or treatment after one session, which means counselors need to be culturally competent enough to develop rapport quickly (Sue & Sue, 2008). In addition to competence is the increased awareness of general racial and gender disparities as far as access to health care that disproportionately affects African Americans (Institute of Medicine, 2003). Community programs offering substance abuse services need to have counselors who match the majority of the cultural population being served. Education and training programs in addiction counseling need to be actively recruiting ethnoculturally diverse students to work within local, state, and regional communities. We want counselors reading this book to recognize that managed care, for example, has caused some good and some difficulty for our field. One good thing we believe is that it has focused us to hone our skills to effect change more quickly and with more precision.

An important distinction must be made between the therapeutic value of culture and an excessive amount of energy and time focused on differences. In our experience, the true sense of what is helpful or not is felt between the client and counselor. Such a distinction (generally) is as follows: Attention to cultural attributes is necessary, but too much focus can limit the attention paid to the addiction. According to Williams, race must be taken into consideration during treatment, yet he has cautioned counselors that race shouldn't become the sole focus of treatment (see Figure 2.1). Although important, he has further stated that addicted clients would rather talk about anything but their chemical use ("Clinicians Add Cultural Element," 1998).

Research has indicated that clients who attend culturally appropriate programs do better in treatment (L. Schmidt, 1996). An important and often overlooked piece is for both the staff and the program components to represent the client population they are serving (L. Schmidt, 1996). One example that highlights such representation might be the desire of African American clients to have African American counselors and staff to relate to culturally. Such suggestions highlight the strong need for counselors and agencies to honor diversity. In doing this, counselors must be aware of their own limited frame of reference, be aware of and acknowledge their clients' racial issues, and work therapeutically with them to explore their experiences (L. Schmidt, 1996).

What this means for educational training programs, treatment facilities, and clinics is the need for ongoing systematic multicultural training along with intentional hiring of counselors from varied cultural and ethnic backgrounds (Smith, 2004; Vacc, DeVaney, & Brendel, 2003). Although the primary focus of treatment is substance abuse, cultural diversity must be factored into creating a safe and supportive setting for client growth. Of course, such a setting may vary depending on the particular needs of the client. Therefore, in some instances, other helpers may be called upon to bridge ethnic, cultural, and racial gaps between the counselor/agency and the client (Ivey & Ivey, 2008). Examples of such community resources include spiritual healers, medicine men, and clergy.

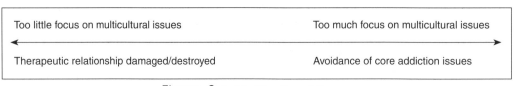

Figure 2.1. Multicultural Focus

Toward Multicultural Competence

The Association for Multicultural Counseling and Development, a division within the American Counseling Association, developed and promotes a set of multicultural competencies for counselors to achieve in order to most effectively help culturally diverse clients. Counselors seeking to understand their own cultural experience and the ethnic background with which they identify is one of the first steps toward achieving multicultural competency (Diller, 2004; Ivey & Ivey, 2008). Counselors need to understand their own cultural values and recognize how they can be projected on clients from other cultural backgrounds. Numerous authors have suggested counselors make an effort toward increasing values and cultural orientation self-awareness while working through the pains of societal oppression, which may impact them personally (Hulnick, 1977; Ivey & Ivey, 2008; Murphy & Dillon, 2008). These personal insights typically yield increased empathy and understanding of the clients they serve. Corey (2005), Diller (2004), and Fukuyama (1990) suggested that counselors envision culture as a whole and pay particular attention to its influence on self, society, and the helping process. They encouraged counselors to obtain a balance between transcultural counseling (i.e., commonalities across cultures) and culture-specific awareness. We have also found in our clinical work that such information cannot be acquired in a class or two, but that learning about different cultures and individuals within the cultures is a life-long journey.

The following are important areas (i.e., culture, ethnicity, ethnoculture, and individualism and collectivism) of understanding for counselors as they become multiculturally aware and competent (Sue & Sue, 2008).

Culture

"Culture consists of commonalities around which people have developed values, norms, family life-styles, social roles, and behaviors in response to historical, political, economic, and social realities" (Christensen, 1989, p. 275). Culture is also described by Devore and Schlesinger (1996) as a concept that is very challenging to define because human groups differ in the way they structure their behavior, worldviews, perspectives on the rhythms and patterns of life, and in their frameworks of the essential nature of the human condition. Culture then is the compilation of values and the patterns in life shared by individuals within a given community (Straussner, 2002). In a broader context culture includes ethnicity, race, and various other factors that help counselors better understand their clients' frame of experience.

Ethnicity

The term *ethnicity* refers to "the sense of commonality transmitted over generations by the family and reinforced by the surrounding community" (McGoldrick, Giordano, & Pearce, 1996, p. 4). Straussner (2002) suggested that the concept of culture is global whereas ethnicity is more specific and refers to the notion that members of an ethnic community share common identity, ideals, aspirations, and a sense of continuity. He further contended that counselors working with substance-abusing clients need to focus on both the specific ethnicity as well as the broader cultural context and become ethnoculturally competent.

Multicultural and Ethnocultural Counseling

Multicultural counseling is identified as any counseling relationship in which the participants represent differing ethnic or minority groups (i.e., counselor and client) (Atkinson, Morten, & Sue, 1993; Smith, 2004; Vacc et al., 2003). Ethnocultural counseling is defined as the ability of a clinician to function effectively in the context of ethnocultural differences. It moves beyond "cultural sensitivity" and includes awareness and acceptance of ethnic and cultural differences which need to be explored respectfully, without judgment, but with curiosity. (Straussner, 2002, p. 35)

We suggest that *all counseling is multicultural counseling* because while sharing commonalities, each individual retains a significant degree of uniqueness. Effective multicultural counseling requires the following:

Acknowledgement and acceptance of differences, regardless of ethnicity, culture, sexual orientation, socioeconomic status, religion, etc.

Respect and reverence of all human beings, while having a genuine stance that is *Without judgment,* because when we judge, we elevate ourselves, and potentially become the oppressor.

With a passionate curiosity in the heart and soul searching for understanding in the spirit of knowing.

Individualism and Collectivism

Individualism refers to a primary focus on the individual as opposed to the group. Collectivism emphasizes the entire group (Murphy & Dillon, 2008; Okun, Fried, & Okun, 1999). Counselors whose backgrounds stem from an individualistic culture may value autonomy and independence rather than the focus on interdependence and the importance of group involvement for survival (Smith, 2004). Individualistic cultures include most of Europe and North America, where hierarchy and power are found through individual efforts and achievement. Collectivism characterizes the cultures of most Asian, Arabic, and African countries. Our work has taught us also that when we mix in family culture, these are not dichotomous poles but rather a continuum. We find that attending to such "unique" aspects of a client is necessary in understanding who he or she really is.

Case Example: The Lost Opportunity

A male European American counselor is working in an outpatient drug and alcohol treatment program with a client who is an African American female addicted to crack cocaine and living with her physically abusive boyfriend. The counselor is not culturally aware and attempts to impose unknowingly onto the client his values of hard work, self-control, and individualism. He infers to his client that she needs to immediately get clean from cocaine, leave her boyfriend, and obtain employment. All of these suggestions, of course, make perfect sense from the worldview of the counselor. What he fails to understand is the environment and culture in which she was and is living. She was raised in a family where physical abuse was common; however, despite such upbringings, she felt loved and taken care of. Her father, who was an alcoholic, was also a financial provider and instilled in the family the importance of staying together. Additionally, the town where she grew up had very few job opportunities, the school system provided minimal education and vocational training, and because she had a large family, she took care of her siblings and at times missed school. To this client, her family and community have been very important in her life thus far.

The counselor's background is quite different. He grew up in a White, middle-class environment with an excellent school system, which provided many occupational training opportunities. Following high school, both parents were supportive and contributed significantly to his education and training to become a counselor. His family believes individual achievement, hard work, and financial stability are truly the measures of success.

Unless the counselor is sensitive, aware, and willing to understand his client's environment, cultural background, and familial rules and values, he will impose his values onto her as well as other clients. His approach, in turn, fosters her already low self-esteem and feelings of hopelessness, which may ultimately contribute to her dropping out of treatment. As well-intentioned as this counselor may be, all of his knowledge about addiction (and suggestions about recovery) may go unheard if she won't return for the next session because of his imposed values. Too many times, a client in such a situation is blamed by the pronouncement, "Well, she just wasn't ready to stop using." Although that may be true, the counselor's approach may be seen to have alienated the client rather than to have begun creating an encouraging and constructive relationship.

Paradoxically, the harder this counselor tries to drive home the points he hopes to make about living a better life, the more apt the client may be to move away from his services, and perhaps counseling altogether. Good intentions are one thing, while effective counseling is another. The apparent missing piece from this case is the counselor spending some important time reflecting on and understanding his own values (and how they may surface with clients).

Spirit of Multicultural Counseling

Awareness of multiple cultures and their unique characteristics allows counselors to develop cultural empathy, which in turn can positively impact therapy (Okun et al., 1999; Pedersen, 2003; Sue & Sue, 2008). Through what is known as an advancing "spirit of counseling," a professional counselor can embrace learning about other cultures while constantly self-examining and reviewing his/her own cultural background (Ivey & Ivey, 2008; Sue & Sue, 2008). It is incumbent upon counselors to be open, curious, and willing to learn how alcohol and drugs are viewed within particular cultures (Stevens & Smith, 2005). For example, in some regions in the world, the primary crop is not soy or corn or wheat, but rather marijuana or poppy plants. Clients from such regions may embrace such "illegal" drugs as a necessary part of their family's and culture's existence. Failing to recognize this may lead the counselor to unintentionally dishonor and disgrace the client. In sum, cultural customs, norms, and traditions vary from country to country and region to region; therefore, counselors need to be ever vigilant about stereotyping clients and cultures.

Cultural competence, otherwise known as *cultural empathy*, is important in understanding where a counselor is in regard to multicultural drug and alcohol counseling (Castro, Proescholdbell, Abeita, & Rodriguez, 1999). What follows are the basic tenets of a model by Castro et al. (1999).

The lowest stage in cultural competence development is *culturally destructive*. Counselors in this stage are characterized by negative approaches and attitudes toward clients of different cultures and are not sensitive to cultural issues. The counselor in the previous vignette serves as a clear example of a culturally destructive counselor. Because we are counselor educators as well as practitioners, classroom discussions with students have educated us on the fact that often times, *destructive* thoughts about groups or cultures may be present in our students. We strongly suggest that counselors explore this aspect of self and work toward addressing hidden or overt attitudes.

The next level is that of *cultural incapacity*, where counselors may separate clients on the basis of culture, believing clients will not benefit from conventional treatment. Because clients may need assistance with language interpretation or other cultural issues, clients may be separated into a remedial form of treatment. Similar segregation also occurs in mental health facilities where higher and lower functioning clients are separated. The recommendation for counselors is to treat clients equally while addressing specific needs of the clients in those groups.

Castro et al. (1999) cited *cultural blindness* as the next stage in which counselors believe everyone is equal and that one size fits all. Such thinking allows counselors to avoid cultural variations. The mantra is, "If everyone is equal, then we don't need to discuss the differences." Sometimes this results from counselors not understanding the impact of culture on treatment, while other times it results from counselors trying to simplify the case to one or two basic issues (as opposed to respecting the multitude of significant variables within each case). Our students have taught us that this belief typically comes from a good place, but can be powerfully blinding to the fabric of the true story of the client.

The next level, *cultural competency*, is where counselors are open and willing to explore cultural differences, mores, norms, and customs, yet their understanding is limited. Cultural competency is attained when counselors are fully aware of the culture in which they are working and feel as though they can truly empathize with the client of that culture.

Finally, *cultural proficiency* (along with the skills and assets in cultural competency) is the result of extensive study, immersion in a variety of cultures, and personal cultural reflection and exploration.

These stages, as outlined by Castro et al. (1999), provide counselors with guidelines for multicultural development so important in effective, ethical, and appropriate treatment. Then counselors can appreciate and embrace culture, ethnicity, and gender in the counseling process as well as their importance in developing a therapeutic relationship.

The rest of this chapter is devoted to the basic understanding of various distinct groups as well as older persons and people with disabilities. A word of caution, however: We do not suggest you compartmentalize the groups that follow; nor do we suggest that reading the following sections counts as advanced study in this area. Clients are unique with myriad variables. A 48-year-old African American, heterosexual male raised in an upper-middle-class neighborhood outside Chicago will have a different worldview than a 48-year-old African American, lesbian woman raised in an upper-middle-class neighborhood outside Chicago. Of course, the differences found between these clients go far beyond sexual orientation and gender. We believe (in most cases) that the best source of understanding the dynamics, strengths, and presence of a specific culture is the client.

With that in mind, in the sections that follow, we explore African American, Latino, Asian American, Pacific Islander, and Native American ethnic groups in relation to counseling and substance abuse. The aspects of counseling women and men and the importance of understanding the differences are critical to effective and ethical care. In addition, the sexual orientation of clients can factor significantly into relapse and recovery efforts.

Note: We offer the following sections as primers for you to start your journey toward increasing your own personal awareness in working with special and diverse populations. We have covered many of the predominant minority groups identified within the dominant White culture. Though the sections differ in length, the spirit of our work is the larger view that all counseling is a multicultural experience.

In working with diverse populations, we have found it important for counselors to understand the following overarching beliefs. Counselors need to know and accept the client and understand the socioeconomic issues of the client (Ivey & Ivey, 2008). Clients must not be perceived stereotypically (Sue & Sue, 2008). In addition, counselors must avoid assuming the acculturation of clients into White, middle-class society (Pedersen, 2003). Rather, they must help clients set goals for themselves in the context of their own lives (Ivey & Ivey, 2008). Counselors must create an open and safe environment, never exposing a client in a group setting but exploring on a one-to-one basis. Professionals should also be aware of and acknowledge cultural pain, which stems from an oppressed society. Finally, counselors who address racial and ethnic issues in treatment enhance the relationship with their clients (Smith, 2004). However, although cultural issues are a layer in good treatment, the main issue is still chemical dependency.

African American Clients and Addiction Treatment

A survey of 200 African Americans in recovery conducted by Roland Williams revealed the following: Of those surveyed, 45% cited race as a factor in substance use relapse. Forty-eight percent believed they have more relapse triggers because they are African American and that those triggers are related to racism. Of the respondents, 39% said they experienced a lot of racism in recovery, 28% said they did not feel welcomed in 12-step meetings and that there were fewer persons of color, and 37% said there were not enough African American role models in recovery. Finally, those surveyed said they had difficulty finding sponsors of color and observed very few counselors of color working in treatment programs specific to clients of color ("Clinicians Add Cultural Element," 1998). It is clear through Williams's survey that the impact of racism and lacking role models can contribute to the relapse cycle.

These results highlight the need for counselors to understand how socioeconomic, racial, and cultural factors play a significant role in client dropout rates. Further, the findings suggest the importance of counselors surfacing and addressing these issues respectfully in the therapeutic relationship. Finally, the results seem to highlight the need for African American clients to have allies, supports, and community resources available throughout the treatment and recovery process. In addition to cultural competence is the issue of access to health care where general racial and gender disparities disproportionately affect African Americans (Institute of Medicine, 2003).

African American Clients and Drinking

Research on drinking patterns with African American clients indicates they have higher abstention rates than European Americans (Pavkov, McGovern, Lyons, & Geffner, 1992). Literature also supports (a) that African Americans and European Americans have similar frequent heavy drinking levels, and (b) that the heavy drinking rates have not declined at a similar rate among African American women and men as among Whites (Pavkov et al., 1992).

Additionally, the variables of age, social class, church attendance, drinking norms, and coping through avoidance may be significant in understanding differences between Whites and African American problem drinking (Jones-Webb, 1998). In 1997 the National Household Survey on Drug Abuse revealed that 53% of African Americans and 68% of European Americans reported alcohol consumption within the past year (Substance Abuse and Mental Health Services Administration, 1999). The biggest difference appeared between African American (48%) and European American (64%) women. Dawson, Grant, Chous, and Pickering (1995), in a longitudinal study, also found lower rates of alcohol use among African Americans as opposed to European Americans. However, there are studies indicating that African Americans have higher numbers of drinking consequences and dependency symptoms than do Whites (Grant, 1997; Herd, 1994). A correlation between church attendance and abstinence has been found among African Americans but not among European Americans (Darrow, Russell, Cooper, Mudar, & Frone, 1992). A 1992 research study examined the influence of stress on alcohol use among African American and European American subjects. The results of the study suggested that African American subjects who coped with their life stresses through the mechanism of avoidance had increased alcohol consumption and subsequent drinking problems as compared with European Americans (Cooper, Russell, Skinner, Frone, & Mudar, 1992). In essence, then, African American clients may benefit greatly from focused attention to spiritual and religious resources (both internal and external).

Clinical Examples

When I (Ford) completed graduate school almost 20 years ago, multicultural and diversity issues went under the category of "special populations" and rarely were given much attention or discussion in class. Even after reviewing a number of the current textbooks in substance abuse, I found that few seem to address the issue of culture and diversity as an imperative in counseling the substance abuser or addicted client. In my own experience I have found this to be not only crucial for the client–counselor relationship but also a very important aspect of relapse prevention and an ethical imperative (American Counseling Association, 2005).

My first employment opportunity was as an outpatient counselor in an alcohol and drug community counseling program that serviced a large and diverse population of clients. The town where I worked as a counselor had very few employment opportunities for clients and even fewer resources when it came to training or entry-level positions. Most of my clients either lived in this small town or out in the country, having limited access to transportation. Most of my clients were African American males between the ages of 18 and 24, many of whom were on probation or parole. One day a week I would travel 75 minutes south, almost into North Carolina, to facilitate two groups in which most of the clients were self-described "country folk." At least twice a week I would go to the city jail or local state hospital to assess clients for treatment services.

What troubled me most was my inability to really understand my clients from a cultural viewpoint. I am a European American male who was raised in a middle-class suburban family and whose exposure to persons of color was minimal. I now found myself with a large caseload, a majority of whom were African Americans. Through much self-exploration, community/client immersion, and a willingness to learn, I strived to be an effective multicultural alcohol and drug community counselor.

I remember one day getting a call from the coordinator of a summer youth camp, asking me if I would be willing to talk with the students in the program about alcohol and drug abuse. I thought to myself what a wonderful opportunity it would be to do some actual prevention with young athletes. So, in my very young, naïve, and European American way, I planned for the presentation.

After arriving in the auditorium, I soon realized how ill prepared I really was when more than 700 students, ranging in ages from 13 to 18, strolled in before lunch for my presentation. After all of the students had taken their seats, I was keenly aware that I was the only White person in the room. At that very moment I realized I knew very little about culture, about my own sensitivity to others, and my own arrogance to think I had anything to say that would be meaningful. I was about to show the students a 40-minute film about a stereotypical White alcoholic family and then follow it up with a short lecture.

Although the audience had politely watched the film and listened to my lecture, I left the auditorium feeling very unprepared and ignorant. For one of the first times in my life, I was acutely aware of what it felt like to be a minority within the majority of a room. That experience has never left me, and I learned that in order for any of my counseling skills or approaches to be at all effective, I needed to listen to my clients and their experiences.

I (Bill) received my master's degree 12 years ago, around the time that the field of counseling started paying closer attention to issues of culture and diversity. Although the curriculums at many programs had not been infused with multicultural concepts, there was a multicultural course as part of the required course work.

When I accepted a position at an inner-city adult rehabilitation agency, I knew going in that I would be the minority. I, a 20-something-year-old White male would be working at an agency that served almost exclusively an African American population of a large city.

Approximately 3 weeks after I started, I was referred a client who needed services in the area of job preparedness. He had struggled over the previous few years at holding a job. He had a history of depression and alcohol abuse.

About 10 minutes into our first session, he looked up at me, peering through his dark sunglasses from underneath his pulled-down baseball cap, and with both hands firmly entrenched in his jacket said, "I don't want to work with you, you're White." I sat back and thought "So, what's my color have to do with anything?" Thanks to this client, I might have not learned so quickly that my color *does* matter. And, that I must be aware of not only what the client presents with but also what I present him (or her) with.

When I shared my experience from the session with my supervisor, the director of rehabilitation, he laughed and said, "You did know you were White, right?" Later that day he handed me a short article that described how many African American clients prefer to work with African American counselors. The article talked about trust, safety, resources, and someone who knows the cultural rules. I was stunned to be made aware so fully of my Whiteness and my perceived culture. In the same brush stroke, I realized when clients looked at me they saw something … perhaps a helper, perhaps someone who has been hurtful. These lessons remain with me today.

African American Clients: Implications for Counseling

According to Castro et al. (1999), there are a number of important factors for counselors to consider when working with African American clients. They have suggested that spirituality, the church, the role of women in the family, and the concept of collectivism are critical in working with African American clients. We have found in our work that each of these entities holds powerful and useful resources for the client and the client's family.

Historically, spirituality and the church were sustaining factors in times of slavery (Robinson, Perry, & Carey, 1995). The church had been and still is a central aspect to the African American community. When counselors refer African American clients to 12-step or other support meetings, the literature suggests they prepare their clients for the possibility of smaller numbers of minority members (Sue & Sue, 2008). Counselors would best serve their clients by knowing which meetings typically have larger minority participation. They could ethically and respectfully explore the spiritual beliefs and what place, if any, the church plays in their clients' lives and use it as a resource to help clients in recovery.

According to the U.S. Bureau of the Census (1996), 46% of African American families in 1994 had a female head of the house without a spouse. It is important for counselors to recognize this, particularly if the client is the designated head of the household. Counselors also need to recognize the importance of the family constellation and seek to involve family members in the treatment process. The family (which includes what many White counselors would term *extended family*) may provide relief for the identified matriarch and allow her time to attend treatment and support meetings. It may also serve to reduce the client's shame and embarrassment and enlist the family as the main support system.

Collectivism is characteristic of an African American worldview. Thus, for many African American clients, existence in the world is perceived in terms of "us" and "community" rather than the individualistic "I." Counselors may do well to refer to this collectivistic approach when discussing the first three steps of AA. The first word in the first step is "We" and not "I," which supports the idea of community and fellowship. The words "Higher Power" and "God" are introduced in Steps 2 and 3, and may fit well with the client's spiritual beliefs.

Latinos

The term *Latino* refers to a person in the Spanish-speaking country-of-origin population and includes Puerto Ricans, Cubans, Mexican Americans, and individuals from Central and South America. The term *Hispanic* is an ethnic label created by the U.S. government's Office of Management and Budget in 1978 to identify persons who trace their ancestry, regardless of race, to Spanish-speaking countries. It is used to this day as a category in the U.S. Census, but has been replaced in popular usage by the preferred term *Latino*, which can be either gender nonspecific as well as male gender specific. Overall this group is the second largest minority population in the United States (Smith, 2004; U.S. Bureau of the

Census, 2000). The largest portion of this group is Mexican Americans, consisting of over 60% of the Hispanic population in the United States. Puerto Ricans comprise the second largest Latino group, accounting for over 3% of all Latinos in the United States. The third largest Hispanic group is that of Cuban and Cuban Americans (Campbell, 1996; Gloria, Ruiz, & Castillo, 2004).

Clinical Example

I (Bill) recently conducted a summer institute for Latino high school students in the areas of career awareness and going to college. In my efforts to reach Latino youth, I enlisted the help of both graduate and undergraduate students in the area. The vast majority of the college students were White. The program went extremely well. When I asked the students to journal about their experience, I was somewhat surprised to read report after report of how the students learned they had "hidden" prejudices and biases with this population. Our question to you, the reader: What do you think of when you consider being referred a Latino client with drug and/or alcohol issues?

Latino Clients: Implications for Counseling

Generally the use of illicit drugs and alcohol appears to increase in proportion to the degree of acculturation (Amaro, Whittaker, Coffman, & Heeren, 1990; Stevens & Smith, 2005). Traditional Latino cultures tend to be conservative. Respect (*respeto*), personal relations (*personalismo*), and trust (*confianza*) are some of the most important values held by Latinos (Gloria et al., 2004). Machismo is a desirable quality for a male characterized by male dominance, sexual prowess, physical strength, and honor (Cuellar, Arnold, & Gonzalez, 1995; Neff, Prihoda, & Hoppe, 1991; Vacc et al., 2003). The feminine complement of machismo values dependence on men, self-sacrifice for husband and family, and discourages striving for personal achievement. This worldview parallels that of a collectivist, who focuses on the needs of the community or group rather than individual achievement. Another Latino cultural aspect is *familism*, which relates to the sense of obligation to, and being connected with, one's family (both immediate and extended; Diller, 2004). Strong familism provides support for family members. Such systemic support potentially provides an environment for the healthy development of coping strategies, which are more adaptive and useful than substance abuse.

Although there is limited research that targets Latinos and drugs and alcohol, in a recent study, Grilo, Becker, Anez, and McGlashan (2004) found that Latino clients with borderline personality disorder (BPD) were underdiagnosed. In their study, the authors found that a strikingly disproportionate number of clients were not accurately diagnosed as having BPD on the basis of the issues they presented with. In particular, those clients having significant diagnostic criteria such as suicidal ideation were diagnosed more often than those meeting the affective instability criterion. Such misdiagnoses may be related to differences associated with cultural rules and expectations.

Being familiar with Latino values facilitates an understanding of the impact of therapeutic interventions on both the individual and family. Also, in consideration of these values, it may be advisable to involve the family, respecting and developing trust with each member. These interactions help the counselor understand machismo and its ramifications as a cultural aspect rather than pathology. Given the size of the Latino group and the population projection mentioned above, counselors would be well-advised to learn the Spanish language. Learning how to speak the language, coupled with an understanding of the strong cultural values, combined with substance abuse knowledge would be a very effective combination for the counselor–client relationship (Clark, 1993).

Asian American and Pacific Islander Clients

In 2000 the U.S. Census Bureau created this category, which combines 10 separate sub-groups. Rank ordered by size, they are Chinese, Filipino, Japanese, Asian Indian, Korean, Vietnamese, Hawaiian, Samoan, Guamanian, and other Asian or Pacific Islander. This entire category is the fastest growing of all the U.S. racial populations (Chang, 2003). Historically, the Chinese were the first group of Asian immigrants to enter the United States in significant numbers. The Chinese immigrants were followed by Japanese immigrants, who gravitated to jobs involving an industrialized lifestyle (Chang, 2003). The Filipinos came to the United States as nationals, when the United States owned the Philippines in the 1990s, followed by the Koreans, and later the Vietnamese (Locke, 1998).

Pan Asian values include family as a significant aspect to social and cultural activities (Diller, 2004). Respect of elders and a hierarchical structure within the family are aspects of the collectivist nature of this culture (Diller, 2004). Emotional and personal restraint, along with discipline and the avoidance of bringing shame to the family at all costs, are important cultural values for this population (Sue & Sue, 2008).

Asian American and Pacific Islanders: Implications for Counseling

Understanding that addiction to chemicals brings about feelings of shame and embarrassment, Asian clients may be doubly impacted by the shame addiction brings, not only to them but also to their families. Counselors also need to realize eye contact as well as expression of emotions may be restricted because of cultural values; thus, counselors need to be sensitive to not pressure Asian clients in these areas. Counselors may find Asian clients more comfortable in expressing feelings individually rather than in a group, particularly if very few group members are from Asian culture. Counselors will benefit their Asian clients by seeking to understand the hierarchy that exists in many Asian families and appreciating the impact this may have on treatment planning.

Wall, Shea, Chan, and Carr (2001) found that adolescents with higher levels of ALDH2 (aldehyde, dehydrogenase gene) were less likely to exhibit alcohol and tobacco use on a regular basis. Their research supports previous studies (Shibuya, Yasunami, & Yoshida, 1989) in connecting potential use patterns with higher levels of ALDH2. Those of Asian descent are more likely to have higher levels of ALDH2. Therefore, this research seems to indicate one of the reasons Asian Americans are less apt to be seen for alcohol issues.

Although genetic dispositions have an effect on the use of drugs and alcohol by clients, no population or group is immune to the powerful effects of these substances. Further, even though members of the Asian or Asian American population exhibit later onset of use and are less likely to develop addictions to substances (Wall et al., 2001), each client must be seen as having individual attributes and needs. The decreased incidence of abuse in this group further complicates clients admitting to a problem and/or going to treatment.

Native American Clients

Native Americans represent 252 different languages, 557 federally recognized tribes, and several hundred state-recognized tribes and many nations (M. T. Garrett, 2003). Today the Native American nations maintain their own government and work with the United States government (M. T. Garrett, 2003). An interesting dichotomy exists within the Native American population in that not only do they have higher rates of alcoholism than the total U.S. population, but they also have a higher rate of abstention (Cutler, 2004).

A number of cultural factors need to be considered when working with Native American clients, which include their valuing harmony with nature rather than trying to control or manipulate it, being in the present rather than in the future, and preferring a natural explanation for events rather than a scientific explanation. Cooperation with others rather than competition, group connections rather than individual status, humility rather than being the center of attention, and the current sharing of wealth and benefits rather than saving for the future are also aspects of Native American culture (M. T. Garrett, 2003; J. T. Garrett & Garrett, 1994; Good Tracks, 1973; Herring, 1990; R. G. Lewis & Gingerich, 1980; Red Horse, 1980; Sanders, 1987; Thomason, 1991). Additionally, spirituality and the involvement with extended family is a very strong cultural aspect within the Native American culture (Cutler, 2004).

Native American Clients: Implications for Counseling

According to Diller (2004) and Szapocznik and Kurtines (1989), counselors who want to work primarily with this cultural group need to immerse themselves in the Native Community in order to develop trust and connection within that community. History has dictated a strong message of mistrust of the White man coming to help the Native person. Overcoming this message will be necessary to developing trust and credibility, the first step in helping individuals suffering from addiction. Spirituality and living in the moment for many Native American clients is second nature, and can significantly enhance the benefits derived from group therapy and the AA principle of living one day at a time. For clients living on a reservation, or who have strong ties to their cultural community, counselors need to explore the resources that already exist (i.e., spiritual leaders, native support groups, traditional healing practices).

Women and Substance Abuse or Dependency

Although there has been more attention to the treatment of women suffering from alcoholism and specific treatment programs, women still are underrepresented in the general treatment population (Hanson & Venturelli, 1998; Tait, 2005; Wilsnack & Wilsnack, 1991). Even though alcohol and drug treatment is available in most communities, typically a larger proportion of patients are men. An effort has been made over the last 15 to 20 years, both by federal funding agencies and treatment programs, to identify and address the roadblocks that may impede addicted women from obtaining treatment. The barriers to women seeking treatment include deep shame, difficulty finding child care, familial and professional denial, enabling, and the issues of being a single mother.

Shame

The double standard still exists whereby societal permission to become intoxicated is granted to men but denied to women. Women who are deemed nurturers (by the family or environment) yet become high on drugs or intoxicated on alcohol set into motion a societal dissonance, which ultimately interferes with women entering treatment. Shame and fear keep many women from engaging in the treatment process (Staub, 2004). Along with this shame come isolation and using drugs and alcohol alone (Gomberg, 1993).

Children

The responsibilities of motherhood can impede women from entering treatment for addiction. Federal monies in the mid-1980s were earmarked for community programs specifically addressing the needs of alcohol and drug addicted women. Additionally, prenatal addiction programs were developed in order to treat addicted pregnant women in the final months of their pregnancies. These initiatives increased the likelihood that women would engage in treatment, knowing that their child/children would be cared for by counselors and medical staff. As a result, mothers could more fully concentrate on their recovery. Such focused attention is necessary for women to ultimately be responsible and nurturing mothers, while breaking the cycle of addiction within the family system.

The day-treatment model allows addicted mothers to return home each night to care for their children. The following morning, mothers return to treatment, thus maintaining continuity within the home rather than entering treatment for 30 days away from home. Unfortunately, the day-treatment model is not present in all communities. Essentially, the daily obligations of motherhood must be taken into consideration when working with addicted women who have children at home. Failing to do so may in fact ensure that fewer women will enter into treatment programs.

Enabling and Family Denial

According to Sandmaier (1992), relatives, professionals, and friends are more willing and likely to see a woman's issues as related more to a mental illness than to alcoholism. Her alcoholism is seen as a secondary problem resulting in inappropriate diagnosis and care. This subtle form of enabling, which places the emphasis on something other than addiction, may be reinforced by those physicians who are more likely to prescribe mood-altering medications to female alcoholics than to male alcoholics (Sandmaier, 1992). This same kind of enabling can also occur within families where the partners do not acknowledge that their relationship is in competition with alcohol and drugs, resulting in minimization, excuses, and denying the existence of a problem.

Single Mothers

According to a study by Jayakody, Danziger, and Pollack (2000), many single mothers on public assistance require both substance abuse and mental health treatment to obtain or maintain jobs and fulfill family obligations. The study provided a picture of behavioral and mental health problems faced by welfare mothers who were not easily employable because of their substance abuse and mental health challenges. Many community mental health and substance abuse resources require minimal or some payment for services. This means that many women may choose to forgo treatment because of the lack of finances (choosing to use their limited funds for family needs, and/or drugs and alcohol). Increasing the accessibility to treatment for these women could facilitate attainment of goals and help create a successful transition from welfare to work. Single mothers who are employed bear the responsibility of being the primary caregiver and sole income producer in the family, which comprises another set of barriers to seeking treatment.

Treatment for Women

Gomberg (1999) suggested that women fare better in treatment programs that include child care, thorough evaluation and treatment of concomitant disorders, as well as support from work and family members. Counselors need to be sensitive to clients' fears and shame of entering treatment and the issues of finances, child care, and appropriate evaluation of trauma, eating disorders, and other co-occurring issues (Staub, 2004). Typically, treatment programs (outpatient or inpatient) remind patients of the importance of attending daily support meetings within the first 90 days of recovery. Counselors, however, need to consider the responsibilities of a single female parent and the challenge in attending support meetings each day. Although recovery tasks and meetings are paramount, maintaining sensitivity to the varied parental tasks is also significant so as to not set them up for failure, only reinforcing those already existing feelings (e.g., shame, regret). Keeping this in mind will allow counselors to help single female parents set realistic recovery goals.

Unique Factors With Women in Treatment

In addition to the role a single mother plays in the family, women differ physiologically from men in that they become more intoxicated while consuming lesser amounts of alcohol (the result of a higher fat to water proportion ratio; "Women and Alcohol," 2003). Additionally, women tend to have a larger number of co-existing disorders or issues, which include trauma, violence, and depression ("Women and Alcohol," 2003). Wilsnack, Klassen, Schur, and Wilsnack (1991) found the rate of childhood sexual abuse among female problem drinkers was more than double that of nonproblem drinkers, which suggests the need for trauma work in the treatment and counseling process. Risk factors for women include a history of alcohol or drug addiction in the family, significant use of chemicals by peers and partner, stress, and depression (Gomberg, 1994). In fact, depression was found in 66% of the women studied by Helzer, Burnam, and McEvoy (1991) preceding drinking problems.

In addition, alcoholic women and those with anxiety disorders have significantly higher scores on eating disorder evaluations (Sinha et al., 1996). According to Gomberg (1993), alcoholic women experience themselves more negatively than nonalcoholic women. This leads alcoholic women to surreptitious drinking and a great deal of shame. Because of the isolative drinking, female drinking tends to go unnoticed until the later stages of the addiction (Manhal-Baugus, 1998; Staub, 2004).

Women are more likely than men to use prescribed psychoactive medications such as minor tranquilizers and sedatives (Ross, 1989). Female drinking has been found to be higher with achievement in education and those of higher income as compared with women of lower income (Celentano & McQueen, 1984). The ethnic group with the largest percentage of female drinkers is European Americans, followed by Native Americans, Hispanics, African Americans, and Asian Americans (Wilson & Williams, 1989). Family history of addiction appears to have a significant influence among men on the development of addiction, which does not seem true for women (Gomberg, 1991). It also seems apparent that women have their first drink later in life than do men (Schuckit, Anthenelli, Bucholz, Hesselbrock, & Tipp, 1995).

A large proportion of women who are addicted to chemicals have a history of depression, trauma, anxiety, and low self-esteem preceding their initial alcohol or drug use (Gomberg, 1999). Although women present with signs of greater severity than do men (e.g., comorbidity, medical consequences, depression, and prescribed psychoactive drugs), women appear to negotiate treatment, in some settings, as well as if not better than do men (Gomberg, 1999).

Failure to address these preexisting issues in the process of addiction treatment will significantly increase the likelihood of relapse, as the drugs or alcohol were primarily used to numb the emotional pain associated with depression, trauma, and anxiety. Furthermore, following such drug/alcohol use, the preexisting issues (e.g., severe depression, suicide, excessive binging and purging with food, cutting on wrists and arms, higher anxiety) may become more pronounced and lead to more alcohol and drug use.

Counselor Awareness

As counselors work with women in recovery, it is important to encourage self-awareness and continuous appreciation of self. Also, counselors should aid women in finding a balance between recovery and other life commitments (Hartman, Staub, & Styer, 2002). The support group Women for Sobriety is presented as an adjunct and alternative to AA. Much of what is written in AA from either their main text, *The Big Book* (AA, 2001), or the 12 Steps, uses the male pronoun. Given that the co-founders were both European American males, the use of *he* or *him* is not inclusive and therefore needs to be discussed with female clients. Some female clients may find it offensive whereas others may not. In any case, an alternative can be Women for Sobriety. If counselors find that their community has no Women for Sobriety meetings, a portion of each session can be dedicated to ways clients may feel more comfortable in AA. Counselors can encourage female clients to read personal stories from *The Big Book* about women in AA getting sober or they can help clients find women's AA meetings. A women's therapy group can also be helpful early in the recovery process. In addition to such specific training, counselors may make recommendations to women in early recovery that they attend women-only support groups, work with a female therapist, and if possible be in a women-only therapy group.

Counselors working in mental health agencies, college counseling centers, or who are school counselors need to be aware of the multiple issues female clients bring to counseling. In addition to alcohol and drug training and education, counselors need to obtain training in (a) dual-diagnosis assessment, (b) trauma issues (assessing for and working with), (c) referral (e.g., specialized sources), and (d) medical issues unique to this population (i.e., amenorrhea, perimenopause, cramps, sexually transmitted diseases [STDs], and pregnancy; Staub, 2004), as these coexisting issues need to be treated simultaneously within a safe, therapeutic environment.

Clinical Example

One client I (Ford) worked with spent 30 days in treatment for alcohol dependency in a relapse specific treatment program. Upon discharge she was referred to me for continued outpatient counseling with the following issues to be addressed: a coexisting diagnosis of depression and concern over unexplored trauma from childhood, posttraumatic stress disorder (PTSD), potential separation and divorce from her husband, recent loss of employment due to her absenteeism from work, and medical problems related to an active eating disorder.

She had been in treatment once before, two previous detoxifications, and one outpatient treatment, all for alcoholism. This was the first time, however, that she was working on relapse prevention issues in treatment. She talked about her reluctance to see a male counselor, at which point I discussed other female counselors in the area for potential referral. She made the decision to continue with me and enter a relapse prevention outpatient group consisting of both men and women. I referred her to a psychiatrist who worked specifically with addicted clients and was certified as an addictionologist, so she could be medically monitored for her depression and antidepressant prescription. She entered the outpatient group and attended three sessions for couples' communication work, at which point I referred her and her husband to a practitioner specializing in couples' therapy. She became employed after 4 months and appeared to be handling the stress of sobriety and work. However, for 6 months she continued to describe her discomfort in sobriety. She attended AA at least twice a week, had a female sponsor in AA, attended group therapy three times per week, was involved in couples work, as well as working full-time. At times she reported feeling overwhelmed and stressed, yet was able to remain sober.

The longer she stayed sober, the more her emotions from childhood surfaced, thus bringing past trauma into her present experience in sobriety and into the counseling sessions. Although she was following her treatment plan, she felt more and more overwhelmed by memories and emotions of terror and sadness. She began to share those feelings in individual counseling, in group, and with her sponsor, but the emotions were too overpowering for her. She started drinking again and at that point was amenable, with her husband's support, to enter an inpatient treatment program that focused on both the trauma that consistently surfaced with lengthy sobriety and her alcoholism.

She stayed in treatment for 4 months and then continued in an extended treatment program where she slowly reintegrated into the community with the support of other women, treatment, and 12-step support meetings.

This case illustrates that treatment focusing *only* on the tools for sobriety without addressing other areas that potentially lead to relapse is not an effective, holistic way of approaching female clients (or any clients for that matter). Although sobriety is the ultimate goal, the case above exemplifies the importance for counselors working with women to have options for referral and training or experience in the multiplicity of issues accompanying sobriety for women.

Male Clients and Substance Abuse or Dependency

The majority of clients in treatment for chemical addiction are men, which makes understanding distinguishing aspects of male clients important for counselors (Cunningham, 2004). Men are more likely than women to develop severe substance dependence (Substance Abuse and Mental Health Services Administration, 2005). Male clients typically report data rather than emotions, making the identification and expression of feelings in treatment important for stress management strategies and relapse prevention. The emotions typically identified by men are those of anger, resentment, or happiness (Cunningham, 2004). The suppression of feelings coupled with the use of drugs and alcohol only further separate men from their emotions. According to Shem and Surrey (1998), men are socialized differently than are women. As boys they typically strengthen their self rather than develop mutual connections. They understand that growth occurs through separation with others and that disconnection (independence) is rewarded by society. The reward for many men reaching adolescence is the opportunity to drink alcohol, which over time can result in men who are significantly distant from their own feelings (Cunningham, 2004). For instance, the use of substances may not only become a coping mechanism to handle internal feelings and stress but it may also become a physical addiction. Feelings of sadness, hurt, and shame are unexpressed, but instead are medicated, thus slowly distancing men from their internal emotional experience.

When men present themselves for treatment and substances begin to leave their bodies, they often experience great difficulty in managing feelings or life crises. Additionally, male clients may experience feelings that have been suppressed for many years. At times they can experience the insecurity and vulnerability of not knowing how to deal with the pressures and feelings associated with everyday life.

If counselors can understand this deep fear and vulnerability within male clients, it can facilitate the beginning of a healing process. Unfortunately, many male clients come across as arrogant, self-willed, controlling, or insensitive, and attempt (and many times succeed) to engage counselors in a nontherapeutic battle of control. Addiction is an illness of disconnection from self and from other relationships (Gideon, 1975). Therefore, counselors need to meet male clients where they are emotionally and empathize with the outward feelings being expressed. Many male clients referred by a third party (i.e., judge, partner, family, job) are many times angry and resentful. Using W. R. Miller and Rollnick's (1991, 2002) motivational interviewing approach found in later chapters of this book can be very helpful with empathy and resistance. Really understanding the anger, bitterness, and simultaneously listening for the fear and then reflecting back that understanding can help male clients feel heard. Because of the difficulty many men have with feelings, Cunningham (2004) uses a statement in sessions with male clients to help them identify feelings: "From listening to your story, I would not be at all surprised that you were feeling _____."
Hearing such a statement might prompt male clients to consider the possibility of having the identified feeling. Such a statement may also help the male client identify and own similar feelings. Cunningham (2004) suggested that the relationship with the therapist can provide the opportunity for clients to begin to trust and open up about feelings and the vulnerability that accompanies the process. This in fact is not unique to counseling male substance abusing clients and is important in all therapeutic relationships.

Counselors need to look beyond the words of male clients and tap into the vulnerability that perpetuates and contributes to continued chemical use. Counselors able to express to men that they know how important and seemingly helpful alcohol has been over the years, create for clients an environment conducive to discussing this powerful connection. Counselors may find empathy, probing, humor, and use of self in the therapeutic relationship vital in developing and maintaining trust. Counselors overly formal and staid, lacking spontaneity and genuineness, will probably be less helpful to the fearful and guarded male client. Male counselors can model healthy and appropriate behavior in individual and in group counseling through consistency (being on time for appointments or following through on commitments), by verbally self-disclosing feelings (appropriately and therapeutically), and by evincing genuine compassion for and interest in clients' lives. Male group facilitators can model exploration of feelings with other men and appropriate discussion with women in a mixed group. For men-only groups, counselors can facilitate discussions about feelings and thoughts concerning sex, control, fear, and intimacy. Sometimes men will joke about these issues in a mixed group; therefore, an all-male group provides the opportunity to engage in more meaningful discussions of these important issues.

Clinical Example

A group I (Ford) facilitated for many years consisted of men who had substantial histories of alcohol and drug treatment, numerous relapses, and counseling to address other issues besides alcohol and drug issues. These men were veterans of the treatment system and could cite chapter and verse from most AA literature sources. However, each one of them had unique and specific issues that led them time and time again back to using drugs or drinking alcohol. Over time I realized this all-men's group had something that was significant to each of their sobrieties. The group was a consistent place and time for each participant to come on a weekly basis to talk and listen to each others' experiences in sobriety and to discuss vulnerable issues of intimacy, feelings of fear and failure, and feelings in general. As a male facilitator I realized my actions and inactions had an impact on the group, whether it was keeping the group members on task or helping explore feelings in the sessions. Many of the men in the group had difficulties maintaining relationships, which resulted in various compulsive behaviors. In addition, many of them had posttraumatic issues either from childhood, having been sexually or physically abused, or from combat situations. Even though each member attended group, had a sponsor in AA or was sober, they all had unique issues relating to their acculturation of being a male in this society and feeling unable to share their vulnerabilities. This particular group provided just that environment, where for the first time, many of them remained clean and sober for substantial periods of time. If a member did relapse and returned to the group, he was met with support, compassion, and genuine care.

In addition to being male, the majority of the group members were identified by their referral sources as impaired professionals, meaning their occupations ranged from doctors, lawyers, or teachers, and were in job jeopardy because of their drug and alcohol use. The feelings of embarrassment, guilt, and shame were overwhelming as was the stigma of being a relapsing client. Over time the healing process of sharing with other men in a group allowed an alternative for the members other than the suppression of feelings.

The next section of this chapter focuses on aspects of sexual orientation that have implications for substance abuse and addiction counseling.

Gay, Lesbian, Bisexual, and Transgendered Clients

Research from as far back as 1977 (Fifield, Latham, & Phillips, 1977) has suggested that gay, lesbian, bisexual, and transgendered (GLBT) individuals are at greater risk for substance use than their heterosexual counterparts. Recent research provides continued evidence for this assertion (Cochran & Cauce, 2006; Hughes & Eliason, 2002). Cabaj (2000) indicated that the gay and lesbian population uses approximately 30% of all types of alcohol/drugs, in contrast with 10–12% in the general population.

The higher incidence of alcohol and drug use among gay and lesbian individuals may be related to the antigay bias in society along with increasing incidents of hate crimes (Klinger & Stein, 1996; Tait, 2005). Although this is not a cause of addiction, it certainly suggests that gay and lesbian individuals may use alcohol or drugs in order to cope with feelings engendered by cultural or societal disapproval. The process of coming out, as well as being gay or lesbian in this society, has two significant obstacles: homophobia (i.e., irrational fear and hatred of a sexual minority group) and the prevalent attitude of heterosexual superiority (Dempsey, 1994; Sears, 1997; Smith, 2004). Heterosexual counselors are not immune to being homophobic or heterosexist and need to address their biases and feelings about this population.

The word *gay* refers "to both gay men and lesbian women" and "reflects more fully the social, cultural, and affective dimensions of this subculture" (Beatty et al., 1999, p. 542). The coming-out process is a series of steps, some moving forward, and then some moving backward (Cabaj, 2000). First the individual, in his or her time and place, becomes aware that his or her sexual orientation is dissimilar to the majority. Recognizing this, the individual integrates the sense of being "different" into self, along with the feelings that accompany this awareness. The individual, as a result of this integration, begins to act on these feelings. Finally, the individual may decide who he or she will let know about their feelings, choices, and sexual orientation.

Another model of gay identity development (Coleman, 1985) delineates a similar process whereby the individual has a sense or feelings of difference, yet may not identify it as same-sex attraction. The next stage is the awareness of same-sex attraction, followed by disclosure to others. From there, the individual experiments with same-sex social and sexual behavior, resulting in initial stable and subsequent relationships. Finally, there is the integration of this awareness into the overall development of the self. Coming out is a nonlinear process, which may take a lifetime to fully accept one's sexuality (Hicks, 2000).

Some children who are gay or lesbian learn to separate or dissociate from their true selves and disconnect, preferring rather to conform to parental expectations (Gibson, 1989). As kids develop, many parents or caregivers are unable to provide adequate support. Because of this, children minimize or ignore those attributes of difference, which ultimately contributes to emotional pain, denial, and fear (Cabaj, 2000). As these children enter adolescence and adulthood, the denial of self for many is overpowering. Over time, they have developed exceptional skills at denying true self, trying instead to constantly conform to familial as well as societal rules. Like many children raised in families where affirmation, acceptance, and love has been conditional, the use of alcohol and drugs certainly can provide feelings of relief to an otherwise anxious and emotionally separated individual. Gay and lesbian people are more prone to use substances for a variety of reasons because of their oppression in society (Hicks, 2000). Cabaj stated, "Many men had their early homosexual sexual experiences while drinking or being high" (2000, p. 12).

As adolescents and adults present for counseling and treatment, counselors will want to be aware that the issue of being gay, lesbian, bisexual, or transgendered is an important aspect to be addressed.

Implications for Counseling

Counselors have a responsibility to provide effective treatment and counseling services to those seeking services, regardless of culture or minority status (Maccio & Doueck, 2002). Counselors must first examine their feelings, biases, and judgments when working with all clients and specifically their own attitudes toward gay and lesbian clients (Maccio & Doueck, 2002). Counselor educators, in particular, need to "increase the awareness of students on the impact of homophobia, heterosexism, and internalized homophobia on the lives of LGB [GLBT] people, and how LGB [GLBT] individuals might cope with minority stress" (Weber, 2008, p. 45). The overwhelming majority of the studies reviewed by Maccio and Doueck indicated that many of the clients appreciated or would have appreciated having providers with the same sexual orientation as themselves. Those counselors who were of the same sexual orientation were rated by clients as being more helpful than the counselors who were not (Maccio & Doueck, 2002). This supports the recommendation earlier in the chapter for the hiring of counselors with the same cultural orientation as the community they serve, and in this case, for hiring counselors of the same sexual orientation. Counselors need to be both supportive and aware of the issues surrounding homosexual clients and the impact these issues can have on sobriety. According to Weber, in order "to achieve recovery from substance abuse and homophobia, an LGB [GLBT] client needs to address his/her own acceptance of self with the support of a gay-affirmative counselor" (2008, p. 44). Agencies, schools, and hospitals can provide information, training, skill development, and advocacy for this invisible population (Maccio & Doueck, 2002).

The initial assessment and subsequent individual sessions not only need to focus on chemical and alcohol use but also on relationship history, current relationships, medical concerns, children, previous marriages and custody issues, domestic violence, as well as bisexual feelings or relationships. Exploring with clients the consequences of homophobic behaviors they have been subjected to and the feelings related to those incidents is very important (McHenry & Korcuska, 2002). Counselors need to maintain a supportive, open, and compassionate approach, as they would with any other client. Unfortunately, some counselors may avoid asking clients about their sexual orientation and behaviors because of their own discomfort. In these instances, such an approach by a counselor may ultimately harm clients.

For counselors working in schools, they should be aware that adolescents who are gay may be threatened, physically harmed, or shunned from their peer group (McHenry & Korcuska, 2002). Suicide rates for the gay adolescent population may be three times that of other adolescents (McHenry & Korcuska, 2002; Rotheram-Borus, Hunter, & Rosario, 1994). Cabaj (2000) suggested that clients who are addicted to alcohol and drugs begin exploring gay and lesbian issues, feelings, and oppression in the early stages of recovery. Important, however, is the support network around the client and the ability of the network to hear and accept what the client is disclosing (McHenry & Korcuska, 2002). Therefore, it is imperative that counselors identify GLBT support meetings, and if possible, direct clients to specialized addiction treatment programs for gay clients. PFLAG (Parents, Friends, and Families of Lesbians and Gays) is a support group for those with a gay or lesbian family member or friend. This nationwide organization can be helpful support for family members in their journey to increased understanding. Clients who are abusers of drugs, not addicts, and who are able to reduce or limit their use of chemicals can explore the impact chemicals have had on coping with their sexual orientation.

Because a significant portion of treatment is conducted in a group setting, it is important for counselors to uphold the confidentiality and privacy of clients who are not yet comfortable or ready to disclose their orientation in the group. The use of motivational interviewing as well as using GLBT resources in the community are important approaches in the delivery of services. In the past few years, significant growth in specialized services for the GLBT population has emerged. Treatment programs such as the Lambda Center (Washington, DC) and the PRIDE Institute (Eden Prairie, MN; Arlington, TX; and Fort Lauderdale, FL) focus on addiction treatment services within the GLBT community.

The Lambda Center, the Psychiatric Institute of Washington, and the Whitman-Walker Clinic have joined together to provide psychiatric, substance abuse, and medical services. The Lambda Center provides both inpatient and outpatient services to the GLBT community. The Whitman-Walker Clinic is one of the nation's largest gay and lesbian health clinics in the United States (Hicks, 2000). The Lambda Center provides services not only to clients but also to the surrounding community, including information on transgender issues, substance abuse, employment discrimination, and domestic violence. Although AA has over 500 gay-friendly support groups around the country and specific chemical dependency programs for gays do exist, there are still too few programs for the number of GLBT clients with chemical dependency problems (Amico & Niesen, 1997).

Human Immunodeficiency Virus (HIV) Diagnosis

Clients enter counseling or treatment for various reasons including substance abuse problems, issues not related to their chemical use, as well as consequences related to their drug and alcohol use. Following assessment, clients may receive three, if not more, diagnoses as a result of the evaluation. The client may be diagnosed with an addiction to alcohol and drugs, a coexisting psychiatric disorder such as depression, and a third diagnosis: HIV positive or AIDS. The issues for the client and counselor to negotiate are multiple and difficult. Even with new drug therapies effectively impeding the initial infection, clients typically see the diagnosis as a death sentence. Issues of mortality, depression, suicidality, retribution, risky behavior, and relapse must be attended to when working with a client who has multiple diagnoses.

Counselors need to assist gay clients to understand internalized homophobia, which can significantly impact self-esteem and worth. Clients internalize the societal hatred, prejudice, and shame of being homosexual and in turn may use alcohol or drugs to cope with those feelings. Although homosexuality is not a cause of the physical addiction, it can be, however, an initial impetus for clients to begin using drugs and alcohol. Counselors can help clients identify their feelings of shame and embarrassment brought on by societal homophobia, which have been internalized by their clients. Counselors can help clients realize these feelings as separate from their homosexuality, for which they need not feel shame.

Other unique issues that counselors may need to address when working with GLBT clients include bars as a means to socialize, the use of "poppers" to enhance sexual pleasure, and conflicts with AA and spirituality. Bars have been one of the main environments in which GLBT individuals socialized that seemed safe and accepting. The use of sexual-enhancing drugs such as poppers potentially heighten the pleasure of orgasm during sex, making this a powerful connection. The initial reaction by many GLBT clients when they see the words *Higher Power* or *God* is reluctance. For many GLBT clients, spirituality has been linked to religion, which, for many, has been a main source of shame regarding their sexual orientation. Counselors need to talk with clients who have negative reactions to these concepts of spirituality.

Clinical Example

One client who I (Ford) worked with for almost a year exemplifies many of the issues presented here. Barry, who was a young, 25-year-old European American male, was referred because of a second drunk driving ticket. He initially came in very upset, minimally resistant, and depressed. Barry had just moved back from New York where he was a bartender, living paycheck to paycheck. It was clear he was living on the edge each night, drinking until 6:00 a.m. and waking up around 4:00 p.m., only to repeat the cycle again each night. He left New York to get away from the late nights, the parties, but more importantly, the breakup from his boyfriend of 3 years. He was very sad, depressed, and reported feeling lonely.

He disclosed to me his sexual orientation after three sessions, feeling, by his report, that he could trust me with this information. The issues that Barry presented were the following: minimization around the severity of his alcohol dependency, the need for psychiatric evaluation for depression, exploring his most recent breakup, as well as his employment uncertainty.

For the next few months he agreed to discontinue drinking and attend support meetings, to be evaluated for depression, and discuss the feelings around his breakup. He reported being abstinent, was taking an antidepressant as prescribed, and was able to share his feelings of sadness and grief over the loss of his relationship. Barry also began to explore employment possibilities within the session. At one point he discussed the multiple sexual partners he had in New York and how he had unprotected sex with many of them, which left him concerned about HIV. He realized, after some discussion, that he wanted to find out and get tested, which he did.

The next session Barry came in with a very down and depressed demeanor, at which point he said that he was told by the health nurse that his test came back positive for HIV. Eventually toward the end of the session he shared with me that he had not been completely sober over the past months, but since this diagnosis, he felt he needed to be honest with me.

I helped Barry through counseling to share his feelings of loss, sadness, anger, rage, and fear. He renegotiated his abstinence contract and agreed that he wanted to attempt to live a clean and sober life since the HIV diagnosis. Three diagnoses—alcohol addiction, depression, and now HIV—were impacting Barry and those whom he loved. His remaining sessions with me were bittersweet. At times he was depressed and very angry, and others quite content and serene with future plans he had for self-employment. After about a year of counseling Barry terminated therapy with me, and I referred him to an aftercare group provided by the driving under the influence (DUI) program. He continued with medical care to treat his HIV and depressive disorder.

As a counselor I felt I provided a safe environment to explore the breakup with his lover and at the same time focused on his drinking and how that played into the breakup and subsequent DUI. I evaluated the symptoms of his depression and referred him to a psychiatrist who was very familiar with addiction medicine. Finally, I talked with him about his decision to be tested for HIV and the results that followed. Additionally, he signed a release of information to his family, and at least twice I met with Barry and his family. With Barry I made three referrals: one to a psychiatrist, the second to a physician working specifically with HIV clients, and the third to an aftercare group. Barry was involved in individual, group, and psychopharmacological therapies, as well as family and AA meetings.

Though we have already integrated diverse populations with each chapter of this text, we felt it critically important to address the special needs of two additional populations that are often overlooked in relation to the use or abuse of drugs and alcohol: older persons and persons with disabilities.

Older Persons

Substance abuse among older persons is typically not identified as a major problem. There is a wide range of speculation among researchers on the degree to which elderly people abuse substances such as alcohol; their estimates vary from 2% to 25% of this population (Benshoff, Harrawood, & Koch, 2003; Menninger, 2002; Ondus, Hujer, Mann, & Mion, 1999; Pennington, Butler, & Eagger, 2000; Rigler, 2000). Regardless of the definitive percentage of abusers in this stage of life, counselors must be aware of the multitude of issues facing elderly populations who become addicted to drugs and/or alcohol.

One place to start in recognizing the uniqueness of this group is in identifying those who started abusing substances before entering late stage life versus those who (for one reason or many) turned to substance use in the twilight of life. Each group requires special attention to the different needs and patterns related to their use.

Generally speaking, those who start using later in life are typically attempting to cope with social, emotional, relational, medical, or pragmatic issues. Dar (2006) suggested that older persons who start using later in life are masking or ineffectively coping with bereavement, loss of friends and social status, loss of occupation, impaired ability to function, family conflict, reduced self-esteem, new or increased severity of physical disabilities, chronic pain, insomnia, sensory deficits, reduced mobility, cognitive impairment, impaired self-care, reduced coping skills, altered financial circumstances, and dislocation from previous accommodation.

Take, for example, a 72-year-old man who recently lost his wife of 45 years. Having been retired for 8 years, he has lost many of his work contacts. He spent the last few years traveling with his wife. Additionally, within the last 6 months he has noticed a dramatic change in his physical capabilities (especially his ability to hold a golf club). Having always enjoyed a cocktail once and awhile, he notices that he sleeps much better when he mixes his prescription arthritis medication with 3 or 4 glasses of cognac each night. Would this change in behavior be noticed? If so, by whom?

The second group to be aware of are those who have had significant relationships with substances throughout their lives. This group typically has more medical issues to deal with as a result of the previous use. Further, in many instances, they have become "wise" to treatment procedures and interventions. Imagine an individual who abused drugs through her 20s and 30s, subsequently turning to alcohol in her 40s and 50s. Now in her late 60s, she has been prescribed several medications to deal with the physical problems that resulted from her drug and alcohol abuse in previous decades. Having learned to "function" while impaired, she has access to powerful medication/illegal drugs/alcohol cocktails. Rigler (2000) found nearly two-thirds of elderly individuals with alcohol problems had high levels of use of alcohol prior to later life. Individuals who successfully survive the rigors of alcoholism in earlier life often have significant mental and physical health complications. Others probably survive to this stage because they have learned to moderate consumption to remain functional in the community and to maintain a semblance of good health (Rigler, 2000).

Levin and Kruger (2000) suggested that misuse and abuse of drugs and alcohol among older persons was not identified or dealt with effectively by both professionals and family members. They argued that, in many cases, individuals in the position to intervene in the use or abuse mistook the changes in the individual as simply being related to aging.

Meyer (2005) identified several reasons for such oversights by professionals. She suggested such failures were due to the professional lacking awareness of the issue, feeling too embarrassed to articulate the concern (on the part of the professional), lacking awareness of the significance of the issue, and believing it is okay to allow older persons to enjoy their senior years. "Although elderly individuals make-up 12.4% of the population, they consume 25% to 30% of all prescription drugs" (Ondus et al., 1999). This is especially important as the baby-boomer generation continues to move toward their silver years (Levin & Kruger, 2000; "Illicit Drug Use," 2002; Ondus et al., 1999).

Persons With Disabilities

Often overlooked, the population consisting of persons with disabilities require special attention when screening for and working with substance abuse issues. Whether working as a school counselor, mental health counselor, or addiction specialist, counselors must recognize the potential risk inherent in this special population. "Research in substance abuse (SA) treatment has demonstrated that persons with disabilities (PWDs) are at substantially higher risk for SA than persons without disabilities. Despite their higher risk, PWDs access SA treatment at a much lower rate than persons without disabilities" (Krahn, Farrell, Gabriel, & Deck, 2006).

In a landmark study by the National Institute on Disability and Rehabilitation Research (NIDRR, 1996), the researchers found a dramatic difference between the use and abuse rates of persons with disabilities and able-bodied persons. "More than half of the respondents [persons with disabilities] drank alcohol in the past 12 months. 14.7% drank once a week. 17.2% reported binge drinking. 32% took alcohol with their medications. 28.4%

scored high on the SMAST [Short Form of the Michigan Alcoholism Screening Test], indicative of substance dependence or abuse. A staggering 33% reported having been victimized (physical violence) in relation to use of drugs and alcohol" (p. 14).

In the same study, 43.3% of those who self-identified as having a current or past substance abuse problem believed that their counselors did not know about it. They were afraid to tell their counselor, thinking the counselor would not understand or would make them do something they did not want to do (NIDRR, 1996). It is critical for counselors to both attend to the warning signs and consider the use pattern of persons with disabilities. Left unattended, a significant portion of the population may experience negative effects, if not abuse or addiction to substances.

Moore and Li (2001) suggested that persons with disabilities exhibit substantially higher rates of significant physical, legal, work, and social issues directly related to their drinking. Li and Ford (1998) found that women with disabilities had higher rates of substance use than women without disabilities.

Youth with disabilities are not exempt from the dramatic data presented above. This population experiences a substantially higher substance abuse risk than their nondisabled peers (McCombs & Moore, 2002). In relation to such a concern is the fact that this group must deal with disability-specific factors for substance abuse including prescribed medications, chronic medical problems, social isolation, coexisting behavioral problems, and disenfranchisement (McCombs & Moore, 2002).

Although no minority group is at significantly greater risk than others in regard to abusing or becoming addicted to substances, there exists the vital role of the counselor to attend to such a possibility. Data, research, and clinical experience suggest the need to *broach* the subject with clients. Using such a therapeutic approach allows the counselor to introduce the topic, discuss the ramifications of use and abuse, and address concerns the client may have in regard to his or her use. The following are examples of broaching comments used in counseling to support the client's movement:

> I know we have been talking a lot in recent sessions about your having to adjust to being in a wheelchair, and I want to talk about whether that has lead to your increase in using drugs or alcohol.

> Many people who lose their vision suddenly find it depressing and difficult. They also may turn to substances to help ease the pain of the loss. What has your use of substances been since finding out you were going to be blind?

> We need to address your comment of having a nightcap to help you sleep. Mixing alcohol with the meds you have been prescribed may help you deal with the loss of your wife, but they might also cause significant problems in the near future related to your health.

Addressing substance issues with any client can be a challenge, especially to those not typically working with this population. However, with the unique challenges that both persons with disabilities and elderly persons face, it is critical that counselors consider the use patterns of clients in these groups. Failing to do so may result in unaddressed issues, missed therapeutic opportunities, and misdiagnosed abuse or addiction issues.

Summary

The aim of this chapter was to help counselors understand how culture, gender, and sexual orientation are important primary factors in treatment planning. There is a significant and crucial link between cultural sensitivity or competence and effective treatment with clients of diverse cultures. Developmental processes for becoming more culturally aware and competent must be explored by counselors. Finally, subsequent chapters of this book have multicultural and diversity-related questions for student reflection and discussion to further expand upon this important topic.

Exploration Questions From Chapter 2

1. What exposure do you have to other races or cultures?
2. How will your cultural background and race impact the counseling that you will do?
3. How will you respond when a client who is not of the same race or cultural background enters your office with a substance abuse issue?
4. Would you prefer to work with male or female clients? Why?
5. What are your stereotypes about men? Women?
6. Describe your balance of collectivism and individualism.
7. What would you do if you were referred a client who spoke very little English while you speak only English? What resources would you look for? How might you try to communicate with this client? What did you use as a guide to your previous answers?

Suggested Activities

1. Create a family tree and begin exploring your family rules, biases, prejudices, and stereotypes. Discuss with other students in small groups how this will impact counseling with clients.
2. Attend a 12-step meeting specifically away from your home and preferably in a populated area, and pay attention to your emotions, prejudice, and stereotypes. Record them in your journal. Discuss this with your classmates in small groups and record them in your journal.
3. Take a moment and reflect on your own culture. What are the rules and guidelines imposed on your culture regarding education, money, relationships, the use of drugs or alcohol, and work? Now, take another culture and do the same exercise. What differences do you notice? How might such differences impact your work with a client from that particular culture?

Types of Drugs and Their Effects

We have found the following to be a general principle: Clients do not ingest drugs with the intention of becoming addicted. Instead, they start using drugs to seek pleasure, out of curiosity, or to avoid painful emotions. If drugs or alcohol did not produce pleasure, a high, or intoxication, humans more than likely would not use them. The problem is that one can get addicted to the feeling, experience cravings, and as a result, will do just about anything for more drugs. According to Adinof (2004), a neurophysiologic process underlies the uncontrolled and compulsive behavior, which defines addiction, where each drug provides the user with a unique experience (pleasure) that helps to maintain the user's relationship with the substance. Because of this, all counselors need a basic understanding of drugs, the impact of drugs on the brain, and the various classifications and signs of drug use.

Many clients who are addicted to drugs report the significant impact drugs and alcohol have played in their coping with life. Addiction counselors seldom if ever hear from clients that they intended on becoming addicted to drugs at the time of their first use. Clients often report, "I started using at age eight to kill the emotional pain I felt when my brother was killed. I watched my father drink, so I thought that would do the trick." As a coping skill, these sentiments make sense for the individual. However, this ineffective coping response oftentimes distorts and reshapes into *the* problem. In other words, the solution becomes the problem, unbeknownst to the client. Simultaneously, while drugs and alcohol act as temporary emotional coping skills, they also create pleasure in the brain. Unfortunately, the high for those abusing and addicted to alcohol and drugs is not without consequence.

It is clear that the counselor has a challenge in working with a client whose behavior serves such strong dual purposes. In fact, as is discussed later in the book, the marrying of these two basic reasons for initial using (coping and pleasure) creates its own unique troubling cycle. And our experience has taught us that this is far more than an academic issue, but rather a challenging and complex yet necessary view of the nature of addiction and abuse. Therefore, although current texts on substance abuse counseling use the drug classification chapter as a way of highlighting categories of drugs and methods of ingestion, this chapter adds basic information to aid counselors in their clinical work. We do recognize the challenge of taking in all of the information that follows. The first time we were introduced to these concepts, it was as if we were learning a new language. Therefore, we have made every effort to help bridge conceptual and language gaps by providing clinical vignettes for students to understand approaches in working with drug abusing and addicted clients. Readers are introduced to the impact drugs have on the brain's neurochemistry, drug categories, the routes of administration, and clinical observations. Case vignettes are also provided for five of the drug categories with questions for students to reflect upon as well as our consultation. As we move forward, it is important for counselors to have a basic understanding of drugs, drug classifications, and withdrawal symptoms of various drugs. We believe that counselors who have a basic understanding of drug use will be able to do the following:

- *Provide clients with appropriate referral options.* During the course of drug and alcohol assessments, counselors determine the category of drug(s) clients are ingesting and provide referrals for varied levels of care based on the amounts and category of drugs, taking into consideration previous treatment attempts. Referral options may include medical facilities to address withdrawal symptoms and cravings for the drug or a medication evaluation, which helps clients with craving management.

  Referral options vary depending on the drug, psychological factors, and use history. For example, a client who is caught smoking cigarettes by her parents for the first time with no history or current psychological issues will have a different referral than a client caught snorting cocaine for the eighth time and who is diagnosed as having a bipolar disorder.

- *Provide appropriate treatment planning.* Determining the type of drug(s) being ingested can significantly help the counselor structure, plan and effect appropriate, useful, and comprehensive treatment. Some self-referred clients may want to diminish their level of use while resisting requests to abstain. In these instances, a treatment plan consisting of abstinence is not what the client wants, nor will it have a good chance for success. Although abstinence may be better suited as a long-term goal, a plan of cutting down will better meet the client where his or her energy is focused. Counselors' understanding of the chemicals being used by clients will help in preparation for appropriate treatment. For instance, clients who state that they want to reduce their use of alcohol and discontinue heroin will need specific medical treatment and supervision during this period. These clients will experience the withdrawal from the heroin and subsequently may increase their intake and/or dependence on alcohol in an attempt to avoid the physical discomfort and pain from the lack of heroin.

- *Help clients understand how drugs potentiate each other.* Often, clients may not understand the effects of combining drugs. Because such interactions may in fact enhance each drug's effect (in some cases proving to be lethal if not chronically debilitating), clients who mix alcohol with barbiturates usually are not aware of the lethality the combination can pose. In this case, one plus one does not equal two, it equals sixteen.

- *Help clients strategize and manage cravings for the drug(s).* Counselors who assess clients for marijuana and cocaine use can discuss with the client how the client plans to manage cravings. For example, a cocaine addict may be visually stimulated by the sight of a lighter (which may be used to light crack cocaine in a pipe). The image of the lighter, which creates a physiological response and a craving for the drug, must be addressed through discussions between counselor and client. One major goal in this part of the process is for clients to develop proactive and healthy methods of coping and become an active and engaged part of *their* treatment process.

- *Help clients prepare for potential withdrawal symptoms.* Counselors who assess that their clients are in need of detoxification should refer for a comprehensive medical evaluation. In some instances though, clients are not always amenable to detoxification services, or they may not meet criteria for admission. Therefore, counselors need to alert and educate their clients to possible withdrawal symptoms and discuss how the client will effectively manage powerful symptoms such as sleep disturbances, irritability, emotional instability, and fatigue while in consultation with a physician.

- *Help clients understand the concept of cross-tolerance and cross-addiction.* Counselors familiar with both of these concepts are better equipped to educate clients on the importance of a chemical-free life. Further, counselors can address the potential for addiction to other drugs. For example, clients addicted to narcotics need to understand the concept of cross-tolerance (drugs within the classification of narcotic will have the same properties [e.g., tolerance, withdrawal] as all the drugs within the category), even though they may have never used another narcotic.
- *Help clients understand and explore drug preference.* In many cases, clients arrive for counseling services with multiple drug use experiences. They may be addicted to three separate drug categories (stimulant, narcotic, depressant) but only see the problem with their use in one of the three categories. Clients may also arrive for services addicted to one drug while using other drugs based on their sense that they are only addicted to the primary drug. For example, a client may state, "My problem is really only with heroin; I can have a few beers now and then though." In this case, the counselor who understands the properties and impact on the brain of each drug category can motivate clients for change and prevention strategies with both of the drugs of choice.
- *Show clients that you have an interest.* No counselor can have expert knowledge of all drugs. However, credibility and trust in the therapeutic relationship and counselor are built when clients realize that counselors have an understanding and appreciation for drug interactions, physical symptoms (craving/withdrawal), and slang terminology. We have found that perhaps the best method for clinicians to learn about drugs and the addiction process (beyond course work, trainings, and readings) is to work with clients who use them.

Clients begin using for a host of reasons (e.g., curiosity, familial/social, peer modeling, spiritual emptiness, or emotional pain). Generally speaking, subsequent to using the drug is a feeling of chemical euphoria. In some instances though, individuals experience negative consequences (vomiting or paranoia) or simply experience no effect at all. Some clients continue to use drugs because they experience pleasure/euphoria and become addicted to the feeling; others use drugs to medicate emotions, psychological issues, or irrational thoughts. Whatever the reason, drug use potentially creates a chemical coping skill that is not easily discontinued and can significantly impact the chemistry of the brain.

Here we want to address one more aspect to this chapter and the significance of making meaning from the following pages. Though we do not at all suggest clients are as easy to understand as cars, the following analogy serves to parallel the need for all counselors to understand chemical issues as being unique in the treatment of clients.

Picture yourself taking your car to a garage because something is wrong with it. Imagine also that you have little knowledge of cars beyond the basics. The shop you take it to uses a machine that "pulls codes" from the computer in your car to tell it what's wrong. The mechanic, however, has really only specialized in brake jobs and mufflers.

He gets the codes from the computer printout and recognizes that it is a problem in the air intake valve (at least that's what the computer is suggesting). The mechanic replaces the front air intake valve, resets your "check engine light," and bills you. You drive off, only to have the light reemerge a few days later. You take it back to the same shop...same mechanic...same code. What now?

Here we can imagine that there are some missing data, information, and root *understanding* of the problem. In some cars, the computer would generate an accurate code. However, because the front air intake is upstream from the rear air intake, the wrong code trips for certain vehicles. Had your mechanic understood the unique circumstances of *your* vehicle, he might have saved you time and resources, and you might not be thinking of never taking your car back to him.

In a similar way, we must understand the true nature of the impact drugs have on the brain to fully recognize the "problem" we are working with, especially clients addicted to drugs and alcohol. Failing to recognize such data leaves us to misinterpret actions, reactions, and intentions by the client. It also can leave the client frustrated and dismayed by our lack of knowledge on the subject. We hope you take some time to digest the following, as we have found it particularly useful in our work with clients.

The Impact of Drugs on the Brain

"It is generally believed that drugs of abuse usurp neural circuitry in the brain that normally controls responses to natural rewards such as food, sex, and social interactions (Chao & Nestler, 2004, p. 114). As drugs enter the body, they impact various bodily functions, most significantly, the brain. The brain and spinal cord make up the central nervous system (CNS). Included in the general nervous system are the autonomic nervous system and the peripheral nervous system. The brain consists of neurons, which facilitate message impulses from neuron to neuron as they travel across the synaptic cleft (Craig, 2004; Goldberg, 1997; Kuhn, Swartzwelder, & Wilson, 2003). Each neuron consists of multiple dendrites, which allow the transmission of nerve impulses to the cell body, but only one axon, which sends the electrical impulse across the synaptic cleft to the receptor cells of the other neuron. It is here where drugs have their most devastating effect.

Naturally occurring chemical substances found in the brain called neurotransmitters facilitate the electrical impulse from the presynaptic neuron (sender) to the postsynaptic neuron (receiver). Depending on the drug ingested into the body, the excitation of the neurotransmitters may either increase or decrease. For example, on the one hand, tranquilizers increase the production of dopamine, creating a slow and calming effect. On the other hand, amphetamines stimulate the neurotransmitter norepinephrine, resulting in agitation and excitation.

Neurotransmitters

While some neurotransmitters act as conduits, some actually inhibit electrical impulses in the brain. Of the 200+ variations of neurotransmitters in the brain (no two are alike), each plays a vital role in sending and the successful receiving of messages. Introducing drugs into the brain complicates and negatively impacts the delicate natural balance of neurotransmitters in the brain.

The following is a list of the major transmitter groups aligned with the effects specific drug use has on neurotransmitter production and facilitation of messages (Craig, 2004; Goldberg, 1997; Kuhn et al., 2003). Though we do not believe you need to commit all of these to memory, we want you to have a clear understanding of the items that are confounded by the use of drugs and alcohol.

- *Serotonin.* Regulates sleep, pain, the temperature of the body, and sensory perception. For example, the use of cocaine increases the production of serotonin, thus effecting sleep, energy, and perception (Craig, 2004; Goldberg, 1997; Kuhn et al., 2003).
- *Gamma-Amniobutyric Acid and Glutamate (GABA).* Produces a relaxed effect. This neurotransmitter slows and inhibits impulses from nerve to nerve and creates a lethargic effect. Alcohol increases the inhibitory activity of GABA receptors and decreases the activity of glutamate receptors, thus suppressing brain activity (Kuhn et al., 2003).
- *Catecholamines.* This category of neurotransmitters includes dopamine, norepinephrine, and epinephrine. These neurotransmitters are produced and reabsorbed by the neuron in a process called reuptake. Drugs such as cocaine and methamphetamines increase the production and eventual depletion of catecholamines, thus producing depressive effects following extensive use of cocaine (Kuhn et al., 2003).

- *Peptides.* A group within peptides, endorphins, is a naturally produced morphine within the human body. Endorphins are released into the body at the onset of pain or involved in a stressful activity. Endorphins can also be released with the introduction of opiates into the body (Kuhn et al., 2003).

Factors Affecting the Response to Drugs

As drug use continues and increased addictive use develops, the brain chemistry changes. According to Craig (2004), three factors affect the client's response to drugs: (a) the client's personal variables, (b) the environmental variables, and (c) the amount of drug ingested into the system.

- *Personal variables.* Within this category Craig (2004) suggested that the client's age, gender, race, nutrition, genetics, and potential disease processes directly correlate with the individual's response to the drug. Additionally, he indicated that the client's expectation (i.e., what the drug does to/for the client and how it impacts the client) and any previous drug experiences each have significant and substantial effects on the client's response to the drugs.
- *Environmental variables.* The physical and social milieu plays a role in the impact drugs have on clients. For example, both family members' use of drugs or alcohol as well as use by the greater community in which the client resides affect clients in their decision to ingest chemicals. These cultures also contribute to the client's continued use of chemicals.
- *Dose.* The amount of the drug significantly contributes to the overall experience of the client. For example, a client ingesting 5 beers will have a different reaction than that of a client snorting 10 lines of cocaine in the same time period. Alcohol is a sedative drug, which slows the heart rate and breathing, whereas cocaine is a stimulant, which serves to increase the client's heart rate and breathing.

The remainder of this chapter provides basic terminology, information on each drug, including method of consumption, clinical observations, and pertinent general information. These sections are followed by a chart with each drug category, commonly associated names, symptoms, and identifying information. Also included are case vignettes, relevant questions, and consultations to guide the reader in considering the cases presented.

Terminology

The following terminology is necessary basic language for all practitioners in communication with and about substance abuse issues. We have found that some clients will use some of the following terminology early in sessions with us to "test" us on our awareness of substance abuse issues:

- *Addiction.* A condition characterized by compulsive drug or alcohol use despite negative consequences, loss of control, and tolerance or withdrawal symptoms (a physiological change).
- *Tolerance (increased/decreased).* Increased tolerance indicates the body's need for increased doses of the drug in order to achieve the desired effect. For instance, individuals who were once intoxicated after consuming 6 beers, and now have the ability to consume 12 beers without feeling intoxicated, have developed tolerance to alcohol. Reverse tolerance generally occurs following many years of drinking/using, where intoxication/high occurs after small drinks/doses. This phenomenon suggests liver damage and the diminished capacity for the body to handle the substance (American Psychiatric Association, 2000).

- *Cross-tolerance.* A physiological tolerance to all the drugs in a designated drug category. For example, clients who are addicted to alcohol and start using other sedative-hypnotics, such as Valium, have a similar tolerance level for the drug (Valium) as they have for alcohol (Kuhn et al., 2003).
- *Cross-addiction.* A physiological condition where individuals are addicted to drugs across various categories. Some clients self-identify as "garbage heads" because they are simultaneously addicted to alcohol (sedative-hypnotics), crack cocaine (stimulant), and heroin (opiate). In this example, clients are cross-addicted to drugs in three separate categories and have cross-tolerance within each category.
- *Abstinence.* Complete and total discontinuation of all mood-altering drugs or alcohol.
- *Recovery.* A growth process within the client, beginning with abstinence and followed by changes in cognitive, emotional, behavioral, and spiritual attitudes.
- *Dry drunk/drug.* Discontinuation of drugs or alcohol, but there are minimal if any changes in cognitive, emotional/behavioral management, or spiritual well-being. Clients exhibiting "dry drunk" behaviors may appear unhappy and angry. They are "dry," or abstinent, but have not developed a cognitive, emotional, behavioral, and spiritual framework to support their abstinence. Their behavior continues to resemble that which they displayed when intoxicated or high; thus, the term *dry drunk/drug.*
- *Withdrawal.* This physiological condition occurs in addicted clients following the discontinuation of drug or alcohol use. Clients who are addicted begin to experience physical problems or discomfort when the drugs or alcohol are processed out of their system.
- *Substance abuse.* A pattern of behavior that occurs when individuals abuse substances, but not yet having met the criteria for addiction or dependence per the *Diagnostic and Statistical Manual* (*DSM-IV-TR*; American Psychiatric Association, 2000).
- *Alcoholism.* Addiction to the drug alcohol.
- *Relapse.* An internal process whereby those who have been abstinent and have made cognitive, emotional, behavioral, and spiritual changes, become out of control (behaviorally, emotionally, and/or cognitively) and conclude the process with the use of drugs or alcohol again (Gorski, 1989).

Federal Drug Administration Schedule of Drugs

The Controlled Substances Act of 1970 (Federal Drug Administration, n.d.) partitioned drugs into five separate categories based on levels of abuse and use for medical purposes and a drug's potential to create physiological or psychic dependence. The Federal Drug Administration was charged with the task of breaking the levels of drugs into five separate schedules of drugs. This legislation was created with an effort to address the growing problem of drug abuse in the United States by providing increased efforts in prevention and rehabilitation, through providing more law enforcement, and by providing a balanced effort of crime penalties for criminal offenses involving drugs (Werth, 2002). These efforts resulted in the scheduling of drugs found below along with associated examples.

- *Schedule I drugs.* These drugs have a high abuse potential and no medical use. Drugs such as LSD, Heroin, peyote, and methaqualone fall into this category. These drugs are not used as prescriptions and have high potential for addiction.
- *Schedule II drugs.* These drugs have a high potential for abuse with both physical and psychological dependence. Drugs in this category include codeine, Demerol, opium, methadone, and cocaine.
- *Schedule III drugs.* In general, these drugs have less frequency of abuse when compared with Schedule I and II drugs. Drugs in this category include PCP, pentobarbital, and some stimulants.

- *Schedule IV drugs.* These drugs have less abuse potential than those drugs found in Schedule III. Drugs in this category include Xanax, Valium, and Librium and are only available through prescriptions.
- *Schedule V drugs.* These have less abuse potential than Schedule IV drugs and include antitussive, antidiarreals, and some codeine compounds. These drugs can be prescribed and also purchased over the counter (OTC).

Drug Categories

The main categories of drugs are: sedative-hypnotics, stimulants, cannabinols, opiates/narcotics, hallucinogens, inhalants, club drugs, steroids, nicotine, OTC, and psychotropic medications. These drug classifications are outlined in Table 3.1 and provide the types of drugs in each category, commonly used slang terms, symptoms of intoxication, and miscellaneous information.

Table 3.1. Drug Classifications

Drug Category	Type of Drugs	Common Names	Symptoms of Intoxication	Miscellaneous
Sedative-Hypnotics (Depressants)	Alcohol, barbiturates (Seconol, Quaaludes), tranquilizers (Valium, Librium, Ativan, Xanax)	Booze, barbs, ludes, tranks, bisquits	Drowsy, slows CNS, confused, uncoordinated movements	Dangerous withdrawal, potential for overdose with alcohol and death
Stimulants	Cocaine, methamphetamines, amphetamines, caffeine, nicotine	C, coke, flake, crack, meth, crystal, crank, black beauties, java, Joe	Talkative, alert, stimulates CNS, paranoid, anxiety increase, decrease in appetite, hyperactive	Depression, severe when stops, suicidal, possible hallucinations
Cannabinols	Marijuana, hash, hash oil	Pot, dope, weed, hash, sheesh, herb, doobie	Decrease in motivation, red eyes, decrease in motor skill ability, increase in hunger, excessive laughing, paranoia	Short-term memory loss, hallucinations
Narcotics (Opiates)	Heroin, Demerol, Dilaudid, morphine, codeine, Percodan, methodone, opium	Junk, smack, oxy, China white, H, horse	Nausea, nodding out, vomiting, watery eyes and nose, insensitive to pain, detached	Significant withdrawal, increased weight loss, increased risk for HIV, Hepatitis C, risk for overdosing and death
Hallucinogens	LSD, mescaline, PCP, MDMA, peyote	Sid, ex, rocket fuel	Impairs judgment, hallucinations, change in perception	Mild withdrawal, difficult to detect in drug screens, violent behavior, unpredictable
Inhalants	Gasoline, aerosols, glue, liquid paper, nitrous oxide	Whippets, nitros, rush	Dizziness, odor of chemicals, severe headaches, blackouts, hallucinations	Risk for brain damage, sudden death, suffocations
Over the Counter (OTC)	Cold medicines with alcohol or acetaminophen	OTCs	Dilated pupils, dry mouth, sleepiness	Possible overdose when mixed with alcohol and other drugs
Steroids	Oxymetholone, oxadrolone	Stacking, pyramiding	Mood swings, paranoia, irritable behavior, violent, voice changes	Increase in transmission for HIV and Hepatitis C

Note. CNS = central nervous system; MDMA = methylenedioxyamphetamine; PCP = phencyclidine.

Sedative-Hypnotics

The category of sedative-hypnotics includes alcohol, barbiturates, nonbarbiturates, and tranquilizers.

Alcohol

The production and consumption of alcohol dates back as early as 1800 B.C. (Stone, 1991). Current statistics indicate that by the time students reach eighth grade, nearly 50% of adolescents have had one drink, while more than 20% of adolescents report having been intoxicated (Johnston, O'Malley, & Bachman, 2001). Statistically, 1 in 10 individuals who drink alcohol will become alcoholics (Kinney & Leaton, 1995). In 2002, over 17 million people in the United States were estimated to suffer from alcohol abuse or dependence (National Institute on Alcohol Abuse and Alcoholism [NIAAA], 2006). Among those who drink, having a family history of alcoholism or drug addiction increases the risk of developing the disorder. Individuals who consume alcohol before age 15 are four times more likely to develop alcohol dependence at some point in their lives compared with those who start drinking at age 20 or older (NIAAA, 2003). Essentially, those individuals who drink earlier, have familial alcoholism, and have high genetic risk are more vulnerable to developing alcoholism than individuals without these factors (NIAAA, 2003).

Alcohol is most commonly consumed orally through liquid. Once consumed, it is immediately absorbed into the lining of the mouth and capillaries in the throat. Almost 20% of alcohol is absorbed into the stomach; the remaining alcohol is absorbed into the small intestines. Essentially one third of an ounce of alcohol is metabolized by the liver per hour (Kinney & Leaton, 1995). A normal, healthy adult who has consumed one beer and waits approximately 1 hour will have metabolized that beer. However, if the same individual continues to drink at a rate of three beers per hour over the course of 5 hours, it will not be metabolized by the liver in that period of time. The liver produces alcohol dehydrogenase (ADH), which breaks down the alcohol into acetaldehyde and is crucial in metabolizing alcohol. From the liver, alcohol is broken into carbon dioxide, carbohydrates, and water. Individuals consuming large quantities of alcohol will expel alcohol through their breath, pores, or frequent urination (Kinney & Leaton, 1995; NIAAA, 1998).

Route of Administration

Although rare, alcohol can also be injected intravenously into the bloodstream. This is a very dangerous method of administration where clients, who are primarily intravenous drug users, use needles instead of oral consumption.

Clinical Observations

Counselors meeting with clients for the first session, when alcohol is included in the referral information, need to use their senses and the referent information provided. For example, clients referred by court for counseling will many times include a blood alcohol level in the referral paperwork (drunk in public/drunk driving). The blood alcohol level indicates what percentage of the clients' blood had alcohol in it when the test was administered. The blood alcohol levels range from zero to .60 (Kuhn et al., 2003). The use of the information in Table 3.2 can help counselors understand the impact alcohol has on reaction time, coordination, voluntary, and involuntary functions of the human body.

Blood alcohol levels provide critical information to clinicians in assessing for tolerance. For instance, if clients state during their evaluation that they drink only once a month, and only two beers at most, and they come to counseling describing a blood alcohol level of .24 at the time of their offense, they are likely underreporting their alcohol use. Individuals who drink only two occasional beers would pass out with a .24 blood alcohol level. This strongly suggests underreporting and needs to be continually evaluated by the clinician.

Table 3.2. Blood Alcohol Impairment

Blood Alcohol Level (mg)	Impairment	State of Being
Zero to .10	Reaction time	Giddy, talkative
.10–.30	Coordination/reflexes	Nauseous, vomiting, visibly intoxicated, slurring speech
.30–.40	Ability to move, voluntary actions of the body	Passed out, danger of death
.40–.60	Shutting down of body systems	Coma
.60–.90	Death, breathing/heart stop	Death

During the evaluation, counselors need to explore the quantity of alcohol consumed at the time of the referring incident. In cases where clients report having consumed 12 beers in an hour and a half and "didn't even feel drunk," then an increased tolerance to alcohol should be considered. As presented earlier, an increased tolerance indicates a physiological adaptation where clients need to use or consume more and more of the drug or alcohol in order to achieve the desired effect.

Observations by counselors of clients' bloodshot eyes, shakiness (potential withdrawal), or yellowing skin (jaundice) may also be indicators of significant alcohol use warranting further exploration.

Individuals under the influence of alcohol will often slur their speech, increase speaking volume when talking, or become argumentative. However, those who present significant personality changes or mood shifts, as well as aggressive behavior while intoxicated, tend to be at higher risk for developing problems with alcohol. Although clients with increased alcohol tolerance, who present for counseling and smell of alcohol, may not appear intoxicated, their thought process and response to questions may seem disconnected and/or inappropriate.

Clinical Examples

On many occasions, I (Ford) have had clients appear for counseling sessions under the influence of alcohol. Sometimes, because of their high tolerance, it was difficult to determine whether they had been drinking/drugging. When trying to determine from clients the amount of alcohol consumed, it is very important to ask specifically what kinds of alcohol they were consuming. Most of the clients I worked with in a small, rural town in Virginia differentiated types of alcohol. For some, beer was not alcohol, nor was wine; only liquor sold at the state store or "ABC alcohol" was defined as true alcohol in their eyes. As a result of understanding this, I obtained a much clearer picture of the true amounts of alcohol that were consumed by clients. Their behavior and affect appeared "normal" with the exception of the faint smell of alcohol. In such cases, a Breathalyzer was very helpful in assessing amounts of alcohol clients still had in their systems.

I (Bill) was working with a Native American client who had been referred for "anger issues" while I was working in a college counseling center. As we discussed what was going on, he talked about how his friends were concerned that he was "changing." He went on to add that he was finding himself drinking more and more beer (even when others weren't drinking). When we charted out his drinking patterns, we discovered he was typically consuming a minimum of 15 beers a day. His reaction to this datum was not anger but rather seemed to be deep regret and sorrow. We discussed resources within his Native American community, and he decided to go back to his reservation "to work on this." The next year he returned to see me to share his story. He had reconnected with his "Indian roots," lost 40 pounds, and was markedly different (spiritually, affectively, and cognitively). Our discovery of his "amount of use" yielded a powerful message that only he could hear.

Drug and Alcohol Screening Methods

Urine drug testing and Breathalyzers can be used *therapeutically* to help clients maintain abstinence. Testing can be provided on-site through the use of small drug test kits or sent to separate testing agencies. At some point, counselors working with addicted clients will probably find themselves having to observe urines as part of their job. Of course, this is not typically considered as a highlight of being a counselor. Minimal training is required in order to operate a Breathalyzer or drug testing kit. However, there are specific guidelines when observing federal probation and parole clients submitting urine samples. For these clients, counselors are required to observe clients as they void into a bottle for testing. Although referents may provide testing services, the possibility that providers (counselors) will be the ones administering the urine tests is most typical, thus placing clinicians in a perceived adversarial position with clients (in essence, a dual relationship). Male clients are observed by male counselors and female clients by female counselors. Clients are creative and capable of employing various methods in order to avoid detection. Methods to elude detection include using urine from other family members and concealing it in plastic bottles or improvised rubber bladders under the arm with plastic tubing. Clients may also resort to drinking, diluting, or contaminating their urine in order to avoid detection.

Resistance can be reduced by informing and educating clients on how testing can be helpful in documenting their abstinence and demonstrating to others in treatment, employers, courts, and families that they are compliant with treatment. Although much of what is important to clients is in jeopardy, they may still use drugs or alcohol despite the possibility of losing relationships, employment, and so on.

Urine testing is a therapeutic tool, not a punishment. Although clients generally view it as a punishment, urine testing can help clients set goals for themselves from week to week and to document and show themselves (most importantly) that they can stop using. If counselors present it in a way to clients that is helpful in nature and not punitive, they can begin to view this as a helpful aspect of their therapy. If at all possible, though, having a third party notify, collect, and coordinate the testing would be best so as to separate collection from therapy.

Withdrawal

Withdrawal from alcohol indicates physical dependency on alcohol. Withdrawal symptoms begin when alcohol is metabolized out of the body (usually within 72 hours). This is the time when clients, despite negative consequences, will crave alcohol and are at increased potential to drink again. This reaction, of course, depends on the amount the client has been drinking, how long, and what other drugs, if any, the client has been taking. Medical monitoring and treatment are essential for individuals in need of detoxification. Alcohol detoxification is a medical protocol whereby the client experiences withdrawal in a safe and supportive medical setting, reducing the risk of seizures, delirium tremens (DTs), or other medical maladies (N. S. Miller & Gold, 1998).

Patients entering detoxification are evaluated by physicians, nurses, and counselors in order to develop medical and psychological treatment plans. Detoxification is usually experienced as very uncomfortable for patients, and as a result, they are administered medications to reduce withdrawal symptoms and the risk of other medical complications (e.g., seizures). Detoxification allows patients to be medically monitored, provided with medications to reduce the symptoms of withdrawal, and to prepare clients to enter or reenter treatment following the detoxification. Detoxification is not treatment, but rather a medical intervention.

Other Sedative-Hypnotic Drugs

In addition to alcohol, which is a sedative drug, there are three other types of drugs/alcohol that fall into this same category: barbiturates, nonbarbiturates, and minor tranquilizers.

Barbiturates

Initially developed as medications to induce sleep, barbiturates today continue to be used as sedating drugs to help those with difficulty sleeping (Goldberg, 1997). Phenobarbital has been used as a transitory medication when detoxifying patients because of its long-acting effects, which minimize the symptoms of withdrawal. Barbiturates and alcohol are in the same sedative-hypnotic drug category and hold the property of cross-tolerance should clients be addicted to one or the other. Consider for example, alcoholic clients who have discontinued their use of alcohol and report to their physicians that they are having difficulty sleeping. It would not be encouraged for clients in this situation to obtain prescriptions for Valium because of the cross-tolerance properties (otherwise clients will replace one drug, alcohol, for another, Valium).

It is not uncommon for clients to use drugs in other categories in conjunction with sedative-hypnotic drugs. Clients become their own pharmacists by ingesting certain drugs to stay awake and obtain energy (stimulants) and ingest other drugs to slow down and relax (sedative-hypnotics). For instance, individuals working third shift (11 pm–7 am) may use amphetamines to remain awake and then consume alcohol and smoke marijuana after work to sleep. Upon awakening, these clients may start their day with coffee (stimulant/caffeine) and then snort cocaine to prepare for the evening shift, thus repeating the cycle. Other drugs in the sedative-hypnotic category include Amytal, Miltown, Seconal, Nembutal, Tranxene, and Serax (Goldberg, 1997; Kuhn et al., 2003).;

Routes of Administration

Sedative-hypnotic drugs can be taken orally in pill form or administered intravenously. Once barbiturates have been taken orally, they are absorbed completely through the small intestines. The drugs course freely through the entire body, providing sedative effects, impacting the neurotransmitter GABA, and slowing down brain activity and breathing (Goldberg, 1997).

Clinical Observations

As with alcohol, counselors need to look for lethargic behavior. Clients may appear confused or exhibit poor judgment (depending on the amount ingested and their level of tolerance). Occasionally, the sound of rattling pills in a bottle or canister are heard when clients move. Clients adept at obtaining prescription drugs may "doctor hop" or feign symptoms in order to obtain prescriptions. These clients typically move to multiple pharmacies to avoid pharmacist suspicion. It is not uncommon for these clients who are addicted to prescription drugs to have multiple physicians and pharmacies.

Clients who engage in simultaneous sedative-hypnotic and alcohol use risk chemically induced comas and potential death. A synergistic effect occurs when one drug potentiates the effects of another. Clients appear drowsy, have a slowed breathing rate, and may lose balance when walking. They may lose their train of thought and have a reduction in response time.

Withdrawal

Withdrawal from some sedative-hypnotic drugs can be lethal. Clients may exhibit a number of withdrawal symptoms (i.e., seizures, hallucinations, vomiting, cramps) when discontinuing their use. It is dangerous for clients to detoxify themselves without medical supervision. During the assessment, it is extremely important for counselors to determine amounts (how many milligrams) and frequencies (number of times) of use along with information about the last time the client used. With drugs in this category (e.g., Seconol), withdrawal symptoms may not be exhibited for a number of weeks. Therefore, a thorough assessment by counselors of the patient's Valium/Seconol usage informs detoxification and treatment protocols aimed at preventing seizures. Twelve weeks or longer may be needed to detoxify and stabilize patients who have been taking benzodiazepines for several years (N. S. Miller & Gold, 1998). Unfortunately, without effective medical care, clients who begin experiencing these withdrawal signs either return to use or drink alcohol in order to avoid the pain and discomfort of withdrawal.

Nonbarbiturates

These drugs (e.g., chloral hydrate, paraldehyde, bromides, meprobromate, and methaqualone) help with sedation while reducing anxiety. Chloral hydrate has been used in the past to treat patients withdrawing from alcohol and heroin. Because of gastric side effects, today it is rarely used. Paraldehyde, like chloral hydrate, was used to treat alcohol withdrawal. It is not currently used for detoxification purposes. Both bromides and meprobromates are rarely, if ever, used for the treatment of alcohol withdrawal.

Minor Tranquilizers: Benzodiazepines

Benzodiazepines, or "benzos," are used medically to help individuals reduce short-term anxiety, sleep problems, and for some, managing seizure disorders (Goldberg, 1997; Hermos, Young, Lawler, Rosenbloom, & Fiore, 2007; Kuhn et al., 2003; National Institute on Drug Abuse [NIDA], 2005b). Network (DAWN) monitors medications and illicit drugs and found that across the United States, two of the most frequently reported prescription medications in drug abuse related cases are benzodiazepines (e.g., diazepam, alprazolam, clonazepam, and lorazepam) and opioids. According to the NIDA in 2002, benzodiazepines accounted for 100,784 mentions that were classified as drug abuse cases (NIDA, 2005b).

Initially, when benzodiazepines such as Librium, Klonopin, Valium, and Halcion were introduced into clinical practice, the thinking was that they had advantages over drugs in this category (barbiturates) in that they significantly reduced anxiety and appeared not to create physical dependence. It is the claim of no physical dependence that has been proven to be unfounded (Ashworth, Gerada, & Dallmeyer, 2002). Because benzodiazepines are prescribed drugs, individuals who are addicted to them find that they will need alternative methods of procurement in order to meet their building tolerance and subsequent withdrawal symptoms. Alternative methods include but are not limited to diverting medication, buying illegally, or stealing prescription pads.

The drugs in the sedative-hypnotic category (barbiturates, nonbarbiturates, and benzodiazepines) all have medical applications and uses. They are also the most common form of drug abuse/addiction in older patients (NIDA, 2005b). Elderly persons take three times as much prescription medication as the general population. Combined with this fact, they are also the most likely to not take medications as directed by prescribing physicians, which makes this a growing segment of the addicted population (NIDA, 2005b).

Case of Jerry
Jerry presents for counseling to work on his depression after being referred by his psychiatrist. Jerry reports lethargy and difficulty in waking up for work and falling asleep twice this past month on the job. He has been seeing his psychiatrist monthly for a year, and more recently was taken off of Valium and placed on antidepressant medication. Jerry states that he has not been able to sleep since he discontinued his Valium use and is angry with his doctor for taking him off of it. Instead, he now drinks 8–10 beers each night, just like he did 5 years ago, before he went on Valium to help him sleep.

Jerry reports that since discontinuing his Valium use, he has felt an increase in his anxiety levels. At times he is agitated, which prevents him from going to sleep. When he drinks alcohol, he occasionally has blackouts and exhibits violent behavior.

Questions for Readers to Ponder
1. On the basis of this information, do you believe Jerry has cross-tolerance to both alcohol and Valium? If so, why? If not, why not?
2. Who might you involve in Jerry's therapy (with written permission, such as a release of information)?
3. On the basis of the information, might Jerry have a sleeping disorder, a preexisting depression, or are these reported symptoms a result of withdrawal?

Consultation to Jerry's Case
Upon meeting with Jerry, we would want to encourage him to involve his psychiatrist in the therapeutic process. Although he may be angry with him or her, Jerry is still compliant with the prescribed medication for now. With Jerry's written permission we would work with his doctor in helping to monitor Jerry's response to the antidepressant medication and potential withdrawal from the Valium and alcohol. We would want to determine from his doctor how Jerry's Valium protocol was tapered and how the complicating factor of Jerry's increased alcohol usage may impact the taper.

It appears to us that Jerry is quite possibly staving off his withdrawal symptoms from Valium by increasing his alcohol use. We would specifically want to evaluate Jerry's Valium consumption over the past few years and obtain a more accurate alcohol consumption history prior to his Valium use. We would continue to evaluate his depression, signs of withdrawal, and alcohol use. Additionally, we would work with him on how to manage and create strategies to deal with his difficulty in sleeping at night without using alcohol or Valium. As presented, Jerry seems to be dependent on Valium and has a history of alcohol abuse, to be further evaluated for dependency (i.e., blackouts, tolerance increase, and personality changes).

Being aware of cross-tolerance with sedative-hypnotic drugs and the potential for withdrawal is important. In this case, given the brief amount of information, it is unclear whether Jerry has a preexisting depression or a documented sleep disorder. We would be fairly certain, after consultation with the physician, that Jerry is dependent on both alcohol and Valium, which would help in making referrals for appropriate treatment (alcohol and drug treatment vs. a sleep disorder clinic). His discontinuation of alcohol and Valium would suggest the signs of withdrawal, which include sleep and fatigue issues and could mimic a sleep disorder. In working with Jerry, these areas would be further explored and evaluated to further refine the treatment plan.

Stimulants: Amphetamine, Methamphetamine, and Cocaine

Drugs in this category impact the CNS by increasing both cardiovascular and respiratory rates. Included in the stimulant drug category are amphetamines (which have medical uses), methamphetamines (which are synthetic, high powered stimulants, twice as strong as pharmaceutical stimulants), and cocaine.

Amphetamines

Amphetamines are considered to be weaker than methamphetamines. Patients consuming amphetamines under medical supervision experience dryness of mouth, headaches, or insomnia (Fawcett & Busch, 1995). Those not under a physician's care obtain the drug illegally and may use it to stay awake (long distance driving) or for endurance events (e.g., work or performance enhancement in athletes).

Routes of Administration
Methamphetamines and amphetamines are ingested orally in pill form, intravenously, smoked, or snorted.

Clinical Observations

Counselors working with clients who are under the influence of amphetamines may observe increased anxious behavior, agitation, flushed face, difficulty sitting for any period of time, and clients may grind their teeth in the session (or report it at night when sleeping). Clients who use stimulant drugs on a regular, nonprescribed basis may report and present mood swings, a combination of depression and anxiety, as well as diminished appetite.

Methamphetamine

Methamphetamines are stimulant drugs possessing high potential for abuse. The NIDA (2002) reported on drug-related episodes in hospital emergency departments from 21 metropolitan areas. Its data suggested that methamphetamine-related episodes increased from approximately 10,400 in 1999 to 13,500 in 2000, a 30% increase.

Methamphetamines are Schedule II drugs and can only be obtained legally through a physician's prescription. Amphetamines are regularly used to treat attention deficit and weight disorders. Slang terminology such as "crank," "speed," "crystal," "meth," and "glass" are used to describe this powerful drug. Once ingested, methamphetamines immediately enter the bloodstream and impact both brain and body functioning. Regular use of methamphetamines creates an anxiety state, prompting the use of other drugs to decrease the anxiety. The use of benzodiazepines, alcohol, and marijuana are typical drugs used by individuals in order to counterbalance the effects of methamphetamines. Methamphetamines and cocaine are both psychostimulant drugs; however, they have a number of significant differences. Cocaine is derived from a plant, whereas methamphetamine is synthetically produced; intoxication from cocaine lasts 20–30 minutes, whereas methamphetamines last 8–24 hours; over half of the drug (cocaine) is removed from the body within an hour of use, whereas with methamphetamines, half is removed within 12 hours; and finally, there are medicinal uses for cocaine as topical anesthetics, whereas methamphetamines have limited if any legitimate uses (Goldberg, 1997; Kuhn et al., 2003).

Cocaine

Addiction to, and abuse of, cocaine continues to be a national problem. Although the rate of cocaine use has decreased since 1985, 1.5 million Americans could be classified as dependent on or abusing cocaine (Substance Abuse and Mental Health Services Administration, 2003).

Cocaine is derived from the coca plant and grown in countries such as Peru and Bolivia, where the coca leaves are chewed for relaxation. Cocaine is also a Schedule II drug with a high potential for abuse. Cocaine addicts report how paraphernalia such as soda cans (used as a makeshift pipe), baking soda (to "cut" or mix with cocaine to create larger amounts for sale), and lighters (to light the pipe with cocaine) can be "triggers" to use cocaine.

Routes of Administration

Cocaine can be smoked in a pipe or a handmade smoking instrument, snorted, injected, or rubbed on gums. Cocaine comes as a white powder in the form of a chloride salt and is very addicting. This form of cocaine can be snorted, rubbed into the gums and mouth, or on occasion dropped in the eyes to create a numbing effect. When cocaine is snorted it goes directly into the nasal passage to the lining of the nose and is directly and quickly absorbed into the bloodstream (Goldberg, 1997; Kuhn et al., 2003).

Residue from snorted cocaine runs down the back of the throat, producing an analgesic/numbing effect. Regular users of cocaine who snort it may report nosebleeds and sinus infections. Problems with vision and runny noses can also occur with regularity, depending on the amount and frequency of cocaine being used.

Freebasing cocaine is another method of using cocaine. Although used less often because of its cost (crack cocaine is much less expensive), it is nonetheless a method of ingesting cocaine. In this form, the drug has not been mixed with a neutralizing acid and therefore can be smoked. Cocaine is placed in a pipe bowl and ignited with a lighter. As it is heated, the smoke is inhaled into the lungs. Many times the pipe glass or lighter becomes extremely hot, resulting in burn marks on fingers and hands. Within 10 seconds of inhaling the cocaine smoke, individuals experience an intense and euphoric high lasting a short period of time (10–15 minutes) as opposed to longer acting drugs (sedative-hypnotics and opiates). Smoke enters the lungs and is absorbed into the bloodstream impacting the pleasure center of the brain, or the ventral tegmental area, creating an intense, euphoric feeling. Following the initial "blast," individuals attempt to seek out another high just as intense and repeat the cycle until all of the cocaine has been consumed, making smoking the quickest route to obtaining a high. Experiments with laboratory rats have found, given a choice between eating and using cocaine, the rats would choose the cocaine consistently and eventually die from starvation (Kuhn et al., 2003).

Cocaine blocks the redistribution of the neurotransmitter dopamine, contributing to the euphoria. However, chronic use of cocaine depletes the neurotransmitter dopamine and impacts energy, sleep, and pleasure. Individuals exhibit depression, irritability, and suicidality with diminished dopamine production.

Street terminology for cocaine includes "C," "blow," "nose candy," and "coke." The potential for cocaine being "cut" or mixed with other substances is a strong possibility. Substances such as cornstarch, baking soda, or talcum powder are mixed with the cocaine to create a larger supply. This increased volume yields greater return on the investment when sold. An "eight ball," or roughly 3 ½ grams of cocaine, could be mixed with baking soda to create a larger portion. This process allows drug dealers to increase profits while maintaining a larger supply for their personal use.

Crack Cocaine

Crack cocaine is made by removing chloride from the freebased cocaine mixture. When crack is heated, the sound of "pop" or "crack" can be heard, thus the name *crack cocaine*. The National Survey on Drug Use and Health (NSDUH; U.S. Department of Health and Human Services, 2008) estimated the number of cocaine users in 2007 to be about 2.1 million, aged 12 years and older. Crack is less expensive to buy than powder cocaine and, because of that, is easier to access. The NIDA (1999) has as a priority the identification of an effective medication to treat cocaine dependence.

Cocaine or crack impacts the brain, heart, lungs, and digestive systems. Increased heart rates and rapid breathing result from cocaine use. Headaches, nausea, and digestive problems are also associated with crack use. Respiratory failure and heart attacks have occurred with professional athletes using cocaine. Intravenous drug users have an increased risk of transmitting or contracting HIV.

Clients who are not forthright about their use of stimulants, and are in active withdrawal, can present symptoms that mimic major depression and/or anxiety disorders. Withdrawal from stimulants is not necessarily life threatening; however, clients may be so depressed that they become suicidal or use other drugs (N. S. Miller & Gold, 1998). According to McGregor et al. (2005), failure to manage methamphetamine withdrawal symptoms during the course of treatment may be a contributing factor in the high rate of relapse during the first few days of postcessation. Clients in withdrawal can present with psychomotor agitation and report problems with sleeping and appetite (Bronson, Swift, & Peers, 2005; Elkashef et al., 2005). They also report having little interest in work, family, or hobbies. A recommended detoxification protocol may include outpatient detoxification in a partial treatment program, followed by intensive outpatient treatment. Physical withdrawal from stimulants can last up to 3 days; however, lethargy, sleep disturbances, and depressive symptoms may linger depending on the amount used by clients. They may return to the use of other drugs or alcohol in order to medicate the discomfort of withdrawal.

Clinical Observations

As with other stimulant drugs, individuals using and abusing cocaine appear agitated, tearful, depressed, and anxious. They may exhibit increased energy, report a decrease in appetite, and have an increased heart rate. Cocaine addicts typically (like most other addicted clients) come in for treatment or counseling following their last binge, which has resulted in a crisis (i.e., loss of job, relationship, legal entanglement) and are in need of help.

It has been our experience that a "window of opportunity" exists between the initial phone call and the appointment. The quicker clinicians are able to schedule appointments the better. The adage of "striking while the iron is hot" certainly applies here. Clients at this point are emotionally and physically vulnerable, many times have run out of their drug, and are about to lose things near and dear to them (e.g., friends, jobs, and money). The longer the delay in scheduling, the less likely they will appear for their appointments, so same-day scheduling with cocaine abusers increases the likelihood clients will show for their first appointment. When clients do arrive, counselors need to be aware of any physical abnormalities (e.g., track marks, visible infections from intravenous use, nosebleeds, or scarring).

Withdrawal

Counselors working with cocaine addicted clients may observe erratic and agitated behaviors when clients are in withdrawal or high on cocaine or crack. Withdrawal from cocaine is not life threatening; however, symptoms of depression, agitation, lethargy, poor appetite, and restlessness may be exhibited by clients following cessation of cocaine (Goldberg, 1997; Kuhn et al., 2003). During withdrawal, it is critical for counselors to thoroughly assess for suicide.

Case of Ted

Ted is a 35-year-old crack/cocaine addict who is referred by his employee assistance program (EAP) at work for evaluation of his depression. The EAP has no knowledge of Ted's chronic cocaine use but is aware he has missed time from work because of self-reported depression. Ted has never been in counseling before and is an African American father of two young children. He has a good job working the night shift as a supervisor for the past 8 years.

Upon arrival, Ted presents symptoms of decreased interest in activities, exhibits strong emotions such as being tearful during the session, reports a loss of appetite, suicidal thoughts, and states he feels tired most of the time. He has an appointment with the psychiatrist for an antidepressant evaluation the following week.

Consultation With Ted's Case

Because Ted's presenting concern is depression, we would focus our initial efforts toward the depressive symptoms along with development of rapport and a therapeutic alliance. As European American counselors with a contractual relation to his employer, we understand and appreciate Ted's potential distrust of us and, perhaps, therapy in general. Sensitivity to these potential concerns is necessary in helping him explore issues in counseling, particularly his chemical use. We would explore possible chemical use and, more specifically, cocaine use. We would want to continually rule out drug and alcohol addiction as an issue. In Ted's case, if cocaine use is not attended to, the result may be prescribed medication for depression (which is secondary to his primary problem of cocaine addiction and would not be receiving significant attention). Essentially, the treatment would be addressing the primary symptom of his cocaine use, not necessarily the primary problem.

If Ted is willing to explore his use, we would work with him on what he might want to change and identify allies he would want to include to help him on his journey (i.e., family, psychiatrist). If he is amenable to treatment, we would help him work with his EAP to receive structured treatment services. However, should he refuse a release of information to the EAP, we would maintain his confidentiality and work with him on depression and changes in his cocaine use. If he continues to use or stop, his depression would be significant, and we would want to talk about and evaluate continually his depression and suicidality. We would encourage him to sign a release to the psychiatrist to help him with medication effectiveness.

Cannabinols

Marijuana and Hashish

In 1999, more than 2 million Americans used marijuana for the first time. In 2001, marijuana was cited as the most commonly used illicit drug in the United States. Worldwide, cannabis is the most widely used illicit psychoactive substance, and it is currently used by an estimated 147 million people, with about 10% of users becoming dependent (United Nations Office on Drugs and Crime, 2004). The marijuana available today can be at least five times more potent than the marijuana of the 1970s. Research suggests that marijuana use precedes tobacco use in adolescents, and there is increasing popularity of mixing tobacco (cigars) and marijuana (smoking blunts; Humfleet & Amos, 2004).

Routes of Administration
Cannabinols, including marijuana and hashish, can be smoked, eaten, or used in tea. The chemical delta-9 tetrohydrocanabinol, or THC, is the potent ingredient in both marijuana and hashish. Marijuana is a plant (cannabis sativa) where the buds and leaves are dried and typically sold in ounce weights. Common names of marijuana include "Mary Jane," "weed," "reefer," "doobie/joint (marijuana cigarette)," "pot," "boom," "spleef," "ganja," and "grass." Depending on the geographic area, each town/city has local terms for marijuana. Marijuana can be smoked in cigarette form, in a pipe or "bowl," or in a bong apparatus. Marijuana cigarettes can also be laced with cocaine and smoked in "woolies" or dipped in PCP (phencyclidine) called "happy sticks."

The marijuana plant is harvested and hung upside down in order for the THC to spread throughout the drying leaves. The leaves are then crushed and rolled into cigarette papers or joints so they can be smoked. The bong is a water pipe where the marijuana is burned in a bowl. The smoke filters through the stem, into the water in the tube to cool the smoke, and then inhaled into the lungs. Marijuana can also be placed into a cigar, which is referred to as "smoking a blunt." It appears that some adolescents believe this combination enhances the effects of the marijuana (Gross, 1998).

Hashish is sold in baggies, wrapped in tin foil, and compressed into small square blocks, which are dark green, black, or light tan in color. In this form it can be soft and easy to cut. It is harvested from the resin scraped from the cannabis sativa plant. It is cut with a knife or razor blade into thin slices, which are then smoked. It can be smoked by placing the hash on the head of a pin, which is then struck into a book or magazine cover, and then lit. The smoke rises into a glass, which is covering the burning hash. When individuals want to inhale the smoke, they lift up the glass and inhale the smoke, sometimes referred to as "hash under glass." Hash can also be consumed through smoking a pipe or bong.

When marijuana is eaten, it needs to be baked in an oven. It can then be combined with foods such as brownie mix. Marijuana brownies slowly digest in the stomach, where the euphoric feeling occurs as a result of the THC being absorbed and processed in the stomach then to the bloodstream and into the brain. Likewise, individuals can brew tea with marijuana leaves and have similar effects from the drug. Some marijuana users, however, report their initial use as noneuphoric, meaning they did not achieve a high or effect from it. Medically, marijuana is used to treat AIDS patients in the later stages and persons with glaucoma or multiple sclerosis. There remains a controversy over these medical uses of marijuana in the United States.

Clinical Observations

Individuals using marijuana may appear sleepy, glassy eyed, and distant. They may smell of marijuana smoke, and during the session lose track of the conversation. They may appear thirsty and continually moistening their lips. Depending on when they last used, they may appear depressed or lethargic.

Individuals referred for treatment by a third party may be requested to submit regular urine tests to screen not only for other drugs but also to monitor abstinence from marijuana, as it takes from days to weeks for the THC to clear out of the system. Chronic pot smokers store THC in fat cells and can be detected for weeks following cessation from the drug. Nanograms are the measurements used to indicate the amount of THC in the body. If the nanogram measurements increase from the baseline reading, it suggests the client has used since the previous test. If nanogram measurements decrease, it suggests the client has been abstinent from marijuana.

Once ingested, the effects last 1 to 3 hours. Individuals smoking marijuana may experience dryness of mouth, reddening of eyes, increased appetite, and a euphoric feeling, sometimes interrupted with feelings of paranoia and fear. Users also experience an increased heart rate and potential shortness of breath. Individuals smoking large quantities of marijuana can experience hallucinations, loss of sensory perception, and at times a feeling of dissociation from the body. Like other drugs, THC impacts the pleasure center of the brain, creating an euphoric affect, which in contrast to cocaine is longer acting. Marijuana also affects (diminishes) short-term memory.

Both the heart and lungs are impacted by marijuana use. Smoking marijuana on a regular basis increases the risk of heart attack. The lungs, as with smoking any substance, are also affected in a negative manner. Marijuana smoke contains 50–70% more carcinogens than cigarette smoking (Stephens, 1999). Chronic marijuana smokers can develop a persistent and hacking cough due to the excessive smoking.

Withdrawal

When chronic, addicted marijuana smokers discontinue their use, withdrawal symptoms of irritability, sleep disturbances, and headaches may occur (Kouri, Pope, & Lukas, 1999). Withdrawal is not life threatening, though cravings can be strong and may preclude individuals from discontinuing on their own without medical intervention, support, and treatment. The three most common withdrawal symptoms found in research conducted by Copersino et al. (2006) were craving for cannabis (66%), irritability (48%), and boredom (45%). Nausea and vomiting were the main symptoms of withdrawal, along with agitation and mood swings in a study by Bronson et al. (2005). In their study, withdrawal symptoms lasted approximately 6 days. Individuals discontinuing marijuana may increase their use of nicotine, if they are smokers. There is also potential for replacement of one drug compensating for the loss of marijuana. For example, clients may begin drinking larger quantities of alcohol.

Counselors need to understand that many clients who enter treatment for alcohol and drug addiction will be ambivalent about their abstinence from marijuana. For example, clients who are addicted to cocaine and have a long-standing history of marijuana use many times will find it difficult to acknowledge their marijuana use as problematic. Patients often resist the recommendation to abstain from marijuana as well as cocaine and all other mood-altering chemicals. They see their problem as cocaine, not marijuana, and therefore tend to minimize the connection between their marijuana use and other drug use. Studies indicate marijuana is the first drug used by clients who then move on to use other drugs (NIDA, 2005c). This suggests that marijuana, for many clients addicted to drugs and alcohol, is a baseline drug that is difficult to abstain from.

Case of Joey

Joey has been smoking marijuana since age 13. He arrives for counseling with the goal of discontinuing his use of pot over the summer. He finished his second year in college, and his grades have suffered (a 3.2 grade point average dropped to a 2.5 in 1 year). He reports daily use and difficulty stopping because of both his cravings and his living arrangements in an apartment where both roommates also smoke marijuana. Though he has discussed his use with both parents, he has minimized to them the extent of his consumption and his experimentation with other drugs. He comes in motivated to change his behavior regarding his marijuana use in particular.

Consultation With Joey's Case

Because Joey is motivated to take action at this time, we would see working with him individually as a viable therapeutic modality. We would prepare him for symptoms of lethargy, irritability, difficulty in sleeping, cravings, and overall lack of clarity in his thinking as he discontinues his marijuana use. For each symptom we would cocreate and develop a management strategy. For instance, we would encourage him to consult a primary physician or use local emergency room services to evaluate his health if he started to exhibit withdrawal symptoms.

In our work together we would help Joey understand that irritability is a normal physiological response. He would be encouraged to avoid caffeinated and highly saturated sugar drinks and foods. In addition, we would suggest that he discuss with his family and friends what he is feeling both emotionally and physically.

If he had difficulty sleeping, the use of light exercise, reading, puzzles, and leisure activities would help fill the time gaps when sleeping is not occurring. When cravings occur, it would be helpful for him to have candy, sugar free gum, or toothpicks to put in his mouth. Cravings can be powerful, and therefore it is important to have support for remaining abstinent. Attendance at support meetings, counseling, and journaling can all be helpful activities to counter the cravings. We would encourage Joey to find new roommates for the upcoming academic year.

Finally, we would suggest that Joey write his thoughts, plans, and goals down on paper so he can have a plan and guide to work from. Throughout the summer we would work to create a contingency plan should he return to using marijuana when he goes back to college.

Opiates/Narcotics

Heroin and OxyContin

The 2007 National Survey on Drug Use and Health (U.S. Department of Health and Human Services, 2008) found that approximately 106,000 persons aged 12 years or older had used heroin for the first time within the past 12 months. Opiates, commonly known as analgesics or narcotic drugs, include Demerol, codeine, morphine, Vicodin, OxyContin, Percodan, Percocet, Talwin, methadone, opium, heroin, LAAM (levomethadyl acetate hydrochloride, also known as levo-alpha-acetylmethadol), and Dilaudid. The primary function of these drugs is to relieve physical pain. With the exception of heroin and opium, all the other drugs are used either for medical treatment or to help prevent withdrawal symptoms. According to Monitoring the Future, a national survey, 1 in every 20 high school seniors had at least tried OxyContin in 2007 (Johnston, O'Malley, Bachman, & Schulenberg, 2008).

Opiates are used by physicians to manage patients' physical pain. Morphine is generally used for postoperative pain and administered intravenously. Codeine is used for coughs and dispensed in liquid form. Opiate drugs block pain messages to the brain and allow individuals not to feel the physical effects of surgery or pain from an injury or accident.

A contemporary drug of abuse is OxyContin. OxyContin can be acquired illegally from drug dealers or legally through physician prescription. Clients addicted to drugs in this category may seek out multiple doctors in order to obtain prescriptions and feign physical pain or migraine headaches in order to obtain an opiate.

Heroin, composed from morphine, is a natural derivative of the Asian poppy plant and is highly addictive. It is the most abused and fastest acting of all opiates (Goldberg, 1997; Kuhn et al., 2003).

Routes of Administration

Heroin can be a white or brown powder and is injected, snorted, or smoked (Loue & Ioan, 2007). The 1995 Drug Abuse Warning Network (DAWN) report indicated that 21 metropolitan areas ranked heroin overdose as the second leading cause of drug overdose deaths. In addition to the risk of overdosing on the drug, there is the risk of HIV or Hepatitis C transmission (NIDA, 2000).

Intravenous drug users of both heroin and cocaine report how the sight of needles or "works" (i.e., needle, rubber tubing) immediately stimulates the brain, creating an excitement and "rush" to use the drug.

Clinical Example

A client of mine (Ford's) described how he would sit on the toilet before he pulled out his heroin because of the immediate onset of diarrhea before he even shot up. Other clients, while in treatment, when discussing the use of needles would become nervous and agitated during group therapy.

Generally, heroin is dissolved in water and heated. The mixture is then pulled into a syringe and shot into the selected vein. Some addicts do what is called a "speedball," or a mixture of heroin and cocaine, in the same injection. Addicts can either inject themselves or have a partner administer the drug. Because the sight of needles for IV drug users can be an instant trigger, recovering IV drug users who work in the health care field (e.g., nurses, doctors, and dentists) find this to be a unique challenge in recovery.

Individuals snorting or smoking heroin may initially believe in the myth that as long as they are not "running," or intravenously injecting the drug, they cannot become addicted. Snorting heroin is similar to snorting cocaine in that the powder is chopped and snorted into the nasal cavity through a drink straw or a rolled tube. A heroin high can last 3 to 6 hours, depending on the strength and how much of the drug is ingested. Although injection of heroin is the predominant method of ingestion, a shift to snorting or sniffing appears to be the trend (NIDA, 2000).

Clinical Observations

Because heroin and other narcotics are analgesics, clinicians will observe a sedative effect. Narcotic drug users can appear glassy-eyed and may even "nod out" (fall asleep) during sessions. Clients in withdrawal from the drug may appear sick, as if suffering from the flu, and may report aches and physical pains. Clients addicted to narcotics appear hypersensitive to physical discomfort, which necessitates immediate attention to these pains. This cycle leads to becoming medication, or "med," seeking during treatment and early recovery.

Clients may seem drowsy and slur their speech when high on narcotics. Their pupils may be dilated and have poor memory. Intravenous drug users may wear long-sleeved clothing to hide track marks made from the needles. Sunglasses are also used to protect the dilation of the eyes. Other clients may have itchy skin, whereas others may have bouts of vomiting.

Withdrawal

Clients in the early hours of withdrawal may appear agitated, perspiring, and in both physical and emotional discomfort. In addition, these clients may report nausea, diarrhea, and loss of appetite, as well as a strong craving for the drug. Those in active withdrawal from heroin may also have the "shakes," or uncontrollable shaking, sweating, and vomiting (Hutcheson, Everitt, Robbins, & Dickinson, 2001). It is important for counselors to refer individuals in this condition to a medical facility as soon as possible. Management of withdrawal may be accomplished with the drugs buprenorphine, Librium, or clonidine (Catapres; N. S. Miller & Gold, 1998).

Methadone

Methadone is a synthetic opiate, which blocks the effects of heroin withdrawal, and can be used during the detoxification process when the patient is tapering off another narcotic. The administration of the methadone is tapered, so when patients are discharged from the medical facility, they are free from the drug.

Methadone maintenance, however, which found its initial popularity in the 1960s, has made resurgence and has become quite popular as a method of treatment for heroin addicts (White, 1998). This treatment modality essentially maintains a level of methadone (a narcotic derivative) in the addict's body to inhibit the patient from experiencing withdrawal symptoms and cravings to use heroin. Patients come to methadone facilities on a scheduled basis and are required to attend therapy and submit urine screens to determine abstinence from other drugs (a requirement of most programs). Patients can be on methadone maintenance from months to years. Methadone maintenance helps addicts by providing a substitute drug, enabling them to lead productive, healthy lives. Studies have indicated a reduction in intravenous drug use and HIV transmission with methadone maintenance programs. (N. S. Miller & Gold, 1998).

Tolerance and Medical Procedures

Clients in treatment for or in continuing recovery from narcotics addiction and who are facing surgery need to alert their physicians of this condition. Because of tolerance, clients need to be very careful following surgery not to have an unlimited supply of narcotics to relieve pain when discharged from the hospital or clinic. Clients and physicians should work together to monitor the pain threshold and, if possible, use nonnarcotic pain relievers following medical procedures. Should clients require medication for pain, there must be careful monitoring (i.e., providing a short-term supply that is itself monitored and has no refills). Another important issue for recovering substance abusers and specifically narcotic addicts is preparation for surgery. Informing physicians and anesthesiologists about their tolerance to medication is important in order for the medical team to provide the appropriate amount of anesthesia needed for surgery.

Case of Steve

Steve was referred by his employer for counseling to address absences from work, chronic back pain, and increasing errors at work. The employer feels counseling will help Steve with his stress levels and back pain.

Steve presented as compliant yet agitated about being referred to counseling. He was reluctant to sign a release of information to the employer (employment is conditional on follow-through with counseling) and, although amenable, was still very guarded with information. This particular day was unseasonably hot, yet Steve wore a flannel shirt and appeared cold during the session. He was also reluctant to remove his dark glasses saying that he had just had an eye appointment and the doctor had dilated his eyes, making them sensitive to the light. Once in the session, Steve reported that he had been given a prescription for a narcotic to alleviate his back pain, and since that time (5 years ago), he continues to take it only when the pain gets really bad.

At times during the session he appeared distracted and aloof when questioned about alcohol or drug use. Steve agreed to come back the following week and begin exploring his back pain, time missed from work, and errors on the job.

Consultation With Steve's Case

There are a number of red flags that Steve presents in this session, which would be important to note. We would want to get a clearer picture from the employer about Steve's work performance, the mistakes he is making at work, and any significant changes in attitude. The combination of being absent from work, having a chronic medical condition, which many times is treated with narcotics, and his behavior in the session would bring about concern that he is minimizing his use of prescription medication.

In future sessions we would encourage Steve to sign a release of information to his attending physician to coordinate services related to Steve's back pain and alternative non-addicting medications or therapies. Being drug and alcohol counselors has made us both optimistic as well as very inquisitive into behaviors in the here and now. We might have asked him if he were hot with the long-sleeved shirt on and been interested in his eye exam, wondering how his eyes looked. The following visit we would again look for and gently explore facets of his behavior, which signaled underreporting of his drug use.

Hallucinogens

Current trends indicate a reduction in experimentation with hallucinogenic drugs (NIDA, 2001). Drugs in this classification include LSD, mescaline, and psilocybin. However, psilocybin, or more commonly referred to as "shrooms" or "magic mushrooms," is the most widely used of these drugs today. Annual prevalence ranges from 1.6% in 8th grade to 4.8% in 12th grade (Johnston et al., 2008).

Lysergic Acid Diethylamide (LSD)

Lysergic acid diethylamide (LSD) produces visual and auditory hallucinations. Common names for LSD include "acid," "sid," "window pane," "blotter acid," "pane," or "dots" (Goldberg, 1997; Kuhn et al., 2003) LSD is found in a fungus called ergot, which is found growing on grains. Also included in this category is peyote, a type of fungus that grows on cacti and organic mushrooms.

Routes of Administration
Acid is most commonly taken orally and referred to as a "hit." A liquid drop of LSD is placed on small tabs on a sheet of paper. The paper dries and is sold in blotter sheets or individually. The small tabs of paper are placed under the tongue and the LSD is absorbed into the bloodstream impacting sight, sound, and smell. Feelings of self-loss or depersonalization and difficulty separating reality from the drug-induced state occur (Gold & McKewen, 1995). A liquid form of the drug can be placed directly on the tongue and mouth or dropped in the eyes with a dropper.

Psilocybin is available fresh or dried and is typically taken orally. The active psilocin (4-hydroxy-N,N-dimethyltryptamine) and psilocybin (4-phosphoryloxy-N,N-dimethyltryptamine) cannot be inactivated by cooking or freezing preparations and therefore may be brewed for tea or added to other foods to mask their bitter flavor. The effects of psilocybin usually occur within 20 minutes of ingestion and last approximately 6 hours.

Clinical Observations
Individuals using hallucinogens appear distant and may report auditory and/or visual hallucinations. A description of light trails or movement of inanimate objects can be a part of the reported experience. There can also be a hypersensitivity to sound and light, along with increased heartbeat (similar to the effects of stimulants).

Clients may exhibit changes in feelings, time, and sensory distortion or delusions. A "bad" trip on acid may consist of feeling terrified, tearful, and being out of control.

The effects can last up to 24 hours, depending on how many "hits" are taken followed by the need for sleep. The symptoms can mimic a schizophrenic episode. Clients may also appear glassy-eyed and laugh inappropriately during sessions.

Withdrawal

There is no pattern of withdrawal, nor is it life-threatening. However, individuals may respond to thoughts and feelings with self-harming behaviors, which may be managed with Haldol or lorazepam (N. S. Miller & Gold, 1998).

Phencyclidine (PCP)

Phencyclidine (PCP) was initially produced in the 1950s as a surgical anesthetic. PCP was linked to difficulty during anesthesia, including the unpredictable and violent effects it had on patients while under the influence. It is often considered a hallucinogenic drug because of the hallucinations it produces, yet it also produces depressant effects like that of a trance state of being. PCP is typically used in a white powder and sniffed or sprinkled on marijuana cigarettes and smoked, the effects of which can produce temporary symptoms of psychosis. This drug, in particular, can evoke violent outbursts from users, and thus is known as "rocket fuel."

Routes of Administration

Initial use of PCP came about in tablet and capsule form. PCP can be injected, snorted, or smoked.

Ketamine

Ketamine is an animal tranquilizer and is used by veterinarians as a liquid anesthetic. It is used illegally by evaporating the liquid and snorting or smoking the powder or forming the residue into a pill. The liquid form is colorless, odorless, and tasteless and produces amnesia. The effects of the drug are similar to PCP, though shorter in duration. It is commonly called "Special K" and can produce terrifying results.

Clinical Observations

Clinicians will observe in their clients using PCP a vacant stare and glassy eyes. Clients may have poor concentration, agitation, numbness, confusion, and high heart rate. Belligerent or volatile behaviors can follow large doses of PCP along with significant personality changes, depression, and paranoia. Individuals under the influence of PCP have also been known to exhibit great strength when attempting to be subdued.

Clients may appear aloof, disoriented, and may exhibit psychotic features, depending on the amount used. Clients may be restless and excessively salivate.

Withdrawal

There are no reported signs or symptoms of withdrawal once one stops using PCP.

Case of Donnie

Donnie is a senior in high school who was to attend college in the fall. Over the weekend he was consuming alcohol and smoked a marijuana cigarette laced with PCP, unbeknownst to him. Donnie reports feeling as though he were in a dream after he smoked the joint. He says to you, the school counselor, that he is really afraid because he doesn't remember much of the evening. What concerns him the most was that he drove that night.

Donnie drinks 2–3 beers on the weekends and smokes pot 1–2 times a month. Since he is 18 and ready to attend college, his parents see nothing wrong with him drinking beer occasionally. They are not aware of what happened over the weekend or his pot use.

Consultation With Donnie

We would support Donnie in every way for coming in on his own, allow his fear to be a motivator, and at the same time, work with him on his choices. We would also talk with him about any residual effects (e.g., flashbacks) of the PCP experience and encourage him to seek medical attention should he require it. Because this is a one-time reported use, and he had a "bad" experience, he may be much more hesitant to smoke pot any time soon. Time spent in counseling could help him connect all three—alcohol, PCP, and marijuana— and the choices he has made in his life thus far around chemicals.

Prevention focuses on his desire to attend college and how choices to use chemicals may impact those decisions. Ultimately we see this session as a crisis intervention, where the focus is on validating his feelings, supporting him through the crisis, and working with him on new decisions regarding future choices with chemicals.

Inhalants

According to NIDA (2004), the rate of abuse for 8th graders was up significantly, whereas 10th and 12th graders continued to decline. Inhalant abuse is mainly found in the younger population and has devastating effects on the brain, liver, kidneys, and heart, even after one use (NIDA, 2004). Inhalants can impact the respiratory, digestive, and central nervous systems. Seizures may also occur, resulting in death.

Inhalants include nitrates, gasoline (benzene), paint thinner (methylene chloride), nitrous oxide anesthesia (or laughing gas, which is used by dentists for patients needing medical procedures), glues (toluene), freon, butane, whip cream canisters (whippets), and spot removers (or any substance that might include the compound toluene, which is found in many glues, paints, or nail polish removers). Once inhaled, it immediately enters the lungs, bloodstream, and brain, where the dopamine system is activated (Goldberg, 1997; Kuhn et al., 2003).

Nitrous Oxide

Nitrous oxide has been a popular inhalant at music festivals where balloons are illegally sold and filled with the "laughing gas." The balloons are slowly opened into the mouth of the user and inhaled. Inhalants are readily accessible, and as a result items such as glue, Liquid Paper, and dry-erase markers in most adolescent drug units are removed.

Routes of Administration

Inhalants are ingested in a number of ways, depending on the compound being inhaled. Many users pour liquid paint thinners or gasoline onto a rag and then place the rag into a paper bag. The bag is placed over their nose and mouth, creating a small airway for only the toxic fumes to enter. After inhaling and exhaling a number of times, the noxious fumes fill the lungs. The chemicals course through the bloodstream and into the brain, creating a high or intoxication, albeit short lived, followed by vomiting, nausea, and/or headaches.

Clinical Observations

A chronic inhalant user seems depressed and somewhat disoriented, with poor short-term memory. Family or friends may report finding hidden paint cans and cloths or bags for inhaling. There is a real and potential danger of hemorrhaging and lowering of the immune system, which leaves the body vulnerable to infections.

Clients may appear speech impaired, off balance, or disoriented when using inhalants or they may vomit. In addition, double vision, muscle fatigue, and a faint ringing in the ears may occur. Counselors may notice chemical compound marks on the face (particularly around the mouth and nose) and smell chemical fumes on the clients clothing and skin during sessions. Chemical stains or spots on clothing plus physical reports from the client of nausea or dizziness are also common. Inhalant users may appear drunk, uncoordinated, giddy, and may pass out.

Withdrawal

Although there does seem to be a tolerance to nitrous oxide, withdrawal is not apparent within this drug category. Many inhalant users may take other drugs or drink alcohol to enhance the effects of inhalants.

Club Drugs

Club drugs such as Rohypnol, methylenedioxyamphetamine (MDMA), and gamma hydroxybutyrate (GHB) are drugs used at club parties, or "raves," to intensify the overall party experience (Gold & McKewen, 1995). Rave parties/dances have been in existence for at least the past 10 years and consist of large numbers of participants in a dance area with strobe lighting, loud music, pounding bass, and large quantities of the drugs listed above. Some club drugs such as Rohypnol can be surreptitiously dissolved in alcoholic drinks, where the effects immobilize individuals consuming the drinks and produce blackouts. During such times, individuals are vulnerable to abuse, and yet may be unable to recall events of the evening.

Rohypnol-Flunitrazepam

Rohypnol is in the benzodiazepine classification. When consumed with alcohol, it immobilizes or paralyzes individuals, thereby preventing them from fighting back from an attack or being sexually assaulted. "Roofies," as the drugs are commonly called, initially gained popularity in the early 1990s and have continued to be abused on many college campuses. Following consumption, this drug induces retrograde amnesia, making it impossible for individuals to recall the events after consumption. Examples of this occur on weekends throughout the United States, when unsuspecting individuals leave their drinks unattended, during which time "roofies" are dissolved. Rohypnol dissolves easier than Valium, making it much more dangerous. Unsuspecting victims consume the drinks and within the next 30 minutes become incapacitated. The following morning they wake up and are unable to recall events the night before. In addition to any abuse suffered, the combination of Rohypnol and alcohol can be lethal.

Routes of Administration
This drug is taken orally in pill form or is dissolved in liquids.

Clinical Observations
Because this drug is in the sedative-hypnotic category, the same observations apply when clients are high (i.e., sedation, poor coordination, and memory loss). Of note for counselors is the possibility of clients being abused (physically or sexually) and either unable to recall or able to discuss the event but reluctant to recount the abuse. Effective counselors respectfully ask clients their thoughts and feelings relating to the abuse and discuss possible options for referral (e.g., clinic, women's center, police).

Withdrawal
If taken on a regular basis, withdrawal symptoms can occur, such as agitation, anxiety, or shakiness.

Methylenedioxyamphetamine, or Ecstasy

Methylenedioxyamphetamine (MDMA), commonly known as ecstasy, combines the effects of stimulants and hallucinogenic drugs, producing rapid breathing and heart rates. Those who ingest ecstasy report feeling connected with those around them. Developed in the early 1900s, its use in the 1980s as a recreational drug forced the Drug Enforcement Agency to classify it as a Schedule I drug (see the schedule of drugs at the beginning of this chapter). In addition to the feeling of connection, the possibility of hallucinogenic effects such as visualizing "trails" or wisps of vapor from light or seeing inanimate walls "breathe" to the beat of music may occur. It produces fewer distortions than LSD and is shorter in duration (2–4 hours). The drug causes the release of excessive amounts of serotonin into the brain (Gold & McKewen, 1995). Prolonged use can result in kidney, liver, and heart failure.

Routes of Administration
Ecstasy is usually taken in oral pill form; however, it can also be made into a powder and be injected or placed in the rectum.

Clinical Observations
At higher doses, ecstasy creates dry mouth, cramping, decrease in appetite, and occasionally a nauseous feeling. Being the primary drug of choice at raves, this drug has become very popular. The drug allows individuals to continue dancing for many hours because of its stimulant quality. At high doses this drug can cause seizures.

Withdrawal
In addition to the desired effects of ecstasy, irritability, agitation, and anxiety have been reported.

Gamma Hydroxybutyrate (GHB)

GHB is a colorless and odorless drug that can be slipped or poured into drinks and is used as a "date rape" drug much like Rohypnol. Used in the early 1990s for muscle building and sold at most health food stores, it was later banned by the FDA because of its effects on the body. This drug can induce seizures, comas, and in higher doses cause death. Its effects can be intensified when used in combination with alcohol. GHB is considered to be a depressant and slows down breathing (as compared with MDMA, which intensifies breathing and pulse rate).

Routes of Administration
GHB is taken as a prescribed drug in the treatment of narcolepsy. As an illicit drug, it is taken orally in pill form or dissolved in liquid.

Clinical Observation
An individual on GHB may appear drowsy or sedated and may experience euphoria. Tolerance to this drug develops after regular and continuous use. This drug is also used by sexual predators to sedate potential victims (usually by dissolving it in alcoholic drinks).

Withdrawal
Significant withdrawal can occur and may include insomnia, anxiety, tremors, sweating, and high blood pressure. Combined with large doses of other drugs, the withdrawal can be quite severe.

Steroids and Anabolic Steroids

Types of Steroids

Anabolic steroids were initially used for medical purposes to help males with hypogonadism, a condition where the testes are not able to produce sufficient testosterone for normal growth. Steroids are also used for treating AIDS patients who are atrophying and getting thinner. During testing of this drug with laboratory animals, researchers discovered that muscle growth occurred, ultimately leading to its use and abuse in bodybuilding.

Steroid abusers may take up to 100 times more steroids than individuals taking steroids for medical purposes. A practice known as "stacking" occurs when abusers ingest multiple steroid and stimulant drugs or painkillers at the same time. "Pyramiding" occurs when abusers begin with low doses of steroids, adding more and more over a 6- to 12-week period. Drugs such as Anadrol® (oxymetholone), Oxandrin® (oxandrolone), Dianabol® (methandrostenolone), Winstrol® (stanozolol), and others can be taken orally. Drugs such as Deca-Durabolin® (nandrolone decanoate), Durabolin® (nandrolone phenpropionate), Depo-Testosterone® (testosterone cypionate), and Equipoise® (boldenone undecylenate) can be injected intra muscularly (NIDA, 2006b).

Routes of Administration

Steroids are taken orally in pill form, rubbed into the skin via ointment, or injected, increasing the possibility of contracting HIV or other blood transmittable diseases. The use of unclean needles or sharing of needles also increases the risk.

Clinical Observations

Abuse of steroids results in significant mood swings as well as aggressive and/or violent behavior. Delusions or paranoid ideation can also be present, culminating in irritable and irrational behaviors (Pope & Katz, 1988). Regular use by men can cause breast enlargement and hair loss. In addition, skin can turn a yellowish color, possibly indicating jaundice. Women who use steroids may report a disruption in their menstrual cycle and begin growing facial hair.

Withdrawal

Individuals who regularly use steroids report withdrawal symptoms that include depression, fatigue, headaches, and insomnia.

Nicotine

In 2006, 29.6% of the U.S. population 12 years and older—72.9 million people—used tobacco at least once in the month before being interviewed. This figure includes 3.3 million young people ages 12 to 17. Sixty-one million Americans were current smokers. Most of them smoked cigarettes as opposed to another form of tobacco (NIDA, 2006a). Since 1996, however, the number of teen smokers has decreased.

Cigarettes, Cigars, Pipes, and Smokeless Tobacco

Nicotine is a colorless liquid that, when smoked, turns a yellowish brown. Nicotine is found in cigarettes, cigars, pipes, and smokeless tobacco. It is absorbed into the mucous membranes, lungs, and bloodstream and then into the brain within 10 seconds. Once in the brain, the chemical epinephrine is released, which in turn stimulates the central nervous system and the adrenal glands, releasing glucose into the body. This has a stimulant effect on the smoker, followed by fatigue and some mild depression. Nicotine enters the body quickly when smoked and stimulates the pleasure center of the brain.

Routes of Administration

Typically nicotine is ingested through smoking cigarettes or other tobacco products. It can also be ingested by chewing tobacco or by "dipping" smokeless tobacco in the mouth. In this method, nicotine is absorbed through the lining of the mouth, into the bloodstream, and then to the brain.

Clinical Observations

A chronic smoker may have dry skin, yellowish stains on the second and third fingers of their smoking hand, and a persistent cough. Multiple-pack smokers find it necessary to smoke every 20 to 30 minutes in order to avoid withdrawal from the drug.

Withdrawal

Withdrawal from nicotine is difficult and therefore relapse is extremely high. Nicotine, once ingested, takes approximately 8–10 seconds to reach the brain and immediately provides stimulation to the body. In essence, not only is it a quick chemical high, but it also is physically uncomfortable when the drug is not being ingested on a regular basis. Withdrawal symptoms can include extreme difficulty in obtaining a continuous night's sleep, severe headaches, stomach upset and diarrhea, irritability, agitation, physical cravings for the drug, and flu-like symptoms. In addition, symptoms of depression such as moodiness, tearfulness, and lethargy are most common in individuals attempting to discontinue its use.

Withdrawal aides such as nicotine gum are used to minimize the withdrawal symptoms. This is accomplished by tapering the use of the gum until the individual is no longer using nicotine. The difficulty for many clients using this method is self-administration, which makes tapering difficult. Others have found success in oral medication to minimize or reduce the physical cravings for nicotine. The use of nicotine patches can help individuals reduce the milligrams of nicotine over the course of time, thus allowing the tapering to be gradual. Others use the "cold turkey" method, just stopping all at once and fighting through the withdrawal without the aide of gum, patches, or oral medication. The use of antidepressant medication has also been used to address the symptoms of depression and neurotransmitter depletion in the brain.

Over the Counter Medications

The use and abuse of OTC medications has become popular with adolescents. They can be used to achieve a high or as an adjunct to increase effects with other drugs. Cough medications and some oral antihistamines cause drowsiness, and if taken in conjunction with alcohol or other drugs, they enhance each other, which increases the possibility of an overdose or internal medical complications. For example, a client who consumes eight beers and two bottles of cough medication containing the chemicals acetaminophen, dextromethorphan, doxylamine, and pseudoephedrine may black out and/or overdose.

Clients in recovery need to discuss OTC chemicals with their physicians. Clients may be under the impression that because these are readily available OTC medications intended to help with colds and flu symptoms, they must be safe. However, because recovering substance abusers have special vulnerability, encouraging clients to consult with their physicians on OTC drug use is necessary in their continued recovery.

Psychotropic Medications

These medications are prescribed by psychiatrists to treat clients suffering from mental disorders (e.g., depression, anxiety, or thought disorders). These medications are not physically addictive and are used in conjunction with dual-diagnosis treatment. They are used to stabilize both mood and behavior.

Psychotropics typically have both generic and brand names. For instance, fluoxetine is the generic name for Prozac. This category of psychotropic medication is used to treat depression and therefore is called an antidepressant. Drugs such as paroxetine (Paxil), sertraline (Zoloft), and imipramine (Tofranil) are all used to elevate and stabilize mood and affect with individuals suffering from depression.

Anxiety disorders can be treated with clonazepam (Klonopin), lorazepam (Ativan), or buspirone (BuSpar). Klonopin and Ativan have addictive potential and therefore are not typically prescribed by psychiatrists or physicians with expertise in addiction medicine. These unique medical personnel are called addictionologists and are very important in the team approach to addiction. Addictionologists typically do not prescribe Ativan to drug-addicted clients but rather may prescribe an antidepressant with no addictive potential.

Clients with mood swings or bipolar disorders might be prescribed carbamazepine (Tegretol), lithium (Lithonate), or valproic acid (Depakene or Depakote). These drugs do not have addictive potential and therefore are used to treat clients with co-occurring disorders. Clients suffering from psychotic disorders may be prescribed Haloperidol (Haldol), risperidone (Risperdal), or olanzapine (Zyprexa), which help clients with auditory and visual hallucinations. Clients suffering from both addiction and attention deficit hyperactivity disorder (ADHD) are often also addicted to cocaine and stimulant drugs. The drugs used to treat this disorder typically are methyphenidate (Ritalin), dextroamphetamine (Dexedrine), or pemoline (Cylert). However, clients may use the prescribed drugs as addictively as the cocaine, thus creating a challenge for physicians, clients, and counselors.

Most psychotropic medications are ingested orally; however, long-acting medication may be injected. Once clients begin the recommended medication protocol, emphasis is placed on clients seeing the prescribing psychiatrist on a regular basis. Unfortunately, clients are not always compliant with medication recommendations and, therefore, can find themselves relapsing back into their mania and/or addiction.

Summary

After reading this chapter students should have a better understanding of the various categories of drugs and the specific drugs in each category. Readers have also been provided examples of what to look for in sessions, along with the different ways drugs affect individuals. Most important, though, for counselors is the knowledge of what clients may experience once they discontinue drug use. Readers should now have a basic understanding of what to look for as a client discontinues use and experiences withdrawal symptoms. This is extremely important information when making referrals for medical or treatment protocols.

Exploration Questions From Chapter 3

1. Based on your reading from this chapter, how will you approach clients who use drugs?
2. What difficulties or challenges do you see when you work with drug-addicted clients?
3. What is your biggest fear in working with drug-addicted clients?
4. How will you address this fear?
5. Discuss with other students how you might implement a drug prevention program in your community or school district.
6. What biases might you have with clients who use drugs? In other words, how would you feel about working with clients who use drugs other than alcohol?
7. How do you feel about drug users who use needles rather than other methods of use?
8. What assumptions might you have with clients of color regarding chemical use?
9. What feelings might you have toward a crack-addicted mother who is pregnant?

Suggested Activities

1. Visit and interview an alcohol and drug counselor. Discuss what he or she does when working with drug-addicted clients. Discuss your experience and record your reactions in your journal.
2. Read the newspaper. Over the course of the week, cut out all the articles relating to drug use (e.g., shootings, overdose). Discuss your experience with a small group.

Assessment, Diagnosis, and Interview Techniques

The preceding chapters provided information needed to prepare counselors for this chapter on assessment with substance-abusing or addicted clients. Assessments of drug and alcohol use, as well as other co-occurring mental health issues, are critical to effective treatment planning (Flynn & Brown, 2008; Nidecker, DiClemente, Bennett, & Bellack, 2008). J. A. Lewis, Dana, and Blevins (1994) suggested that although many counselors are not addiction specialists, they need to develop skills in dealing with problems created by substance abuse. It is imperative for counselors to both acknowledge and understand basic substance abuse/dependency and mental health symptomotology as critical pieces in the assessment procedure. Accurate assessment techniques provide useful problem-specific and contextual data to the counselor, while allowing the opportunity for the client to develop a therapeutic relationship with the counselor (Martin & Moore, 1995). Various complicating factors (e.g., suicidal ideation, internal motivation, and resistance) can significantly impact client progress in counseling. It follows then that such case-specific factors need to be both recognized and addressed during the initial sessions with clients.

This chapter examines the counselor as a facilitative gatekeeper (Lawton, 1981) and focuses on the components of a comprehensive assessment, which includes a thorough alcohol and drug evaluation using the *Diagnostic and Statistical Manual of Mental Disorders* (4th ed., text rev., *DSM-IV-TR*; American Psychiatric Association, 2000) criteria and other alcohol and drug assessment tools/instruments. A comprehensive assessment also evaluates for suicide and clients' mental status and is included in this chapter (Pipes & Davenport, 1999). We believe that the counseling approach to assessment can be enhanced by motivational interviewing (MI; W. R. Miller & Rollnick, 2002), and therefore we devote the last section of the chapter to that model. Ultimately, the combination of MI with the other ideas in this chapter can result in an appropriate assessment and subsequent referral.

It is critical to remember that the overall assessment process does not end in one session; in fact, according to Milton Erickson, "Assessment is ongoing; it occurs throughout therapy" (as cited in Geary, 2001, p. 1). Counselors continue obtaining as much information as possible in order to design continuous clinical interventions and effective treatment strategies.

The Counselor as a Facilitative Gatekeeper

Dr. Marcia Lawton was the director of the Graduate Program in Alcohol and Drug Education Rehabilitation Program at Virginia Commonwealth University from the mid 1970s until the mid 1990s. This program was a first of its kind in the United States, which prepared counselors to become alcohol and drug specialists. I (Ford) was fortunate to have graduated from that program and was mentored by Dr. Lawton in my early professional career. Although her concept is dated, I found her concept of the *facilitative gatekeeper* transferable to generalist counselors and is therefore why we've included it in this chapter. Counselors are considered to be facilitative gatekeepers when they play a significant role in helping clients obtain appropriate treatment for substance abuse. The components of the concept are information gathering, assessment, referral, prevention and education, and tracking and follow-up (Lawton, 1981).

Information Gathering

The first aspect, *information gathering*, occurs as counselors collect and organize information from clients and other referral sources. The gathering process starts with the first contact, when counselors are listening for and observing signs of alcohol and drug use in their clients as well as other mental health disorders. Simultaneously, counselors are evaluating client motivation, environmental support, and potential complicating factors that might impact the counseling relationship. For example, John, a counselor, has a 15-minute break between his counseling sessions and decides to return a phone call from a potential client seeking services. John calls the number and allows the phone to ring four times until it is answered by a female voice. In the short time she responds with "hello," he hears children yelling and a loud television playing in the background. "May I please speak to Jessica?" She acknowledges that she is Jessica. At that point John introduces himself and discusses the reason for her initiating the call.

A brief phone interaction like this can provide useful data while initiating the development of a therapeutic relationship. John discovered that Jessica was referred for counseling as a result of a second drunk driving ticket while out "partying" with other friends. During the conversation, she shared how overwhelming it was to be the single mother of two children ages 3 and 5, and how this made it difficult to set an appointment. At the end of the phone call she became very agitated and angry with John about the time and financial commitment to counseling and seemed ambivalent about counseling. However, she was willing to make the appointment and was minimally aware of how her drinking was creating problems in her life.

The information John gathered from this interaction provided him with a brief understanding of Jessica's situation at home. John heard from her how being a single parent of two young children is stressful and that she is ambivalent about counseling. Further, her second drunk driving ticket statistically suggests that she consumes alcohol more than just occasionally. Also, even though she has some possible skepticism about the counseling process, at some level she displayed some insight into her drinking behavior. This initial information gathering provides an opportunity for counselors to communicate empathy with clients.

Assessment

The second aspect of the facilitative gate-keeping role is *assessment*. Although similar to information gathering, assessment is structured and occurs when counselors take information from clients (both verbally and nonverbally) during the assessment and develop a preliminary alcohol and drug diagnosis from which treatment and counseling options are recommended. Appendix 4.A at the end of this chapter contains an outline of questions to assess alcohol and drug use along with other medical, legal, familial, emotional, and vocational issues.

Let us return to our client Jessica. She arrives for the appointment and discusses her current situation at home raising her two children and how lonely she feels. She becomes tearful and states how rarely she goes out with friends. Later in the session, however, Jessica describes how she goes out every weekend with her girlfriends for drinks. In addition to the inconsistencies in her drinking history, her blood alcohol content was .22, which she states was inaccurate because she did not feel intoxicated. When asked about her childhood she revealed little, although she appeared pained. She reported her last use of alcohol (three glasses of wine) occurred 1 week before her appointment. At the end of the session she reported that counseling was "not that bad" and that she was willing to return the following week.

The information gathered during the previous phone contact and this session suggests Jessica is minimizing her alcohol use and may use alcohol as a method of stress relief. Additionally, it appears Jessica has an increased tolerance to alcohol. Further, her understanding of the impact on her two children is minimal. At this point a preliminary diagnosis would at the very least place her in the alcohol abuse category. The counselor should further explore the symptoms of dependency found later in this chapter.

Referral (How, When, and Where)

The third aspect to the facilitative gate-keeping role is *referral*. Once information is gathered and assessed, the counselor makes a clinical decision on what to do clinically with the client and where to refer (Lawton, 1981). Counselors need to understand how to refer clients, be familiar with the resources in the community and surrounding area, and recognize when to refer clients. In chapter 6 we go into more detail about levels of care and the variety of treatment resources, but before that, counselors need to understand the how, when, and where of referring.

- *How.* Once clients have entered into counseling, it is the counselor's responsibility to work within the limits of their competence (American Counseling Association, 2005). A client assessment by a community counselor may reveal a significant alcohol addiction; however, the client may be self-referred and not sure that he or she is ready for addiction treatment. At some point in the counseling process, the client may realize through attempts to control or through increasing consequences that treatment is needed and will be motivated for change. The counselor needs to know how to set up the admission, check the funding source for the client (i.e., state, federal, or managed care), and how to transport the client. The actual process of how a client is referred to treatment can take many hours and phone calls.
- *When.* Counselors provide assessments and referral to addiction counselors for intensive work on the alcohol and drug use. In certain states such as Pennsylvania, treatment can only be provided by a state licensed facility specializing in addiction treatment (Pennsylvania Department of Health, 1999). As a result, counselors in a mental health setting refer clients to addiction programs first and then work with those clients following their alcohol and drug treatment.
- *Where.* Counselors need to find out all the possible treatment programs in the community, around the state, and the funding sources. Actually visiting the outpatient and inpatient facilities and meeting the counselors creates a working relationship with the community. Being aware of which psychiatrists are knowledgeable about addiction and substance abuse is critical for counselors and clients. Counselors must know the programs that address co-occurring disorders (e.g., sexual addiction, gambling, eating disorders) to best provide resources for clients.

Managed Care and the Referral Process

For counselors working in agencies or hospital settings, the assessment process and development of treatment plans are important for a multitude of reasons. The primary reason is the care and treatment of the client. Second is the issue of reimbursement from insurance companies and funding sources. Counselors in these settings need to be both thorough and expeditious in their assessment. The time allotted by many managed care companies to obtain general assessment information and developing a treatment plan is relatively brief—usually one session. Such mandates create a unique challenge for counselors in the development of a therapeutic relationship. With the advent of managed care, inpatient stays have decreased (Davis & Meier, 2001). Generally, acute patients enter detoxification and stabilize and are immediately referred to intensive outpatient treatment. Many 28-day treatment programs (once en vogue) went out of business in the early 1990s because they were not funded to provide varying lengths of stay. Sadly, within the span of 3 years, I (Ford) observed four well-established inpatient treatment programs close and at least five intensive outpatient programs open. Those clients who were able to stay the full 28 days for inpatient treatment were either funded at a contracted per diem rate by counties or were able to pay out of pocket for treatment. Managed care was no longer reimbursing for full 28-day inpatient treatment. "While a strong case can be made to transition more care from inpatient to outpatient settings, a need for a strong inpatient network in every locale is likely to remain for such problems as substance abuse and chronic mental illness" (Davis & Meier, 2001, p. 11).

The initial impetus of these changes had profound effects on the alcohol and drug treatment industry. Also, in the late 1980s and early 1990s, licensure for counselors was becoming more important and essential for reimbursement. As of 2006, counselors held over 635,000 jobs with a projected increase to 771,000 jobs by 2016 (Bureau of Labor Statistics, 2008). Many alcohol and drug counselors who had 10 years or more of recovery, were certified addiction counselors, and had bachelor's degrees in counseling or human services suddenly found themselves doing educational lectures and performing less counseling. Managed care was only reimbursing services for those individuals who were licensed as counselors, psychologists, or social workers. Ironically, those who had the most specialized experience and training were unable to be reimbursed for their specialty in addictions.

With this information, let's return to our client Jessica. The following week Jessica returned smelling of alcohol. It was clear to John that Jessica was in need of treatment. She was referred for detoxification evaluation and continued treatment services. The need for referral to detoxification became clear to John after only a few sessions with Jessica. He initially suspected that her drinking was more than abusive and that her recent intoxication at his office was a blatant cry for help, necessitating a medical referral.

Prevention and Education

Jessica signs a release of information (ROI) to her parents before entering detoxification in order for them to take care of her children. She also gives permission for the counselor to speak with her parents regarding her condition. At this point, the counselor can provide education to her parents as well as prevention efforts with her children (Lawton, 1981). In Jessica's case, the options for treatment and referral could have been discussed at the first meeting along with information on alcohol abuse and alcoholism.

Tracking and Follow-Up

Once Jessica is referred to the detoxification center, the counselor should follow up to determine compliance (Lawton, 1981) and to determine what help she might need after the detoxification efforts. Further, counselors can make themselves available at any point in the follow-up process. In Jessica's case, the referral to detoxification could be streamlined through an ROI, which would allow follow-up contact with the hospital.

Students find the description of the facilitative gate-keeping role helpful in understanding how they, as generalist counselors, have the potential to be significant components in counseling.

Components of a Comprehensive Assessment

A thorough assessment begins with information pertaining to the events leading up to the referral; in other words, "Why here?" "Why now?" Getting the specifics of the *precipitating event(s)* provides information on the client's defensiveness, awareness, and understanding of what has brought him or her to counseling. It is also important to determine the referral source. Some referral sources spend a great deal of time preparing clients for counseling while others do not, resulting in more time for counselors to orient clients to counseling. Many times paperwork for assessments is filled out by clients prior to arrival for the appointment or 30 min before their appointment. As such, more time can be devoted to clients needs. Depending on the therapeutic setting, clients typically present with a host of issues (e.g., depression, relationship problems, anxiety) not necessarily related to alcohol or drug use. Counselors thereby are challenged to determine over the course of the assessment process whether or not alcohol or drugs are connected to the presenting problem. Counselors should ponder two questions, "Is the presenting problem a symptom of the chemical use (e.g., tardiness and/or absence from work because of hangover or intoxication), or is the presenting problem unrelated to chemical use (e.g., depression)?"

Alcohol and Drug Evaluation

Obtaining accurate information from clients regarding their alcohol and drug use can be quite challenging because of two significant factors: the defense system and dishonesty. A thorough alcohol and drug history includes the client's first use (age), last use (when date), types of drugs used, the pattern of use (daily, weekends, etc.), and methods of ingestion (as discussed in chapter 3). It is important to obtain responses to all categories of drugs and determine if a substance abuse or addiction problem exists. Questions during the assessment are most helpful when presented in an open-ended format. For example, "Have you been drinking alcohol these last 3 weeks?" is a close-ended question where the response is either "yes" or "no." In addition to the close-ended nature of the question, the description of alcohol for clients needs to be clarified by the counselor. For example, beer and wine may not be considered alcohol to some clients. This means counselors need to include all the variations (i.e., beer, wine, liquor) in an open-ended format. The open question now sounds like this, "If you would be willing, could you tell me a little bit about your use of beer, wine, and liquor over the last 2 months?" Not only is it open-ended but it also specifically asks about all the alcohol amounts within the past month.

DSM-IV-TR

Effective alcohol and drug intake forms contain questions that parallel the symptoms found in the next few pages per the *DSM-IV-TR*, making the assessment of substance abuse and dependency helpful for counselors. The alcohol and drug assessment data provided by clients, as well as information from other referral sources (e.g., hospital, probation), potentially provide important ancillary information for counselors as they make their preliminary diagnoses. The more information counselors have from family members, referral sources, hospitals, and prior therapy or treatment providers, the better likelihood of developing an effective treatment plan. As with any assessment procedure, successful understanding is facilitated through the use of multiple methods over time. The following pages present the overall *DSM-IV-TR* criteria from which clinicians are able to diagnose alcohol and drug abuse or dependency.

The *DSM-IV-TR* provides counselors with consistent language, allowing for a common understanding among practitioners. A *DSM-IV-TR* diagnosis is also required for insurance reimbursement; therefore, it is essential for counselors to be familiar with *DSM-IV-TR* criteria for the diagnosis of substance dependency and abuse. The *DSM-IV-TR* provides criteria for each drug category (e.g., stimulants, hallucinogens, sedative-hypnotics) and contains information that helps counselors diagnose more specifically. So instead of "chemical dependency" a client can be diagnosed as having alcohol, cocaine, and/or cannabis dependence. Because of the length of each drug category in the *DSM-IV-TR*, we present the primary symptoms of both dependency and abuse and strongly encourage counselors to read the *DSM-IV-TR* section on substance abuse and dependency for additional information.

DSM-IV-TR Criteria for Diagnosis of Substance Dependency

The *DSM-IV-TR* describes dependency as a maladaptive pattern of substance use, which leads to clinically significant impairment or distress, as manifested by three (or more) of the following criteria occurring at any time in the same 12-month period:

1. tolerance, as defined by either of the following:
   a. a need for markedly increased amounts of the substance to achieve intoxication or desired effect
   b. markedly diminished effect with continued use of the same amount of substance
2. withdrawal, as manifested by either of the following:
   a. the characteristic withdrawal syndrome for the substance (counselor needs to refer to Criteria A and B of the criteria sets for withdrawal from the specific substance in the *DSM-IV-TR*)
   b. the same (or closely related) substance is taken to relieve or avoid withdrawal symptoms
3. the substance is often taken in larger amounts or over a longer period than was intended
4. there is a persistent desire or unsuccessful efforts to cut down or control substance use
5. a great deal of time is spent in activities necessary to obtain the substance (e.g., visiting multiple doctors or driving long distances), use the substance (e.g., chain-smoking), or recover from its effects
6. important social, occupational, or recreational activities are given up or reduced because of substance use
7. the substance use is continued despite knowledge of having a persistent or recurrent physical or psychological problem that is likely to have been caused or exacerbated by the substance (e.g., current cocaine use despite recognition of cocaine-induced depression, or continued drinking despite recognition that an ulcer was made worse by alcohol consumption)

Specify if

With physiological dependence: evidence of tolerance or withdrawal (i.e., either Item 1 or 2 present)

Without physiological dependence: no evidence of tolerance or withdrawal (i.e., neither Item 1 nor 2 is present)

Course Specifiers

- Early full remission
- Early partial remission
- Sustained full remission
- Sustained partial remission
- On agonist therapy (antabuse)
- In a controlled environment (incarcerated/treatment)

Substance dependence can be diagnosed with or without physiological dependence. With physiological dependence, clients present evidence of increased or decreased tolerance or withdrawal (physiological signs discussed in chapter 3). The characterization of the client without physiological dependence infers no evidence of tolerance or withdrawal.

- *Early full remission* specifies for at least 1 month and no less than 12 months, no criteria for substance abuse or dependence have been met.
- *Early partial remission* for at least 1 month and no less than 12 months, one or more of the criteria for substance abuse or dependency have been met. However, the full criteria for dependency have not been met.
- *Sustained full remission* infers that no criteria for substance abuse or dependency have been met during a time period of 12 months or more.
- *Sustained partial remission* means the full criteria for substance dependency has not been met; however, one or more of the criteria for dependency have been met.
- *Agonist therapy* is used when clients are on medication (methadone) and meet no criteria for dependency or abuse with that medication for at least 1 month. Those who are taking Antabuse also would apply for this specifier. Antabuse is a self-administered medication that makes those who drink alcohol violently ill. Some clients take Antabuse as an aversion therapy strategy in conjunction with support meetings and treatment groups or alone.
- The *controlled environment* specifies if the client has been incarcerated or in an inpatient unit where, theoretically, clients are not exposed to drugs or alcohol.

DSM-IV-TR Criteria for Substance Abuse

The criteria for substance abuse in the *DSM-IV-TR* are different as they are devoid of criteria for tolerance or withdrawal.

A. Maladaptive pattern of substance use leading to clinically significant impairment or distress, as manifested by one (or more) of the following, occurring within a 12-month period:
    1. recurrent substance use, resulting in a failure to fulfill major role obligations at work, school, or home (e.g., repeated absences or poor work performance related to substance use; substance-related absences, suspensions, or expulsions from school; neglect of children or household)
    2. recurrent substance use in situations in which it is physically hazardous (e.g., driving an automobile or operating a machine when impaired by substance use)
    3. recurrent substance-related legal problems (e.g., arrests for substance-related disorderly conduct)
    4. continued substance use despite having persistent or recurrent social or interpersonal problems caused or exacerbated by the effects of the substance (e.g., arguments with spouse about consequences of intoxication, physical fights)
B. The symptoms have never met the criteria for Substance Dependence for this class of substance.

Note. From the *Diagnostic and Statistical Manual of Mental Disorders*, fourth edition, text revision (pp. 197–199), 2000, Washington, DC: American Psychiatric Association. Copyright 2000 by American Psychiatric Association. Reprinted with permission.

Adolescent Substance Abuse Assessment

The challenge in evaluating substance abuse problems with adolescents is differentiating between normal adolescent behavior and change from alcohol and drug use or abuse. The following questions can help counselors differentiate as well as use the substance abuse assessment tools:

1. Has the student's behavior changed significantly in class over time? For example, the student has begun talking back to the teacher or the student appears lethargic or hyperactive in school (which differs significantly from his or her known behavioral presentation).
2. Has the student's attitude changed? For example, by teacher report, the student's behavior the prior year was easygoing, and this year the student is combative; the student displays a significant drop in interest regarding extracurricular activities.

3. Does the student have bloodshot eyes?
4. Has the student's attire and peer association changed?
5. What activities has the student engaged in, both in the past and currently?
6. Has the student been tardy or absent from classes?
7. Has the student's interest in school declined?
8. Does the student appear to be high or intoxicated?
9. Has the student's grade point average dropped significantly?
10. What is the student's attitude and behavior during the interview? Is he or she blaming or not taking responsibility for actions?

The difficulty in assessing adolescent substance abuse is that the behavior of adolescents can mimic alcohol- and drug-using behavior. Adolescence is a time of developing autonomy, testing limits, and finding one's identity in the world. Therefore, acting out behavior and defensiveness can be a normal aspect of adolescent development. Many times school counselors have sufficient understanding of the clients coming into their offices based on their experience in the school environment. This depends, however, on the size of the school. In cases of large school settings, corroborating information is helpful in providing a thorough assessment.

Additional resources for information regarding student behavior, affect, and attitudinal changes include administrators, school psychologists, school social workers, therapeutic staff support workers, teachers (especially homeroom teachers), coaches, and parents. In some cases, the changes observed by one individual can be minimal at best, but when combined with the observations of several other key personnel they can paint a clearer picture of significant change that should be assessed.

Alcohol and Drug Assessment Instruments

In addition to the counselor's evaluation, there are a number of instruments available to use with clients in order to make a diagnosis of drug or alcohol abuse and/or dependency and to determine those who are at high risk to develop an addiction.

Relapse Calendar

The relapse calendar was introduced by Terence Gorski (1989) as a tool for evaluating clients who have relapsed. The calendar is used primarily with clients who identify themselves as addicts or alcoholics and who have relapsed into active addiction. With this assessment tool, counselors can document how long individuals have been in recovery and what behaviors they enacted during their recovery in order to remain sober and clean. The relapse calendar also helps counselors investigate why clients stopped using drugs and alcohol each time and what led to the relapse. Additionally, counselors find out what has occurred during this relapse (consequences) and why they are seeking counseling and treatment at this time.

Counselors make a time line to chart the above information from when clients stopped using, how long they stopped, and when they started using again. Counselors document the patterns of the relapse on a grid and explore with clients the significant life events that may have occurred during their life (e.g., deaths, births, and marriages). This calendar provides a visual description for both clients and counselors of the clients' relapse histories and aids in creating prevention strategies. Counselors can use the calendar by drawing a curvy line to show when the clients' use occurred and a straight line to indicate abstinence or recovery attempts. It is important for the counselor to explore what led a client to return to use as well as to consider what contributed to relapse. Life events, traumas or loss, and consequences of chemical use can all be marked on this calendar, thus cocreating a visual map for the client and a point from which effective treatment planning can take place. Figure 4.1 is a sample of the relapse calendar, which can be used during the initial assessment and subsequent sessions with clients. The counselor and the client complete this form in hopes of identifying warning signs, areas of strength, and potential relapse themes.

CAGE

This acronym represents a brief screening instrument used in conjunction with data collection during the assessment. This screening tool was first introduced in 1970 by Ewing and Rouse. The instrument provides counselors with initial information on clients' alcohol use.

C—Have you ever felt a need to *cut* down on your drinking?
A—Have you ever felt *annoyed* by someone criticizing your drinking?
G—Have you ever felt *guilty* about your drinking?
E—Have you ever had an *eye opener* or drank in the morning to steady your nerves?

Responding "yes" to two or more of these questions indicates the likelihood of an alcohol problem. This series of questions focuses primarily on alcohol and not on drug use.

Michigan Alcohol Screening Test (MAST)

The MAST (Laux, Newman, & Brown, 2004) consists of 24 items and takes about 10–15 minutes to complete. Items are scored with a 0 for nondrinking, or a 1, 2, or 5 for an affirmative response to drinking. A sample question is, "Have you ever attended a meeting of Alcoholics Anonymous?" If the individual responds "yes," 5 points are given; if the person responds "no," 0 points are given. The total possible score is 53, with a score of 0–4 being considered nonalcoholic, 5–6 suggesting an alcohol problem, and 7–9 being considered alcoholic. A score of 10–20 is considered a moderate alcoholic, and above 20 points is considered a severe alcoholic. The test was created to only measure alcohol use, and a drawback is that it is relatively easy to fake (Fisher & Harrison, 2005; Laux et al., 2004).

Substance Abuse Subtle Screening Inventory-3 (SASSI-3)

This instrument was created by Glen Miller (1983) and has both an adult and an adolescent version, each with separate norms for evaluating results. The first revision was in 1994, and in 1997 the SASSI-3 was released. Differences exist in that some of the items, decision rules,

Jan.	Feb.	Mar.	Apr.	May	June	July	Aug.	Sept.	Oct.	Nov.	Dec.

Figure 4.1. Relapse Calendar

and subscales were added or replaced. The SASSI-2 added a correctional scale to measure recidivism in the criminal justice system, and the random-answering scale was added to identify random responses. The supplemental addiction measure was replaced by the defensiveness scale. The SASSI-3 is widely used in college counseling and mental health agencies and takes about 10–15 minutes to administer (Laux, Salyers, & Kotova, 2005).

The initial form had 52 items and then was increased to 62 items; it now has 67 true–false items on the adult version and 55 items on the adolescent version. A review by Kerr (1994) suggested that the SASSI does a good job of identifying individuals with a dependency to alcohol and drugs. Although it does not diagnose substance abuse, only dependence, it does suggest the possibility of substance abuse problems.

Alcohol Use Disorders Identification Test (AUDIT)

The AUDIT (Babor, De La Fuente, Saunders, & Grant, 1992) is a standardized diagnostic alcohol and drug test that was developed by the World Health Organization and is able to screen separately for hazardous, harmful, and dependence-related symptoms associated with alcohol (Saunders, Aasland, Babor, De La Fuente, & Grant, 1993). Many of the earlier screening instruments mainly focused on the presence of alcohol dependence, whereas the distinct advantage of AUDIT is its capability of highlighting drinking behavior all along the continuum from alcohol misuse to hazardous drinking. AUDIT has been used increasingly with a variety of populations within a number of settings (Donovan, Kivlahan, Doyle, Longabaugh, & Greenfield, 2006; A. Schmidt, Barry, & Fleming, 1995).

Drug Use Screening Inventory–Revised (DUSI-R)

The DUSI-R has an adolescent version, which assesses both alcohol and drug use patterns. The inventory has 159 true–false questions and provides data for 10 functional adolescent problem areas: alcohol and drug use, physical health, mental health, family relations, peer relationships, educational status, vocational status, social skills, leisure activities, and aggressive or delinquent behaviors. This inventory has been shown to have good reliability and validity (Kirisci, Mezzich, & Tarter, 1995).

A continuous concern for many school counselors, in particular, is working with substance-abusing and addicted adolescents. The school counselor is truly a gatekeeper with an important place in the continuum of assessment and referral. Some school systems have a Student Assistance Program, which specifically focuses on alcohol- and drug-abusing students. Counselors may determine that a student's behavior is a symptom of significant dysfunction in the family, and that he or she is acting out through chemical use. Alternately, the counselor may determine that the student is both acting out because of family dysfunction and has an addiction to alcohol and drugs.

Psychological Information

It is necessary for counselors to obtain a history of psychological issues, previous counseling, treatment for mental health or substance abuse disorders, or use of psychotropic medication.

Co-Occurring Disorders Assessment

Along with the evaluation of substance abuse symptoms, counselors also need to assess for other psychiatric disorders, which are crucial in effective treatment planning and referral. The term *co-occurring disorder* suggests that a client has met the criteria for two disorders on Axis I, one being a substance abuse/dependency disorder and the other a mental illness (Evans & Sullivan, 1990). The most significant challenges many times are not the client but rather with agencies and their funding sources. Historically and currently, funding for substance abuse treatment and mental health treatment in many states is separate. Health insurance companies also separate mental health and substance abuse benefits. Such differentiation creates a substantial gap in both treatment services for clients and the perception of these problems. Unfortunately, clients are caught in the middle and have the potential to fall through service gaps. A comprehensive assessment can help create an effective treatment protocol and blend services within the community. Dr. Ronald Kessler, principal investigator of the National Comorbidity Survey—Replication study, and colleagues determined that about half of Americans will meet the criteria for a *DSM-IV* diagnosis of a mental disorder over the course of their lifetimes, with first onset usually in childhood or adolescence. Lifetime prevalence for the different classes of disorders were anxiety disorder, 28.8%; mood disorders, 20.8%; impulse control disorders, 24.8%; substance use disorders, 14.6%; and any disorder, 46.4% (Kessler et al., 2005).

The major mental disorders outlined here that may co-occur with substance abuse disorders include, but are not limited to, anxiety disorders, major depressive disorders, bipolar disorder, and schizophrenia. In treatment, co-occurring disorders are addressed simultaneously (A. J. Brooks, Malfait, Brooke, Gallagher, & Penn, 2007).

Anxiety Disorders

Within the category of anxiety disorders are generalized anxiety disorder, posttraumatic stress disorder, social phobia, panic attacks, obsessive–compulsive disorder, and agoraphobia. Anxious clients tend to be future focused to think about events that may or may not materialize and exhibit excessive worrying. In response to such thinking, anxious patients often report somatic symptoms (e.g., headaches, migraines, and/or backaches) and present as hypervigilant in the session (Evans & Sullivan, 1990). Comorbidity among mental disorders appears to be the norm, particularly for mood and anxiety disorders. This comorbidity significantly impacts the treatment approach, prognosis, and outcome (McDermut, Mattia, & Zimmerman, 2001).

Clients with an anxiety disorder may have been evaluated by a psychiatrist for "nerves" and may already be taking an anxiolytic medication (Ativan or Xanax). These medications are used to reduce the anxious feelings. In addition to the prescribed medication, clients may also be using alcohol (a sedative-hypnotic) to anesthetize the thoughts and feelings.

The challenge for counselors in a college, school, inpatient, or outpatient setting is to separate anxiety as a mental illness from chemically induced anxiety. Depending on the diagnosis, clients may need detoxification or relaxation techniques. These measures illustrate why the need for accurate diagnosing in an outpatient setting is so significant for appropriate client referral.

Counselors need to evaluate clients for symptoms of mental disorders before their first use of alcohol or drugs. This helps differentiate the effects of substance abuse from the preexisting features of mental illness.

For example, a counselor may, in working with a 27-year-old client, determine that before his alcohol use at age 12, he was very anxious as a child and "on edge" because of his father's raging behavior when intoxicated. The client reports that most of his childhood was spent feeling terrorized and upset. In turn, these feelings resulted in bed wetting, difficulty in school, feeling the need to be very reclusive, and experiencing anxiety with peers. This information, along with the client's alcohol use, can help structure a treatment plan that addresses both his potential alcohol abuse *and* his anxiety disorder. The counselor works with him on treating *both* issues, not treating one and then the other but treating them simultaneously. A referral to alcohol and drug treatment along with a referral to a psychiatrist for a medication evaluation is appropriate. Given the psychiatrist is knowledgeable in addiction medicine, he or she would hopefully prescribe a nonaddicting medication to reduce the symptoms of anxiety. The medication, along with group or individual treatment and relaxation techniques, would address this client's dual diagnosis.

Major Depression

Clients suffering from major depression may present as sad or tearful and exhibit low energy or agitation during the interview. Typically, these clients are cognitively focused on the past, eliciting feelings of guilt, remorse, and shame. They may report thoughts of suicide or feelings of hopelessness. Behaviorally, these clients may report difficulty sleeping (falling asleep or awakening), eating (loss of appetite), or maintaining energy (lethargic). Depressed clients tend to isolate and are unable to discuss their emotions with family or friends (Evans & Sullivan, 1990).

The difficulty in diagnosing major depression is confounded by the possibility that clients may be drinking excessive amounts of alcohol or using drugs on a daily basis. Such use patterns typically yield similar side effects as the behaviors associated with major depression (difficulty sleeping, loss of appetite, and lethargy). According to Star, Bober, and Gold (2005), other challenges exist with depressed adolescent clients who present with symptoms of depression (usually in the form of irritability) and can overlap or mimic symptoms of problem alcohol and drug use.

Appetites may be suppressed as a result of the alcohol use, and isolation may be due to the feelings of guilt and shame regarding drug use. Completing a thorough depression history can reveal, in many cases, a preexisting depressive disorder, which clients medicate with drugs and alcohol.

Suicide Assessment

During the initial assessment and subsequent visits, suicidal and homicidal ideation and gestures need to be evaluated. Deutsch (1984) and Farber (1983) surveyed therapists' perceptions of client behavior and what was most stressful to them. They found that clients making suicidal statements was the number one stressor to counselors. According to Bryan and Rudd (2006), the mention of suicide by clients uniformly increases anxiety in clinicians. Blumenthal, Bell, Neumann, Schuttler, and Vogel (1989) found that 33% of suicides were correlated with alcohol use. Whereas psychological autopsies have shown that psychiatric illness is the primary antecedent in 90–100% of completed suicides, substance abuse and alcohol are found in 20–50% of cases. Therefore, it is second only to a depressive disorder in the contribution to suicide (Jenkins, 2007). Because of the high lethality associated with alcohol and drug clients, we provide questions that counselors need to explore with clients below (Pipes & Davenport, 1999).

1. *Have you ever had thoughts of suicide?* What is significant here is the use of the word *suicide* and not "thoughts of ending it all" or "thoughts of checking out for good." Providing clarity eliminates confusion. If clients have had thoughts, find out in what form and when, how long ago, and what did they do. When they were thinking of suicide, were they sober and clean, or were they drinking or using a substance?
2. *Does the client have any current or past attempts at suicide?* Again, determine if they did attempt and whether they were drinking or using alcohol or drugs. Find out how they attempted to kill themselves before (e.g., pills, rope, knives, overdosing, driving) and whether they have a current plan. If so, do they have the means (e.g., gun at home, ample supply of pills at home) to implement or carry out that plan?
3. *Have you ever had treatment for depression (inpatient, outpatient, psychopharmacological treatment)?* It is important to ask clients if they have ever been hospitalized (either voluntarily or involuntarily) for depression or if they have ever been in counsel-

ing before. Also important is for the counselor to inquire whether or not they have ever been on medication for depression. Determine the client's response to treatment and, if possible, obtain an ROI to communicate with any past treatment professionals or current psychiatrists.

4. *Is there a family history of depression?* Determine if anyone in the family has ever struggled with depression, ever been in treatment, or ever been on medication for depression. Included in this information is what response they had to treatment. Also probe into when family members were first diagnosed and if anyone in the family attempted suicide and when. The lethality increases when family members have committed suicide, and therefore client safety becomes paramount.

5. *Does the client present any current symptoms of depression?* The counselor needs to be familiar with the symptoms of depression in order to assess this aspect of current functioning. The symptoms include loss of appetite and weight (20 pounds or more), tearfulness, difficulty sleeping, anhedonia, thoughts of suicide, and how he or she is coping with the current symptoms. Within this evaluation the counselor needs to look for signs of closure from the client's perspective. For example, does the client share about how he or she is giving away personal items or furniture?

6. *What is the client's ability to adapt to changes in life?* Does the client have an ability to cope with change and adapt to abrupt movements in life? Is the client rigid and unbending or does he or she have the ability to work with changes?

7. *What is the client's social support network?* Is the client living alone or with a partner, siblings, friends, or parents? Is the support network readily accessible, and are they concerned at this time about the depression? Have they ever been concerned about the depression in the past?

8. *What are the client's strengths?* Help explore with clients their strengths and resources and how suicide would impact and effect those who they care about. Help clients increase awareness of how suicide would affect the lives of others.

Another method to assess depression is through the use of the Beck Depression Inventory (Beck, Steer, & Brown, 1996). Beyond this assessment tool, a referral for a psychiatric evaluation and consultation may be necessary. Discussion with peers and direct supervisor(s) is of major importance in coping with the stresses involved with working with suicidal clients.

Working With Suicidal Clients Who Use Alcohol and Drugs

If suicide is a stressful issue for counselors, the combination of suicide and substance use can magnify stress exponentially for counselors. Counselors are ethically and legally bound to work with clients to help explore their suicidal feelings while protecting and preserving their lives (American Counseling Association, 2005). On the basis of our experience working with this population, we suggest that most clients (at least at some point in time) have thoughts of suicide. The increase in suicidal depression is many times juxtaposed with the depleting drug supply or mounting of possible or experienced consequences. The overall depression and anxiety related to a depleted drug supply, along with the mounting consequences, can significantly increase the feelings of depression and hopelessness. It is during this critical time when clients perceive their options as limited and ranging from committing suicide, being incarcerated, going insane, or reaching out for help. Counselors who work with substance-abusing clients during these *lowest* times should know that, ironically, they are also times of greatest opportunity for clients to break the cycle of addiction and take action. This transformation to action and surrender is further explored in the chapter on spirituality.

Counselors should seek consultation and supervision when working with this population and, most important, with suicidal clients (this is both for the protection and therapeutic value for the client as well as the protection of the counselor and agency, school, or organization). Determining the level of treatment for a suicidal, substance-abusing client can be overwhelming for any counselor, and especially for new counselors. Assessing clients for the appropriate level of care takes training, practice, and skill. The following are identifiable referrals for suicidal, substance-abusing clients:

1. *Hospitalization.* Does the client verbalize in the session that he or she needs intensive help and treatment? Do you feel the client needs more structure than outpatient treatment provides? Are you concerned that the client will need continuous monitoring? Is the client willing to go to inpatient treatment on his or her own volition? Does the client need to be involuntarily committed, and how does that process occur in your state or region?
2. *Can the client work therapeutically in outpatient counseling through the development of a counselor–client no-harm contract?* In your clinical assessment (after consultation with supervisor and peers), can the client work therapeutically with you in outpatient treatment? Is he or she willing to follow a referral to a psychiatrist for medication evaluation? Is there willingness to attend therapy sessions more regularly? Is he or she willing to attend support groups?

If the client is amenable to working in outpatient counseling and agrees to the above, the client may be able to follow an outpatient protocol versus an inpatient referral. However, the importance of peer consultation and supervisor input is critical. In these consultative and supervision discussions, make sure you use counselors who have experience working with addicted populations.

1. *Is the client willing to have significant others remove items in the household that are lethal in nature (e.g., guns, razor blades, drugs or pills, keys to a vehicle)?* If so, have the client contact them while he or she is in the office. Discuss further the no-self-harm contract, involving as many support individuals as possible. One gauge point is whether or not you request family and friends to meet at your office to discuss the contract. If they are unwilling, this may be a significant piece of information about the follow through and support on the contract. (Of course you must keep in mind any work and travel restrictions for family and friends.)

Although suicide contracts are used in a majority of mental health settings, legally the contract can come under scrutiny (Remley, 2001). From the courts' perspective, if the counselor was concerned enough to have the client sign a contract, and he or she did commit suicide, the family could sue the clinician on the grounds that if the counselor felt strongly enough to do a contract, why didn't the counselor involuntarily commit the client to a hospital for treatment?

Bipolar Disorder

Clients with bipolar disorder present symptoms of mania or euphoria and a history of severe depression. During the manic phase, they have racing thoughts, and their behavior may appear grandiose. Clients may also present as loud and inappropriate during the counseling session. The behavior of clients using cocaine and heroin can mimic bipolar disorder. For instance, when clients are high on cocaine, their behaviors and thoughts may be racing and inappropriate, even grandiose. When they are using heroin, their affect and behavior may appear down and low energy (Evans & Sullivan, 1990).

Schizophrenia

Individuals diagnosed as having schizophrenia may present as confused or having bizarre delusions and hallucinations. They may also report feeling depressed and/or anxious and have difficulty concentrating. Their behaviors appear disorganized and eccentric, which may include poor hygiene and grooming. These individuals are somewhat withdrawn, and if they are employed, they may have a low-stress job.

Counselors need to recognize schizophrenia as a brain disorder requiring medication for management of the symptoms. Unfortunately, clients may use alcohol or drugs to combat the side effects of the medications used to treat schizophrenia, thus creating an additional problem. Even though clients may not be dependent on alcohol or drugs, the amounts used can impact the effectiveness of the psychotropic medication the clients are taking (Evans & Sullivan, 1990). Medication compliance and abstinence from alcohol and drugs are the challenging treatment goals for clients. The importance of counselors working within a team of health care and helping professionals is important. Psychiatrists continually monitor clients' medication protocol, while counselors work on social and job skills with clients, in addition to medication compliance and substance abstinence.

Clinical Example

One of the first clients I (Ford) worked with presented for counseling with a reported history of cocaine addiction. Upon further exploration, however, I found that his self-reported cocaine use was minimal. Throughout the session he smiled and at times inappropriately laughed. As he engaged in outpatient alcohol and drug treatment, it became clear he had a dual diagnosis. After an evaluation with the psychiatrist, he was diagnosed as schizophrenic and abused cocaine but was not cocaine dependent.

An important aspect of the assessment process includes regular urine screens to ascertain what (if any) drugs or amounts of alcohol clients are consuming. Counselors can request a urine or drug test from clients in a number of ways. If clients are mandated for treatment, the counselor can frame the drug screening as a method in which to document abstinence. The screening also helps clients maintain honesty throughout the counseling relationship. Counselors framing the drug-testing process in a therapeutic fashion, rather than a punitive one, can help clients become amenable to screening. The challenge in an outpatient counseling setting is the lack of a controlled environment to ensure that the client is not using alcohol or drugs. The use of random drug and alcohol screenings can aid clients and counselors in evaluating the possible mental disorders without the confounding variable of the drugs or alcohol.

The use of drug screens, referent information, prior treatment, or family information increases the opportunity for counselors to assess for concomitant disorders in their clients. Clients addicted to alcohol or drugs and who are depressed need encouragement to consider remaining abstinent in order for the antidepressant medication to be effective. Clients who continue to use or drink and take psychotropic medication will negate the therapeutic value of the antidepressant medication, and depression will reoccur.

A current mental status examination determines if clients are oriented to person, place, and time, and a suicide assessment evaluates client safety (a significant number of addicted clients report suicidal ideation during the course of their addiction). In 2004, suicide was the 11th leading cause of death in the U.S., accounting for 32,439 deaths. It was also the 8th leading cause of death for males and the 16th leading cause of death for females in 2004 (Centers for Disease Control and Prevention, 2004). Because of these numbers, counselors need to be aware and understand the symptoms of depression, as well as other Axis I mental health disorders.

Mental Status Evaluation (MSE)

In addition to the suicide assessment, counselors should conduct a brief MSE with their clients. Staff psychiatrists or psychologists normally conduct this type of examination; however, it can be clinically useful for counselors during the assessment process. Additionally, especially with this population, the MSE may be useful from time to time during sessions to assess for ongoing use (Pipes & Davenport, 1999).

The MSE has five sections: the evaluation of clients' behavior, thinking, feeling, data gathering, and symptomotology (Pipes & Davenport, 1999).

1. *Behavior.* How do clients appear and how do they interact during the evaluation? Are they slovenly dressed? Do they act childish during the interview? Is there a marked change in the behavior patterns you have come to associate with them?
2. *Thinking.* How sound are clients' abilities to judge situations? How clear is their thought process? Memory? Orientation to person, place, and time? Are they insightful? How do they function internally versus externally?
3. *Feeling.* Can clients express affect? Are they labile? Is there an exaggerated change in their normal affect?
4. *Data Gathering.* How are clients at gathering information and sensory stimuli?
5. *Symptoms.* Are there Axis I symptoms or Axis II personality disorder symptoms?

In addition to the above areas of evaluation, the medical, social (family, relationships), occupational, education, legal, and military service are also of significant importance to evaluate. This comprehensive evaluation supports counselors in better understanding the environment, which is important in cocreating an effective treatment plan.

Medical Information

Along with obtaining information from clients on the frequency, amounts, and types of alcohol and drug use, determining the methods of ingestion is also critical in understanding both the nature of the problem and the possible medical complications. Additionally, counselors may have clients who report having chronic migraines, nosebleeds, and weight loss. A referral to a physician for a complete physical examination would be appropriate during the course of counseling clients with such symptoms.

This section of assessment includes obtaining a medical history, previous or current medications, and physical impairments. Some agencies require their clients to obtain a physical examination before counseling services or agree to one while in counseling. During this aspect of the assessment, the counselor also explores medical family history (e.g., alcoholism, drug addiction, illnesses, chronic conditions) and addresses any presented or suspected medical problems. Client access to a physician is significant in order to facilitate a comprehensive assessment. Collaboratively, physicians and counselors work to create an effective strategy for treatment and/or referrals. If clients already have a designated physician, a referral to their personal doctor is appropriate.

Social/Family/Relationships

As discussed in earlier chapters, the consideration of cultural and environmental support for clients is critical. What kinds of support do the clients have? Do they have close friends? Are they close with their families? Are they, or have they ever been, in a significant intimate relationship? Counselors want to use support networks and incorporate them into the treatment planning.

Occupational Information

In exploring the work history of clients, counselors are seeking a better understanding of any gaps or changes in work, which are related to alcohol or drug use, and other effects on the workplace such as tardiness and absenteeism. Work can be impacted in many ways: being intoxicated on the job, accidents, missing the day after payday on a regular basis, stealing from coworkers, selling drugs on the job site, low productivity because of hangovers, or other medical complications due to drug and alcohol use, just to name a few. Additionally, relational issues may become enflamed as use increases or stops. Attention to relationships the client has at work is necessary in understanding this piece of the context of his or her current life situation.

Education

Determining the highest level of education (i.e., high school, college, graduate school, trade school, community college) can help identify how clients' drug and alcohol use has impacted education and training. A counselor can further explore this with the client by asking the following questions: Have you ever dropped out of school or training because of your drug or alcohol use? Have you ever been asked to leave an institution or training program because of your use? Have your grades suffered as a result of your use?

Legal Involvement

It is imperative to ask clients if they have any upcoming court dates, if they are or ever have been on parole or probation, if they have a prior criminal history (both as a juvenile and an adult), and if they spent any significant amounts of time incarcerated. Exploring a client's legal history highlights possible issues that can be addressed in counseling. For instance, the client who has been arrested twice for exposing himself under the influence in a local playground would also need therapy addressing sexual impulses, feelings, and appropriate displays of behavior. A client who has been arrested, both as a teen and an adult for assault under the influence, will need to address anger identification and expression. Additionally, crimes committed when not under the influence could reveal antisocial or conduct disorders that will probably exacerbate or be exacerbated by the use or abuse of drugs and/or alcohol.

Military Service

When assessing a client's military history it is important to ask specific questions such as the following: In what branch of the military have you served or are you serving? How long were or are you serving? What was or is your specialty training in the service? Have you ever been in combat conditions? (If so, where and for how long?) Additionally, the counselor needs to explore the client's chemical or alcohol use while in the military. Finally, ask whether or not they are still on active duty or in a reservist unit. If they were discharged, was it honorable, honorable under general conditions, or dishonorable? If the discharge was less than honorable or dishonorable, inquire and determine whether alcohol or drugs were related to the discharge status.

For those individuals who have been in combat conditions, this aspect of military experience is important to explore. Probing questions that assess sleep patterns, startle responses (when the client appears to be somewhere else and then returns with a sudden startled reaction), and reports of flashbacks can be used to assess posttraumatic stress disorder (PTSD). For some, the use of alcohol and drugs helps medicate the stress of trauma symptoms stemming from this disorder.

Counseling Approach to Assessment: Motivational Interviewing (MI)

The task of assessing for alcohol and drug problems in and of itself is a challenge. Many clients who come in for assessment are not necessarily clear that there is a problem, and the reason for the referral may be from a third party. That said, defenses with the client are usually quite high. The use of MI (W. R. Miller & Rollnick, 2002) in the evaluation process can help to reduce defenses and at the same time help the client and clinician with referral and treatment options.

The initial task of MI is to develop a rapport with the client and listen to the presenting issue(s). The second task is to help enhance client motivation, and the third task is to work with the resistance the client may bring to the session. Those clients who are referred by third-party sources (e.g., parole officer, employment assistance program, teachers) generally come to the session prepared to do "battle" with the counselor. The MI approach helps in disarming the resistance and allows clients to feel heard and understood, so meaningful therapeutic work can be accomplished. This MI approach works particularly well with substance abusing clients when used in combination with Prochaska and DiClementes's (1984) stages of change and the transtheoretical model of behavioral change (Prochaska & DiClemente, 1982, 1984), as discussed in chapter 5.

Along with the information presented thus far, counselors need to explore client resistance and ambivalence along with their own resistance. According to W. R. Miller and Rollnick (2002), "It is how you respond to client resistance that makes the difference, and that distinguishes MI from other approaches. If resistance is increasing during counseling, it is very likely in response to something that you are doing" (p. 99).

In our clinical work we have observed that clients arrive to counseling in a variety of ways, with unique internal resources and motivations. Some clients appear highly motivated, whereas others seem ambivalent about change. Unfortunately, counselors often blame clients for being noncompliant or resistant and fail to recognize their role in the perceived client reactance. With this in mind, W. R. Miller and Rollnick (2002) proposed six responses to clients that they believe are *not* helpful in promoting growth and only contribute to clients' resistance (p. 50).

1. *Arguing for change.* This occurs when the counselor attempts to persuade clients to make changes from their stated position. This is an internal process, not just the words the counselor uses but the actual view they have of the client and the process itself. These arguments can be overt or covert in nature. When aware of this approach, the counselor should work to understand his or her irrational reason for this positioning (e.g., "If the client doesn't change, I have failed; I must get them to see that they must change").

2. *Assuming the expert role.* This is when the counselor presents as "knowing it all" and tends to answer questions directly as opposed to feeding them back to the client for exploration. A significant concern here is the answer to the question, Why does the counselor feel the need to know it all? Counselors should explore with their supervisor the impact such a stance may have on their clients (e.g., an adolescent may be substantially revolted by a counselor saying "I've been there and know just what you are going through").

3. *Criticizing, shaming, and/or blaming.* Historically, some treatment programs used the approach of breaking down client ego through criticism and blame, only to increase the defenses of the client. Unfortunately, the client would be blamed for the lack of progress and many times be discharged unsuccessfully for noncompliance. In point of fact, such a positioning by a program or counselor may also cause the client to remove therapy from his or her list of useful resources (sometimes for the rest of his/her life).

4. *Labeling.* This occurs when counselors attempt to focus on diagnostic labels such as "they are borderline" and "they are a drunk" as opposed to exploring the feelings related to the client's trauma or addiction to alcohol and drugs. Counselors who are more concerned with the diagnostic labels miss the actual experience with clients. In some instances, the use of negative labeling substantially limits the therapeutic veins

the counselor may see for the client. If one is only known as a "borderline," many of the client's positive aspects may be missed by the counselor. Further, whether the applied label was determined or created by the counselor or through formal assessments (e.g., Minnesota Multiphasic Personality Inventory), it may actually be inaccurate.

5. *Being in a hurry.* With increasing volumes of paperwork that originates during the assessment, either because of insurance or licensure needs, counselors may be less thorough or brief in their interactions with clients. Clients, unfortunately, feel the brevity of the process and may therefore offer little in the way of information and motivation to the counselor. Counselors are wise to recall both the need for presence with the client and the mantra of groups like Alcoholics Anonymous that suggests "one day at a time."

6. *Claiming preeminence.* This occurs when counselors believe they understand what their clients need better than the clients, thus placing themselves in the expert role. This stance runs the risk of feeding a counselor's ego at the expense of clients' needs.

W. R. Miller and Rollnick (2002) suggested that various aspects of these six areas can be appropriate at times (p. 51). For example, it is important to determine an accurate diagnosis for a medication evaluation referral or for the selection of treatment interventions. Although it is helpful to use the diagnosis as a piece of the evaluation process, it is not helpful to look at the client as "only" a diagnosis.

MI is directive, client-centered, and elicits behavior change by helping clients explore and resolve ambivalence (W. R. Miller & Rollnick, 2002). MI is collaborative, evocative, and autonomous. In other words, it allows for client–clinician collaboration as opposed to confrontation and drawing (forcing) out feelings and thoughts from the client. Matta (2004) suggested that MI encourages and supports the autonomy of the client. This therapeutic vantage point minimizes the client's reactance and opposition to the authority (or perceived authority) of the clinician. Further, this positioning generates personal responsibility and is not coercive (Matta, 2004).

W. R. Miller and Rollnick (2002) proposed a four-principle approach to both honor and work with perceived client ambivalence and resistance to change. The four basic principles of MI are expressing empathy, developing a discrepancy, rolling with resistance, and support self-efficacy. A discussion of each principle follows.

Expressing Empathy

- Genuine acceptance allows change and reflective listening.

The importance of empathy as a base for client growth stems from the work of Carl Rogers (1957). Clients who genuinely feel understood by counselors are less resistant and more open to the counseling process. The following is a brief dialogue demonstrating empathy:

Client: I am so angry at being here right now, I could just spit.
Counselor: You really feel frustrated at this process and having to be here today. It is as if no one has really listened to your experience and what you have been through to get here.

As a result of this exchange, the client can begin to feel understood and therefore feel less resistant to the counseling process.

Developing a Discrepancy

- Accurate reflection of the awareness of consequences builds rapport and helps the client envision how actions and behaviors do result in outcomes (positive or negative).
- Pointing out discrepancies between goals and behaviors encourages client growth.

Counselors want to support any awareness clients might have regarding consequences and the relationship to their behaviors. Simultaneously, counselors also want to explore with clients their values and goals and how the use of drugs and alcohol impact them.

Client: Yeah, this is the second time I've been referred to you for counseling because of my drug use. I almost lost my job last year, but came to counseling with you to save it. Now my employer says if I don't follow through with treatment and I use drugs again, I will lose my job.

Counselor: I remember last time you talked with me about how important your job was to you and how hard you worked to get that position. It sounds as though you love your job, and again your drug use is jeopardizing what you've worked so hard for.

Through this brief dialogue, the client can become aware of how his drug use is jeopardizing that which he values greatly.

Rolling With Resistance

- Don't argue with your client.
- Use supervision to process your reactions to the client.
- Use empathy to join with the client.
- Practice being in the moment and truly hearing what the client is trying to express.
- Encourage new perspectives; however, do not impose them on the client.
- Embrace the client's story while supporting alternatives and possible new stories.
- If recommendations are made or suggested, determine how the client feels about them.
- Respectfully work with the client on the possibility of new directions.

The following responses by the counselor reflect the support, empathy, and deep concern for clients' well-being and emotional pain:

Counselor Response: I am wondering how you are feeling about some of the suggestions I made today?

Or

Counselor Response: It really sounds as though you've given this a great deal of thought.

Support Self-Efficacy

- Express hopeful and optimistic attitude for change. This starts with an internal recognition on the part of the counselor of true hope.
- Make affirmation statements to the client.
- Notice and comment on strengths and positive movement by the client.
- Express optimism for change to the client.
- Understand that change is inevitable, it is only a matter of time and to what degree the change will occur.

Many times clients are ambivalent and borrow hope or optimism from their counselors. It is important for counselors to encourage and support the aspects in the clients' behavior and thought processes that indicate change.

Counselor: You know, Tim, it has taken a lot for you to come in today, based on all of the things you have told me. And over the course of our time together, I am getting a sense that although there is a part of you that does not want to be here, there is an even larger aspect of who you are that is motivated to change the direction of your life and the choices you have been making.

Types of Referrals

As part of the assessment process, counselors need to be knowledgeable of the referral sources for clients in order to appropriately plan for their therapeutic process. The most common referrals to counselors originate from inpatient co-occurring treatment programs, alcohol and drug treatment programs, self-referrals, court, relapsing clients, and those clients suffering from mental illness. A brief description of each is outlined in the following paragraphs:

1. *Post inpatient co-occurring disorders treatment.* These clients are referred to outpatient drug and alcohol programs to treat their addictions as well as concomitant mental health services to treat their mental disorders. Counselors providing mental health counseling need to be knowledgeable in drug and alcohol abuse and addiction and the complicating factors with mental health clients. In accordance with the American Counseling Association's (2005) ethical guidelines, contact must be made between the two counselors to provide for a continuum of care.

2. *Clients who have completed drug and alcohol treatment.* These clients have completed a program (inpatient or outpatient) and may be referred to counselors following treatment in order to work on issues relating to family of origin, intimacy issues, gender issues, and so on.

3. *Self-referred clients—motivated.* These clients come in for counseling or therapy unrelated to drug and alcohol use. The counselor, following assessment, determines that the client needs to be further assessed by a certified drug and alcohol specialist. For example, a school counselor meets with a student who comes in for counseling because he is depressed. The counselor determines that part of his depression is alleviated by substantial consumption of alcohol. The client becomes willing to work with a student assistance counselor on his alcohol usage and to explore feelings that contribute to his use.

4. *Self-referred client—resistant.* Similar to the above example, yet different, is the client's unwillingness to address the alcohol use and the impact it may be having on his depression. The client wants to focus on "other issues" and not the alcohol and drug consumption. The client may, in fact, want to discontinue counseling services when drug or alcohol issues are brought up by the counselor.

5. *Court-mandated referral.* These clients are initially referred by the court, are typically resistant, and may be referred for counseling to address multiple issues, such as anger management and alcohol abuse. Counselors need to assess and address the resistance and anger.

6. *Relapsing client referral.* This describes clients who have been in a recovery process and return to active addiction by using drugs or alcohol. These clients generally return to counseling following a crisis related to their drug or alcohol use and may subsequently enter a treatment program.

7. *Referral of chronically mentally ill client.* This client is not addicted to drugs or alcohol but rather is on a regimented protocol of psychotropic medication and is either using or abusing alcohol and drugs. The use of drugs and alcohol severely impacts the effectiveness of other medications, either because the client discontinues his or her medication or because there is an interaction between medication and drugs and alcohol. The client is not appropriate for alcohol and drug treatment, yet is in need of specialized approaches to deal with the mental illness and the substance abuse (Drake, Bartels, Teague, Noordsy, & Clark, 1993). Holmes et al. (2006) indicated the need for a collaborative and integrated system of delivery for community resistant clients.

In each one of these referral types, the MI approach can be used, along with the stages of change model. Ultimately, the MI approach allows more information to be revealed and helps with the treatment planning process.

Treatment Planning

Treatment planning is the process of outlining goals and objectives for the counseling process. This is accomplished by harnessing assessment information, making a preliminary diagnosis, and outlining a course of action for clients to address the diagnosis (Jongsma & Peterson, 1999). Clients with a co-occurring disorder of schizophrenia and alcoholism might have a treatment plan consisting of (a) abstaining from alcohol, (b) regularly using psychotropic medication for their schizophrenia, and (c) developing a social support network. Clients should be involved in the development of their treatment plan, and a copy should be provided for review throughout counseling.

Using a Therapeutic Team Approach

Schools, colleges, and community mental health counselors need to identify and create a clinical team comprising members who (a) are certified as alcohol and drug specialists, (b) can provide psychiatric consultation and ongoing care, and (c) have access to local outpatient and inpatient alcohol and drug treatment programs. Included in the team approach is collaboration with programs offering co-occurring treatment. Questions to consider in such collaborations include

1. Are there local detoxification units, and where are they located?
2. Are there contract funds for medical detoxification care, and who is the contact person?

The majority of counselors are not alcohol and drug specialists; however, they can be part of the treatment continuum. Our message here, then, is that counselors do not have to work with this population alone. Hopefully there are alcohol and drug specialists to consult with and treatment programs to refer to within the general vicinity.

Summary

This chapter described the important facilitative gatekeeper role played in responding to substance-abusing clients. The assessment process along with a mental status exam and suicide evaluation provide the reader with an idea of the information needed to proceed with a suicidal client. MI provides a strategy on how to therapeutically approach client resistance. The *DSM-IV-TR* symptoms of chemical dependency and abuse and clients with co-occurring disorders were also outlined. Finally, the impact of managed care on reimbursement, treatment planning, and access to care was discussed along with the how, where, and when of the referral process.

Exploration Questions From Chapter 4

1. How do you see yourself as a gatekeeper with respect to drug and alcohol clients?
2. What concerns do you have in working with dually diagnosed clients?
3. What steps might you take when working with a suicidal, addicted client?
4. Identify three referral sources for adolescent and adult addiction treatment in your area.
5. Describe how you would obtain information for the intake assessment while developing a counseling relationship? How might you use MI approaches?
6. How could resistance be a multicultural issue?
7. How might you use MI to address multicultural issues?

Suggested Activities

1. With a partner, role-play with a client who is dually diagnosed and suicidal. Following the role-play, discuss thoughts, emotions, and approaches with the role-playing client.
2. Read through and become familiar with the *DSM-IV-TR* and sit in on treatment team meetings with the psychiatrist or discuss other possible diagnoses with the treatment staff.

Appendix 4.A
Sample Assessment Questions

Medical Information

Review the following and check those that are appropriate:

___Under a doctor's care in the past year
___Had a drug or medication problem
___Taken an overdose of medicine or drugs
___Taken medicine to calm nerves
___Heart problems in family
___Had periods of overactivity for more than 3 days
___Family members who have had cancer
___Drink more than 5 cups/glasses of caffeinated soda/coffee daily
___Family member(s) suffered from diabetes
___Gained or lost more than 20 pounds within past month
___Had violent outbursts of temper
___Had a head injury
___Had sexual problems, pain, or lack of feeling
___Been sexually assaulted
___Been under abnormal stress

Check the following that apply:

___High blood pressure	___Stomach disorders
___Heart disease	___Frequent diarrhea
___Rheumatic fever	___Excessive laxative use
___Breathing problems	___Diabetes
___Swelling of ankles	___Thyroid disturbance
___Dizzy spells	___Anemia
___Excessive sweating	___Slow healing when cut
___Nervous breakdown	___Abnormal bleeding
___Nervous attacks	___Liver disease
___Epileptic seizures	___Infectious hepatitis
___Blackouts/fainting	___Allergies
___Memory loss	___Childhood diseases
___Difficulty concentrating	___Birth defects
___Sleeping problems	___Arthritis
___Eye problems	___Severe disability
___Migraines/severe headaches	___Muscle stiffness
___Menopause	___Dry mouth or lips
___Miscarriages	___Frequent colds
___Pregnancy within past year	___Coughing up blood
___Menstrual problems	___Nagging cough
___Kidney and bladder problems	___Herpes or other sexually transmitted diseases (STDs)

Withdrawal History

Tremors	___No	___Current	___History of
Blackouts	___No	___Current	___History of
Seizures	___No	___Current	___History of
Delirium tremens	___No	___Current	___History of
Hallucinations	___No	___Current	___History of
Depression	___No	___Current	___History of
Anxiety or panic	___No	___Current	___History of
Heart palpitations	___No	___Current	___History of
Rapid heart beat	___No	___Current	___History of
Muscle cramps	___No	___Current	___History of
Agitation	___No	___Current	___History of
Insomnia	___No	___Current	___History of
Vomiting	___No	___Current	___History of
Headaches	___No	___Current	___History of
Dehydration	___No	___Current	___History of
Muscle twitches	___No	___Current	___History of

Symptoms

___Chemical taken in larger amounts/more than intended
___Attempts to control chemical use
___Time spent obtaining/taking/recovering from effects of chemical
___Frequent intoxication or withdrawal from chemical
___Social/occupational/recreational interests given up due to use
___Continued use despite negative consequences
___Substance taken in order to avoid withdrawal

List any specific illness for which you are now being treated.

List any illness for which you were treated within the past year.

List any prescription or nonprescription medications you have taken within the past year.

List any drug allergies or medications that cause you side effects.

List any medications you have taken that did not help.

List any psychiatric hospitalizations (hospital/name/date/reason for admission).

List any outpatient counseling you have had.

Current physician.

Overall assessment of personal health: ___excellent ___good ___fair ___poor

Psychosocial Diagnostic Questions

Describe why you are seeking help at this particular time.

Who referred you and for what reasons?

Check all those that apply:

___Panic feelings	___Trouble making decisions	___Suicidal thoughts
___Trouble concentrating	___Feeling inferior	___Difficulty sleeping

___Lonely/depressed   ___Nightmares   ___Tired
___Problems relaxing   ___Memory problems   ___Fainting spells
___History of seizures   ___Shy with others   ___Seeing white flashes
___Hear buzzing in ear   ___Paranoid   ___Moody

Past or current legal history: Include any prior arrests both as a juvenile and an adult.

Are you currently being supervised by a probation officer?

Describe your driving history: drunk driving tickets, how many, current status of license?

Substance History

Chemical

Alcohol	____age of first use	____/____frequency/amount (past)	____last use
		____/____frequency/amount (current)	
Amphetamine	____age of first use	____/____frequency/amount (past)	____last use
		____/____frequency/amount (current)	
Cannabis	____age of first use	____/____frequency/amount (past)	____last use
		____/____frequency/amount (current)	
Cocaine	____age of first use	____/____frequency/amount (past)	____last use
		____/____frequency/amount (current)	
Sedatives	____age of first use	____/____frequency/amount (past)	____last use
		____/____frequency/amount (current)	
Hallucinogens	____age of first use	____/____frequency/amount (past)	____last use
		____/____frequency/amount (current)	
Inhalants	____age of first use	____/____frequency/amount (past)	____last use
		____/____frequency/amount (current)	
Opioids	____age of first use	____/____frequency/amount (past)	____last use
		____/____frequency/amount (current)	

What is your drug of preference?

Do you drink or use drugs with others or alone?

Has any person with whom you have a close relationship ever told you that you drink or use drugs too much? If yes, please state the name and the relationship to that person.

Would you consider yourself a social user, problem user, or addict/alcoholic?

If you feel your chemical use is a problem, at what age did you feel it became problematic?

Relapse History

a. *12-step support group involvement*   ___yes   ___no
   Established a home group   ___yes   ___no
   Obtained a sponsor   ___yes   ___no
   Meetings per week   ___
   Actively worked steps   ___yes   ___no
b. *Previous treatment programs*   ___yes   ___no
   Abstinence following treatment (length)   ___
   Family involvement   ___yes   ___no
   Length of stay in facility/outpatient   ____
c. *Previous relapses*
   How many and when   ____   ____
   Detoxifications   ____   ____

Suicide/Homicide/Self-Mutilation

Have you ever harmed yourself or thought about harming yourself?

Are you currently thinking of suicide or have plans to do so?

Regarding past suicidal thoughts or plans, what was occurring at the time?

Were you intoxicated at the time of attempt?

Any history of self-mutilation?

Do you have thoughts of harming or killing another individual? Have you thought of this before? Please describe.

Mental Status

a. Appearance and behavior
b. Speech
c. Thought content
d. Delusions
e. Hallucinations
f. Mood
g. Affect
h. Orientation
i. Recent and remote memory
j. Judgment
k. Insight into problem

Developmental Chemical Evaluation

Early childhood
What kind of an individual was your father? mother?

Did you know both of them or were you raised by grandparents/relatives or in a foster home?

What kind of relationship did your parents have?

How was your relationship with either parent?

Do you have any brothers or sisters?

Provide three words that would describe you as a child.

What was your earliest recollection as a child?

Chemical use in childhood
Did either parent use alcohol or drugs?

If so, how did their use impact your childhood?

High school
Did you attend high school?

Describe two memorable experiences in high school that impacts your life today.

What kind of support network did/do you have?

Chemical use in high school
Did/do you use chemicals in high school?

How has it impacted your life?

Military

What significant experiences occurred during this stage in your life?

Did you serve in a combat area?

Have you had difficulties since that time?

What were/are the positive and negative aspects about this time in your life?

Chemical use in the military

How much did you drink or use?

How often, what kind, and how did you use?

What are/were the benefits of your use?

Any problems related to your use?

Family relationships

List your intimate love relationship(s), length of relationship, and reasons why ended.

Did/does your chemical use impact these relationships and, if so, in what way?

Is there any family history of addiction or mental illness? If so, who and what diagnosis?

Social

List and describe all of your friends, how long you have known them, and if any have ended because of your chemical use.

Continuum of Nonuse to Addiction:
A Biopsychosocial Understanding

In this chapter the etiology of addiction from a biopsychosocial framework is examined while applying a continuum model ranging from nonuse to addiction. Incorporating a biopsychosocial understanding includes the holistic conceptualization of the interplay among genetic, cultural, social, and spiritual components. Research suggests that addiction is a multifaceted issue with no singular solution but rather has multiple causes. Understanding and working with the etiology of addiction is complicated and at times controversial. With this understood, we describe and outline the continuum of nonuse to addiction along with strategies for prevention and intervention at various points along the continuum. Case vignettes at the end of this chapter guide students in the process of conceptualizing and applying therapeutic processes with clients.

We have two major themes encased within this chapter: causality and the continuum of use. Our primary purpose lies within our belief that these constructs inform one another to such a high degree that compartmentalizing them into separate chapters might miss the mark into helping counselors recognize the significant overlap. For example, your understanding of the nature of the cause of abuse or addiction *will* significantly impact your approach to caring for the client. And because, as we discuss later in this chapter, individuals respond in different ways to ingested substances, your recognition of the needs of the client in each stage along the continuum will be substantially affected by your personal theory of the development and maintenance of the problem.

Biopsychosocial Framework

The biopsychosocial framework combines biological aspects of addiction with psychological precepts. These constructs are further merged with the social/cultural/environmental background of the individual to better describe a multiclustered etiology. This perspective considers the genetic predisposition on the development of addiction along with the social/cultural and psychological risk factors that have been documented in longitudinal studies. We address the medical model and explanation of the disease concept, ideas on the psychology of addiction, the moral model or temperance movement, as well as cultural and ecological considerations. In addition, the spiritual underpinnings of addiction are introduced as an etiological factor in the development of alcohol and drug addictions.

The Disease Concept

In the 1950s the World Health Organization showed support for the classification and conceptualization of alcoholism as a disease. In 1956 the American Medical Association passed a resolution declaring alcoholism a disease; this classification identified alcoholics as sick (White, 1998). The work of Marty Mann had a profound impact on attitudes toward alcoholism and the treatment of alcoholics. As a recovering alcoholic she founded the National Committee for Education on Alcoholism (NCEA) in 1944, which later became the National Council on Alcoholism. The first goal of NCEA was to frame alcoholism as a disease. The significant political, educational, and systemic work of Marty Mann laid the groundwork for this declaration to occur.

E. M. Jellinek's research (1952, 1960) framed alcoholism as a symptomatic and progressive disease. His theory argued that alcoholics present a predictable set of symptoms beginning with increasing tolerance, followed by a loss of control, leading ultimately to a premature death (if left untreated). Flawed research methods placed Jellinek's theory of progression in question. However, since that time, a rather persuasive body of literature has emerged that supports genetics or predisposed influences as potentially significant influences in the unfolding of addiction (Cloninger, Bohman, & Sigvardsson, 1981; Hiroi & Agatsuma, 2005; Schuckit, 1994).

While some researchers view addiction as being influenced primarily by the environment, other researchers support the theory that genetic predisposition, or "loading," with some individuals is so strong that from their very first drink, their drinking can be understood as alcoholic (Goodwin, 1989; Jellinek, 1960). The comparison of alcoholism to the disease of diabetes often helps clinicians and clients alike to understand the components found in a disease process. Five components can be applied to most disease processes: primary, progressive, chronic, potentially fatal, and symptomatic (Fisher & Harrison, 2005; Stolberg, 2006; White, 1998).

Primary

In the disease model, the focus of treatment is on the addiction, which is viewed as the primary or main clinical problem. For instance, a client may be referred to counseling to deal with feelings related to job loss, relationship problems, and difficulty sleeping. However, if the primary problem creating the job loss, relationship problems, and sleep difficulties is alcoholism, then alcoholism should be the main focus of treatment. If alcoholism is not addressed as a primary issue, the secondary problems or symptoms of the alcoholism will continue to intensify.

Progressive

Although Jellinek's (1952) research has been questioned regarding progression of symptoms, those who have worked with alcohol- and drug-addicted clients would concur that addiction becomes progressively worse over time as clients continue to ingest alcohol and drugs.

Chronic

Once an individual develops an addiction (becomes an addict), there is no "cure." In other words, once individuals drink alcoholically, their disease remains a chronic condition in perpetuity (Royce, 1989). This inference is also made with drug users in that once addicted to drugs, a chronic condition exists.

Potentially Fatal

Individuals addicted to drugs and alcohol who continue to consume alcohol and drugs will eventually succumb to (i.e., be overcome by) their addiction. Fatality from addiction occurs in a variety of ways and is not always identified as the primary cause of death. Death can occur through overdose, liver failure, HIV infection and subsequent AIDS-related illnesses, hepatitis, gunshot wounds, car accidents, suicide, or falling down stairs.

Symptomatic

The medical model is a physical, symptomatic disease process treated as an illness similar to patients with diabetes or heart disease. Clients addicted to drugs and alcohol present symptoms indicative of excessive, compulsive, and out-of-control use. The negative consequences that occur as a result of the addiction are considered to be symptoms by the *Diagnostic and Statistical Manual of Mental Disorders* (4th ed., text rev., *DSM-IV-TR*; American Psychiatric Association, 2000). Counselors approaching addiction from the medical model perspective observe clients as having a disease, which needs primary attention and focus in treatment. The medical model adheres to the disease concept of addiction and is the explanation most readily recognized by addiction treatment programs in the United States. In this model, addiction is understood as a chronic condition present until death. Addiction is considered to be potentially fatal if left untreated. As with any diagnosable illness, symptoms of the condition help clinicians evaluate, diagnose, and plan for appropriate treatment (American Psychiatric Association, 2000). Although the disease model originally described alcohol, the process of drug addiction is similar in that it is the primary focus.

Because the addiction process is difficult to understand, we use the following metaphor of glow sticks to help readers comprehend the physiological changes that occur in addiction. Glow sticks are chemically filled, transparent tubes used by motorists to provide illumination in the dark (during emergency situations, such as breakdowns on the side of the road at night). In their dormant state, the chemicals in the sticks are in separate compartments. However, when the sticks are broken in half, the chemicals mix, creating a powerful, chemically induced artificial light. Once a glow stick has been broken and the chemicals mix, the chemical makeup of the stick changes, never to return to its original state. As with the glow stick, the medical model suggests that once the process of a disease such as addiction is fully activated in an individual predisposed (e.g., genetically) to the disease, changes occur within the individual that can never be reversed. Once predisposed, individuals consuming alcohol and drugs who cross the line into addictive alcohol and drug use cannot return to their original state of controlled, nonconsequential drinking or drug consumption.

Genetic Components and Biological Aspects

Research over the past 20 years has provided substantial evidence that supports a strong genetic component to alcoholism. Cloninger, Sigvardsson, and Bohman (1996) found that when both biological parents were alcoholic, 33.3% of boys and 9.1% of girls adopted into nonalcoholic families were likely to become alcoholics themselves.

Cloninger et al. (1981) identified two types of alcoholics from their research: Type I and Type II alcoholics. Type I alcoholics are more likely to develop alcohol problems later on in life and are more harm-avoidance prone. Type II alcoholics, however, tend to be more violent and develop their alcoholism much earlier in life (i.e., late teens or early adulthood). This type appears to be more involved in antisocial behavior and criminal activity. Follow-up studies by Cloninger et al. (1996) confirmed their initial research in the early 1980s and supported Type I and Type II as valid classifications.

Research conducted by Blum et al. (1990) suggested that the dopamine D-2 receptor gene was significant in the predisposition of alcoholism. Although the research initially appeared to support the biochemistry predisposition to alcoholism hypothesis, subsequent research has not supported Blum's initial findings. To date, research has not conclusively detected a singular gene that predisposes an individual to addiction.

Psychological Aspects and Defense System

It is important for counselors to understand the defense systems of their clients and how such reactions impact the counseling process. What makes working with alcohol and drug issues a challenge for counselors is the presence of a burgeoning denial system. Working with the denial system of addicted persons is unlike any other clinical challenge. Cognitive distortions such as denial, rationalization, minimization, blaming, intellectualization, justification, and explaining are common in this population. The client's defensive system has been developed over time in order to protect his or her feelings related to the consequences of alcohol and drug use. An important construct here is that the development and maintenance of defenses is cyclical. The cycle begins with increasing drug and alcohol use. The more drugs and alcohol that addicted clients consume, the more they will experience negative consequences. This, in turn, leads to clients developing increasingly stronger defenses in order to protect them from the emotions related to the negative consequences of their alcohol and drug use. Essentially, defenses help addicted clients from experiencing the realness of their behaviors, which, of course, most people around them can see quite clearly (think Johari's window).

Denial

As addiction develops and subsequently unfolds, so too does an intricate system of denial. Individuals raised in addicted homes have already developed a denial system before their first use of drugs or alcohol. For example, Joey's father is an active alcoholic who drinks daily after he arrives home from work. When his father drinks, his father gets angry and threatens to hit Joey and his mother. When Joey goes to school, he hides his emotions, and when asked how things are going at home, he smiles and says "fine," when in reality he is terrified and sad. His system of repression and self-denial of feelings are the potential underpinnings of self-dishonesty and disconnection from his internal experience (Black, 1981).

It should be clearly noted that the denial system is not the same as dishonesty. Individuals in a denial process believe what they are saying is the truth. Individuals who are dishonest, however, are aware of their dishonesty, deception, and manipulation. Those in denial believe within themselves that what they are saying is the truth, which makes working with denial in the addictive process so challenging. As use increases from abusive to addictive consumption, they are not aware of the significant impact drugs and alcohol have in their lives. The more dependent individuals become on the drug, the more the defense system needs to justify, rationalize, and minimize their continued use. Below are examples of the extensive defense system created over time by addicted clients.

Rationalization

This is a defense that "rationally" describes "irrational" behavior and thinking. For example, Phil has been in counseling for 2 months because of anxiety. He describes how his most recent binge with alcohol was related to being passed over for a promotion at work. He provides the counselor (really trying to rationalize to himself) with an explanation of why he got drunk over the weekend. He believes wholeheartedly that his alcohol use was justified. However, because of his denial, he is unable to see that the reason he was passed over for the promotion at work was because of his constant tardiness resulting from hangovers.

Minimization

This is a classic defense mechanism that, in the minds of those addicted to drugs and alcohol, reduces the consequences of their use (both cognitively and emotionally). For example, Kathy is a 15-year-old student caught by her parents for smoking pot. She presents to her counselor that she "doesn't smoke that much" and what her parents caught her with was "only a joint." In reality, Kathy smokes pot daily, up to three joints, and drinks 8–10 beers on the weekends. The defense of minimization hides the frequency and the amount Kathy uses in order to present to others that her alcohol and drug use are under control and are not a problem.

Blaming

Blame is also a common defense used by addicted clients. The blame can be cast toward the systems that referred them to counseling (i.e., parental systems, school systems, or anyone involved in that person's life who intervened or caught them in the midst of being out of control). I (Ford) worked a great deal with drunk-driving clients, many of whom had accumulated up to 5–7 drunk-driving tickets. Initially clients blamed the police officers who had pulled them over (many times the same officer). Additionally, when these clients were reminded of the session fee, they would launch into a dissertation about how the system was biased and unjust and that everyone was in it for the money. What clients were unable to see at the time was how they were blaming everyone else for their alcohol-related consequences (including court costs, counseling fees, etc.).

Intellectualization

When a client asks the question "why?" a lot, you probably have someone who uses the defense of intellectualization. When addicted clients try to figure out "why" they are not able to stop using or "why did it happen to me?" or "why am I an alcoholic?" a great deal of time is spent at the cognitive level. Although researching and understanding their addiction is important, the use of intellectualization keeps clients separated from the experience of how it feels to be out of control with their use.

Clinical Example

I (Ford) had a client years ago who had obtained his third driving under the influence (DUI) penalty and had a very high blood alcohol level. He spent time in his initial session very methodically sharing with me his reasoning why his blood alcohol level (BAL) was so high. He believed it was high because the alcohol swab used to clean the spot on his arm where they took the blood sample contaminated the reading and therefore increased his BAL. In his mind, he very clearly believed his situation was due to the swab when the reality, of course, was that he had obtained a third DUI, with two other BALs higher than the current one. He also neglected to acknowledge his consumption of almost a pint of liquor and 10 beers the night of this DUI.

Justification and Explaining

Similar to the defense of blaming, addicted clients justify their behaviors. For instance, a client in counseling at the request of his wife, because of his continuous use of marijuana, explains to his counselor that his marijuana use has become an issue for his wife because she is going through a stressful situation at work. His use is really not the problem; the "real" problem is her stress level and her inability to cope with her feelings. This client is not only redirecting the attention, but he is also projecting his own feelings of being out of control onto his wife and justifying/explaining his use of marijuana.

Defenses are used unconsciously. The picture the clients are unconsciously trying to create is that their use of drugs and alcohol is not out of control, supporting their illusion of control. Clients may possess any combination of defenses to avoid experiencing the emotional pain related to their use. Behind the defenses lies a great deal of emotional pain. Emotions of terror, sadness, shame, extreme guilt, and self-loathing hide behind the exterior of the defensive walls. Paradoxically, the more addicted clients are out of control, the more intense and creative the defense system becomes, making it challenging for counselors. Because in such cases the defenses are generally quite intense and are reinforced by continuous alcohol and drug use, group therapy is the modality of choice. Under the scrutiny (and support) of other group members, the defenses can be systematically challenged, helping clients recognize ineffective defensive positioning.

When clients begin seeing themselves (and their behaviors) in the actions of others, there is a possibility for their defenses to let down. As this process unfolds, counselors will want to help clients explore their emotions as they relate to the consequences of their drug and alcohol use. This deep exploration is critical for clients to recognize that their drug and/or alcohol use is out of control and consequential.

For some helping professionals, a question emerges regarding what needs to be addressed first with addicted clients: the addiction to drugs and alcohol or the emotional pain associated with childhood conflicts that may have contributed to the client's first use of drugs and alcohol. We strongly suggest that both are important factors to work with in the recovery process. Clients need to see the reality of their use of drugs and alcohol. Clients need to explore experiences (and the associated thoughts and emotions) that influenced their first use of drugs or alcohol. Emotions left unchecked will resurface and potentially contribute to a relapse, if not addressed in counseling. Additionally, however, counselors who focus solely on childhood conflicts and parental relationships as the *cause* or *root* of the client's addiction fail to address the entire problem. Although it is important how the clients are in relationship to significant others and family, it is not the cause of their addiction. Some counselors mistakenly believe that allowing clients to talk about how angry they are at their parents or upbringing will, by itself, decrease the desire and compulsion to drink or use drugs.

There is research, however, to suggest that behavioral disorders early in life can be predictors of alcoholism in adulthood. One study found conduct-disordered behavior as a predictor of men developing alcoholism in adulthood (Robins, 1966). It is difficult, however, to predict which childhood behaviors consistently contribute to adult alcoholism. A study by Zucker and Gomberg (1986) suggested that antisocial behaviors and the lack of achievement-related activities in youth have been related to adult alcoholism. Additionally, as discussed in previous chapters, clients may suffer from depression or other concomitant psychiatric disorders.

This three-pronged description of addiction emanating from a combination of genetics, psychological composition, and social/cultural impacts helps clients as well as counselors with understanding potential origins of addiction. Because addiction to drugs and alcohol are different for each client, a holistic understanding is necessary.

Temperance Movement: A Moral Model

During the temperance (1830s) and prohibition periods (1919), the prevalent view of alcoholism was that it was sinful behavior and reflected a lack of willpower (J. Jung, 1994). The early temperance movement shifted from alcohol moderation to total abstinence, which played a significant role in the belief that total, complete abstinence was necessary for alcoholics to reform (White, 1998). The American Society for the Promotion of Temperance asserted that the main goal for those already abstinent was to continue with abstinence and suggested that for those not reformed, death would be the penalty. The plan was to prevent new alcoholics from developing and allowing those already in the throes of their alcoholism to simply die (White, 1998). Alcoholics were blamed for their condition, and little compassion was provided to those considered to be "skid row." Ironically, the moral judgment excluded the reality that many of those addicted to alcohol were employed and respected community members, thus reinforcing, even today, that the vision of an alcoholic is a person who is homeless and unemployed (White, 1998).

In 1842 Abraham Lincoln suggested, as he spoke to the Illinois Washingtonian Society, that there were physical causes of alcoholism. The Washingtonian Society emerged during the declining years of the temperance movement. The Washingtonian Society was organized and set out to recruit new members in bars and clubs. The only requirement for membership in this society was a pledge for abstinence, a precursor to the requirement in Alcoholics Anonymous (White, 1998). The Martha Washington Society was created for women in need of support for their alcoholism and for the wives and children of alcoholics.

The moral model considers addiction to be a matter of choice or free will. The model suggests that individuals who are addicted to drugs and alcohol have chosen to do so and therefore willfully get into trouble from their use. This approach to understanding addiction does not believe in a disease process, rather, it views chemical use as a moral problem or sin. This model has typically been used by religious organizations to explain or understand the addictive process. Though historically popular with the criminal justice system, a change in corrections philosophy has introduced the concept of drug courts and diversion programs to refer addicts and alcoholics to appropriate treatment. The moral model is rarely used by traditional treatment programs (Fisher & Harrison, 2005).

Cultural, Social, and Environmental Aspects

Stanton Peele (1989), a critic of the disease model of addiction, believes that culture plays a significant role in the development of addiction, citing the low rates of alcoholism in the Jewish and Chinese populations. Alan Marlatt (1996), another critic of the disease model, views addiction as a social learning process whereby individuals learn by observing others using alcohol or drugs. Social learning theory suggests that individuals learn about the expectancies of alcohol and drugs through observation (Bandura, 1969). If, for example, adolescents observe family members and peers using alcohol to reduce stress and cope with difficult feelings, social learning suggests these adolescents would expect alcohol to lower inhibitions and successfully help them to cope with stressors too. Conversely, if these same adolescents observe negative consequences from drinking, then they would probably have minimal expectations for alcohol.

Collins, Parks, and Marlatt (1985) conducted research examining consumption rates between model participants and observers. Their research determined that the more sociable the model participants were, the more the observers drank. They also found that the more unsociable the model participants were, regardless of their level of drinking, the more the observers drank. In this case, however, it was believed they drank because of the tension in the room. This supports Bandura (1977) in his belief that an individual's level of self-efficacy impacts the motivation for engaging in that behavior. This is evident in the American college environment where the media, celebrities, and social organizations (e.g., fraternities and sororities) impact client consumption.

Ecological Considerations

According to Bronfenbrenner (1988), human development is impacted by the immediate systems in which we live as well as by broader ecological forces. Counseling from this perspective broadens the focus of intervention from the individual to the concentric circles of influence around the client. Social and cultural influences are important in understanding where societal, familial, and environmental relationships have an impact (Matto, 2004). For example, a client living in a small town with minimal employment opportunities, who has a significant history of addiction in the family, and who engages with peers who use drugs and alcohol will be significantly affected by each social sphere. Each of these spheres or concentric circles is described in Bronfenbrenner's four systems, which include the microsystem, mesosystem, exosystem, and macrosystem.

- *Microsystem.* This system significantly impacts clients (home) and determines how they interpersonally relate with one another. Counselors need to consider the impact this system has on clients and their emotional well-being and contribution to alcohol and drug use. Family systems with active alcohol and drug addiction have significant influence on the behaviors and choices of children who are raised in such an environment.

- *Mesosystem.* This system looks at the link between two or more settings where clients live and interact. For example, consider an individual who is involved in collegiate athletics where alcohol use is encouraged and is from a family environment where alcohol use was permitted. Both have an impact on this student's decision to use alcohol.
- *Exosystem.* This system impacts clients through formal and informal structures ultimately impacting the microsystem. An example of this is the workplace, a social club, or network such as a community club or sorority/fraternity and how these structures impact the microsystem of the individual. The impact is through peer pressure and the individual's need to be accepted and liked by peers, ultimately fearing rejection. Therefore, the need to be accepted by peers overrides the decision to not drink alcohol or use drugs.
- *Macrosystem.* These are multiple systems impacting directly and indirectly the development of individuals. Legal or political systems have direct impact on individuals and their abililty to grow as human beings.

Spiritual Aspects

The spiritual approach to understanding addiction sprang from the fellowship of Alcoholics Anonymous in 1935, by cofounders Bill Wilson and Dr. Bob Smith. In addition, support for their approach originated from Dr. Carl Jung, who suggested treating alcoholism with spirit in a letter to Bill Wilson by quoting the Latin phrase *spiritus contra spiritum,* which means "treating the spirit with spirits." He believed addiction was a spiritual condition needing spiritual "cures." In order for alcoholics to truly transform their lives they needed to be in a spiritual or religious atmosphere (Jung, 1974). Alcoholics Anonymous (2005) presents addiction as a spiritual disease, or "soul sickness," that emanates from an existential emptiness and disconnection. Additionally, Alcoholics Anonymous suggests that alcoholism is a physical illness and supports the medical model of alcoholism.

In summary, the biopsychosocial and spiritual understanding takes into consideration that addiction is multifaceted. A client may have abused drugs and alcohol for many years, only to cross the line into addiction around the age of 35, whereas another client who started drinking at the age of 16 drank alcoholically from the very first drink. We can hypothesize that the first client may have had less of a genetic influence, whereas the second client may have had a strong genetic predisposition. The next segment of this chapter helps counselors understand the continuum of nonuse to addiction and how this process unfolds.

A Description of the Continuum of Nonuse to Addiction

Here we shift from theorized epistemologies regarding the root causes of abuse or addiction to the pragmatic steps along the path of nonuse to addiction. Though each individual has unique reasons for using drugs and/or alcohol, there is a consistent set of general factors that we have recognized in our work with clients.

The process of how one becomes addicted to alcohol and drugs is multifaceted. Because the process involves multiple influences, counselors need to understand the continuum by which a percentage of individuals will move from nonuse of alcohol and drugs to addiction. While the minority of adolescents and young adults do not ever use alcohol or drugs of any kind, the majority do. The reasons why individuals begin drinking or using drugs depends on a variety of factors, which include curiosity, peer acceptance, spiritual emptiness, and coping with emotional pain, to name a few.

Curiosity

Remember when your parents said to you as a child, "Don't touch that!" or "Stay out of the sun," and you didn't listen? In fact, many of you reading this book did the exact opposite—either out of curiosity or defiance. Add to this a parent who does not heed his or her own direction and only reinforces that which he/she is saying not to do. Drug and alcohol use in many ways is similar, where the curiosity to smoke a cigarette is only enhanced by parents who smoke and say not to do what they do, thus piquing the curiosity, which is reinforced. The response is, "Well, if they are doing drugs, it must be okay." Not only is there modeled acceptance but there is also curiosity of what it might feel like to smoke a cigarette or a joint of marijuana.

Peer Acceptance

Acceptance from peers in adolescence is of primary importance. Many adolescents find athletics, academics, and other extracurricular activities places for peer development and acceptance. Students who already feel alone, disconnected, and outside of the social circle may begin to feel accepted and connected to a culture involving drug and alcohol use. In this sense, the drug- and alcohol-using culture provides acceptance and understanding, establishing a powerful connection between drug and alcohol use and peer relationships (Fowler et al., 2007).

Spiritual Emptiness

A third idea posited by some practitioners in the addiction field relates the use of drugs to an unconscious movement toward the spiritual. Stanislav Grof (1987b), whose initial research was with hallucinogens in the 1960s, believed that much of the attraction to drugs and alcohol initially is a thirst to fill a spiritual emptiness. He contended that loneliness and desperation (which may be symptomatic of this spiritual emptiness) engender a desire to connect to a greater process. The existential emptiness and search for meaning, connection, and self-definition is temporarily assuaged with chemical euphoria. While the drugs are medicating the pained soul, however, they interfere with and substantially affect the natural process of growth.

Emotional Pain

A fourth reason an individual may begin using drugs or alcohol is to reduce or eliminate emotional pain. Those who begin using drugs and alcohol at an early age tend to have active addiction in their immediate families. A 12-year-old who has witnessed her father high every night for the past 5 years learns quickly how drugs are used to medicate. Her self-esteem at some level is impacted by his unavailability, creating emotional pain. If or when she begins drinking or using drugs, she will more than likely feel temporary relief from the emotional pain, a relief that not only registers in the brain but also reinforces using as a coping mechanism.

Many of the clients with whom we've worked described their first drug and alcohol experiences as moments when they felt connected with others. These momentary connections diffused feeling ostracized or different. The use of drugs and alcohol seemingly opened doors to popularity, connection, and chemically induced self-esteem. In addition, chemicals provided a mood-altering experience unlike any natural feeling they had ever experienced. The combination of the altered state along with peer connections after years of isolation (for some), created a powerful salve to emotional pain. This physiological experience, coupled with the observation of active addiction in their homes, contributed to the development of an addictive process.

The description above is a common experience for many budding addicts or alcoholics. The initial use is so significant that they continue using drugs or drinking alcohol in order to recapture that initial experience. Very early on in the addicts' using or drinking career, a number of significant lessons are learned. The first lesson is that the ingested drugs or alcohol create euphoric feelings each time they are used. The second lesson reinforces that the more they drink alcohol and use drugs, the better they feel, resulting in the creation of a repetitive learning cycle (Johnson, 1980). The intention for those using drugs and alcohol, however, is not to become addicted to the chemicals; on the contrary, the intention is to be in control of their use and at the same time be able to enjoy the effects of the drugs without consequence.

Interestingly, the addictive cycle does not occur with all individuals who start drinking or using drugs. Some individuals may experiment with or try various drugs or alcohol without developing the strong and significant connection that those who become addicted experience. Individuals experimenting with drugs or alcohol may find they abuse them, yet do not build any significant tolerance. Further, some may find that even though they abuse drugs or alcohol, they have no compulsivity to use drugs or alcohol.

It is important for counselors to assess where clients may fall in relation to the continuum of nonuse to addiction. The *DSM-IV-TR* (American Psychiatric Association, 2000) delineates abusive drinking and drugging from dependent or alcoholic drinking or drugging on the basis of three significant criteria: tolerance (increasing or decreasing), withdrawal, and compulsive use despite negative consequences. Additionally, clients may exhibit signs of withdrawal. There are those, however, who may use and abuse chemicals, yet never develop increased tolerance or cross the line into addiction.

For instance, clients with a predisposition to alcoholism may fall into the category of Type II alcoholics, where their tolerance tends to build very quickly. As their tolerance increases, so does the amount of the drugs or alcohol they ingest. The more chemicals used by clients, the greater the possibility for negative consequences. As a result, the negative consequences are used as symptoms of social, occupational, and emotional impairment as found in the *DSM-IV-TR*. A baseline consistency for alcohol and drug addictions is excessive use.

For those who begin to experience negative consequences as a result of use many times question why they started using drugs or drinking alcohol in the first place. With respect to understanding the beginning phases of the continuum, it is helpful to know from clients what their initial reasons were for usage that took them out of the nonuse category.

Clinical Example

I (Ford) remember a client who stopped using marijuana and cocaine ask this very question only to relapse later for the same initial reasons. He said he started using drugs at age 10 because he was angry and hurt from the violence he witnessed in his home. He became afraid and used drugs to feel normal and safe, only to resume drug use in adulthood to counter the anger, hurt, and fear. The responses to these questions give clinicians and clients a better understanding of areas in their lives that would be high risk for using drugs again.

When clients are identified as having potential or current problems with alcohol or drugs, counselors should examine where on the continuum of nonuse to addiction that clients might be, based on the presentation of their information and referring data. Possible questions posed by counselors include,

- Are the clients using alcohol and experimenting with drugs?
- Are they abusing alcohol and becoming intoxicated every couple of months?
- Are the clients hiding their drug use?
- Are they blacking out each time they drink?
- Are personality changes occurring with your clients when using?

The responses to these questions help counselors identify *where* the person may be on the continuum, which ultimately helps in prevention strategies and treatment matching. For example, placing clients who are already on the dependency side of the continuum in an education group with first-time offenders would not be an appropriate referral. Rather, these clients would be better served if they were referred to a structured alcohol and drug program. Likewise, clients who briefly have used alcohol would not be appropriate for an outpatient alcohol and drug treatment program. Matching prevention and treatment recommendations with client placement on the continuum also takes into consideration the client's stage of change. In some cases, clients may either not be ready to change or are not interested in abstinence. It becomes quite challenging for counselors when these factors are added to by the client wanting something to change or the client being addicted with no awareness of the problem.

Given these client possibilities regarding change, the following discussion examines how the stages of change are applied in this continuum.

Stages of Change: A Transtheoretical Model of Understanding

Having now recognized the possible causes of abuse or addiction, it is important to underscore the general categories and stages of change. Along each stage of the following model, the counselor's perspective on the root causes of the problem will also help to understand the needs of the client. Although we will provide a richer description of each stage in following chapters, we believe counselors must attend to their personal theories of change (anchored in what caused the problem) as they consider treatment steps and options for clients.

Prochaska, DiClemente, and Norcross (1992) examined two primary constructs: how people changed and the application to addictive behaviors. Prior work by Prochaska and DiClemente (1982, 1984, 1986) resulted in a stages-of-change model that was developed after reviewing addiction literature and conducting research. For alcohol- and drug-addicted clients, these stages are useful in determining motivation and treatment preparation. These stages inform counselors working with ambivalent clients who abuse drugs and alcohol and who have been referred to counseling by a third party (e.g., principal, judge, or parent). The stages of change are precontemplation, contemplation, preparation, action, and maintenance (Prochaska et al., 1992).

- *Precontemplation.* In this stage, individuals are not considering changing their behavior. For example, a client in this stage might say, "I know I received a DUI, but I was caught for speeding. I wasn't drunk and I don't have a problem." This client does not connect the consequence with drinking and instead blames it on speeding. The client is not at a point of understanding a need to take action concerning alcohol use.
- *Contemplation.* According to Prochaska and DiClemente (1986), this stage includes increased awareness with a developed motivation and willingness to change. Returning to the example above, the same individual obtains a second DUI 2 years after the first one. At this point the individual recognizes, "Wow, my drinking is really getting me into trouble. I may lose my license and my job because of this DUI. I think I might have a problem with it. I'm not an alcoholic though, alcoholics drink everyday." This person is beginning to understand drinking as problematic and is aware of the consequences (i.e., second DUI).
- *Preparation.* As a result of this second DUI, he is referred for an assessment, which recommends him to outpatient treatment requiring abstinence. At this point the client is ready to stop drinking and prepares himself mentally by visualizing what will need to occur for him not to drink and how, importantly, his life will change.
- *Action.* This aspect of change indicates behavioral action taken. Upon entering the outpatient program, he discontinues drinking and attends support meetings. He stops going to bars and removes all of the alcohol from his house. He has moved from "I don't think I have a problem (precontemplation)" to "I have a problem (contemplation) and I am doing something about it" (preparation and action). Clients are idiosyncratic in what motivates them to initiate action. It could be a third DUI, a suspension from school, or a lost relationship that is the impetus for the internal motivation culminating in subsequent change.

- *Maintenance.* Once clients take action, it is important for new behaviors to continue and be "maintained." This client, when discharged successfully from treatment, has the arduous task of maintaining abstinence, attending support meetings, and living life without the use of alcohol or drugs. The goal is for the action to be rigorously maintained.

Counselors play a significant role in transiting clients from one stage to another. Although Prochaska and DiClemente (1986) questioned the specific reasons people change, they argued that helping professionals can be a significant and important part of the change process. They also believe that this process is cyclical. Clients can begin at any stage and move both forward and backward in the process. Should individuals relapse, they may return to contemplation and continue drinking, move immediately into action and discontinue drinking, or move back to precontemplation and be reinforced by the denial system.

The stages of change can also be applied to younger clients referred for behavioral problems where alcohol or drugs may be a part of the referral. Clients referred may not exhibit signs of addiction, however, they may meet criteria for abuse. After meeting with clients who use or abuse alcohol or drugs, instead of referring them to outpatient treatment they could benefit from a number of options in a comprehensive prevention program.

A Comprehensive Prevention Program

A comprehensive, six-pronged program developed by the Center for Substance Abuse and Prevention outlines specific ways to help prevent and intervene in clients' chemical use (Hogan, Gabrielsen, Luna, & Grothaus, 2003). The program's design addresses core areas in which clients may need information, activities, or referrals. The six components of the program are information dissemination, prevention education, alternative activities, community-based processes, environmental approaches, and problem identification and referral. In conjunction, a comprehensive program such as this can be used in a school system, college setting, or community setting.

- *Information dissemination.* This component of the program provides information, Web sites, and pamphlets and acts as a clearinghouse. Information is disseminated through the media (e.g., radio, television, Internet, mailings, and newspapers) and provides a speakers' bureau for community and regional discussions. Information provided to parents or guardians highlights actions they can take if they suspect chemical use with their child or signs of chemical use. Additionally, the various forms and types of drugs could be presented at community forums and reinforced by scriptograph pamphlets.
- *Prevention education.* Research supports early, proactive prevention efforts targeting schools and before the actual drug or alcohol use starts. Programs within the schools focus on identifying and coping with feelings, talking about feelings to others, exploring activities, or learning about self-esteem through games. This type of program does not focus specifically on drug and alcohol information, but rather on the well-being of children and alternative activities to build and create self-esteem.
- *Alternative activities.* Many college campuses use this strategy of funding weekend programming and generating multiple activities to offer an alternative to social activities that include or are based on using alcohol or drugs. Activities may include bingo, coffee house singing, poetry readings, karaoke nights, movies, live bands or DJs, comedians, or rock climbing walls. The concept is for college students to be provided with activities from which to choose.
- *Community-based processes.* This approach to prevention focuses interaction and collaboration within the community. Examples of community planning members in-

clude local school district representatives, beer distributors, community bar owners, law enforcement personnel, and chamber of commerce representatives. This method of community approach addresses concerns while coordinating efforts to create specific community strategies that address alcohol or drug use among the youth in the area. Outcome data have demonstrated the potential effectiveness within university and college communities (Hingson, Heeren, Zakocs, Kopstein, & Wechsler, 2002).

- *Environmental approaches to prevention.* This aspect of prevention challenges the norms of the community. For instance, many colleges and universities distribute an assessment instrument called the CORE survey (Presley, Meilman, & Lyeria, 1994). This instrument assesses the drug and alcohol use behaviors of the university/college community and compares these data with other similar institutions around the country. Statistics from this survey are used to dispel myths and encourage the creation of healthier norms. An example of this is the belief by students that "everybody gets drunk on the weekends." Statistics from the CORE survey may suggest that only 20% of the students on campus drink five or more drinks a week, thereby challenging the cultural beliefs surrounding alcohol use. The statistical information is also used on campus in social marketing strategies through advertisements and eye-catching posters. Posters along with sponsored parties by university clubs can support a sober lifestyle and alternative activities (Hogan et al., 2003). Counselors need to examine clients from a community counseling and multicultural perspective. Bensley and Wu (1991) found that after a confrontational message from a counselor advocating for abstinence, students responded by actually drinking more alcohol. This suggests that establishing a helping alliance versus an adversarial stance yields a more favorable outcome (Parks, 2002).

- *Problem identification and referral.* As communities increase awareness through prevention programming, the number of referrals for assessment simultaneously increases. With increased referrals comes the need for a central referral location to provide an organized approach to referring clients for treatment, education, and/or counseling. The following is a model of prevention that focuses primarily on education and referral.

A Model of Prevention, Education, and Referral: Application in the Continuum

Taking into consideration the stages of change model and components of a comprehensive prevention program, the following example demonstrates how they are applied in the continuum of nonuse to addiction in a university drug and alcohol program.

The example used here is a program at the university where we teach and has been in existence for the past 10 years. Students who violate the alcohol and drug policy on campus are referred to the program by the judicial system. Students who violate off-campus laws are referred by the district justice. Following the referral, students are preassessed by graduate student volunteers who were previously trained in assessment and psychoeducational group skill facilitation. The volunteers meet individually with students for an hour during which they are administered the Substance Abuse Subtle Screening Inventory (SASSI; G. A. Miller, 1983) and E-Chug (an online program that creates a client profile regarding drinking behaviors; Walters, Vader, & Harris, 2007). Also during this meeting, the clients are asked questions regarding their alcohol and drug use.

Following preassessments, recommendations are made to the client depending on the severity of his or her drug or alcohol use, family history, SASSI, and E-Chug results (computerized assessment tool). The possible options for referral are CD-ROM, education groups, early intervention groups, and a professional assessment for treatment. Occasionally there is no formal referral for any services. The volunteer then meets with the same student for a second appointment and presents the results and recommendations.

- *CD-ROM.* This is an interactive program students complete online. This option is used with those who have been found in the presence of alcohol but were not consuming alcohol at the time of the citation. Typically there is minimal drinking or drug history or evidence of family addiction problems for those referred to the CD-ROM program.
- *Education groups.* These groups meet for 3 consecutive weeks, 2–3 hours each session, during which students are provided basic information on drugs and alcohol, how the violations impact their potential careers, and healthy choices. This education group is for students who were drinking or intoxicated at the time of the citation. These students may be abusing alcohol but are not presenting data warranting them a referral for treatment or the early intervention group.
- *Early intervention group (EIG).* This group meets for three sessions. For clients who are in need of a strategy beyond an education group and not yet ready for a treatment group, an EIG can address their needs. The goal of the EIG is to provide a group experience for at-risk clients to evaluate, discuss, and express their life choices and to learn about the stages of change and the choices they make regarding alcohol and drugs. The group is not a treatment group, nor is it an abstinence-based group. Although members are encouraged to contract with the group to reduce alcohol and drug use, it is not required. This group also prepares some students for treatment services in outpatient or inpatient treatment. The group consists of 10–12 members deemed at-risk for developing dependency on drugs or alcohol. The early intervention groups are psychoeducational in nature, thus helping clients obtain information, communicate, and share feelings. Students referred to this group have had multiple drug or alcohol offenses, have a family history of alcohol or drug abuse, and are presenting minimal symptoms of dependency. However, these students do not meet the criteria to enter a structured outpatient treatment group. A significant difference with this group as opposed to a treatment group is the issue of abstinence. Clients in alcohol and drug treatment meet the criteria for alcohol or drug addiction, whereas individuals in the EIG may not. Those in EIG explore at-risk behaviors with drugs and alcohol and are encouraged to evaluate their usage each week, particularly the weekends. Discussions focus on control, what they experience positively as well as negatively when it comes to alcohol and drug use, and if they are able to reduce the amounts they are using. Treatment groups, on the other hand, focus primarily on making choices and changes to foster and support the goal of abstinence.

  On occasion, clients get into trouble with chemicals while participating in the EIG. Students are then assessed to determine whether a professional evaluation is warranted. Some clients attend both the education and the EIG in order to have the basic drug and alcohol information as well as the experience of the psycho-educational group.

  Early intervention groups can be developed and used in college, high school, and community settings. Preliminary assessment, group participation, and screening are necessary components of this process. Groups are closed (once the group starts, no one will be added until the completion of the group cycle). The groups are cofacilitated by counseling students with experience in alcohol and drug abuse and addiction and who have been trained as group facilitators. Following closure from these groups, some participants are referred for individual counseling or professional assessment for treatment.
- *Professional assessment.* Students who are referred for professional assessment are presenting numerous symptoms of dependency and have significant life-threatening consequences related to their use. These students typically attend a treatment group provided by a local outpatient treatment program or enter an inpatient unit if criteria are met. Multiple referrals are also made to the university's counseling center or aftercare meetings on campus to reintegrate students into college/university life.

Case Application: Using the Continuum Model

So far we have examined the continuum of nonuse, abuse, and addiction along with a model of prevention. The next step is to consider how to integrate the continuum in helping clients. The following cases are presented and emphasize each client's placement on the continuum, the impact of Bronfenbrenner's ecological systems, and the stage of change each client presents.

Case of Sandy

Sandy is an 8-year-old White female in elementary school who is having difficulty with concentration in class. Her graded work has resulted in increasingly poorer scores. Sandy, who is usually very social with her peers, seems sad and withdrawn. When teachers have asked if she was okay, she tended to respond with, "I'm doing fine. I'm just a little tired, that's all."

Out of her teacher's concern for the drop in grades and sad affect, Sandy was referred to the school counselor. The school counselor met with Sandy five times and asked for permission to contact her parents and invite them for a session. Sandy agreed, and the counselor made a phone call and spoke briefly to the mother. The conversation began with the mother sounding rushed and then indicated to the counselor how she would not be able to come in because of her work. The conversation ended with no appointment being made and the counselor feeling as though the mother was avoiding something at home.

At that point the counselor had no reason to believe alcohol or drugs would be involved; however, it was important for the counselor to keep it in mind as a possible issue at home. Although Sandy may not be drinking or using drugs, there is a strong possibility that one of the parents may drink too much or use other chemicals.

Let's look at how this could work with the continuum, the ecological approach, the possible prevention or intervention strategies, and the stage of change Sandy and her parents may be in at this point.

Continuum

After having met with Sandy each week for a month, the counselor determines that Sandy is not an alcohol or drug user; however, Sandy does reveal to the counselor that her father "drinks every night and then gets loud and then falls asleep." In sessions, Sandy says her father is probably an alcoholic and that he doesn't remember what he says or does each night when they are all sitting at the kitchen table. The counselor speculates, on the basis of Sandy's report, that the father's drinking is on the dependency side of the continuum. Understanding this will help the counselor determine how the drinking is significantly impacting Sandy in her schoolwork and her ability to sleep at night.

Ecological Approach

The counselor begins to examine the systems that are significantly impacting Sandy, which is primarily her family. Second to this is school, and third is her involvement in young Christian life. The counselor could help Sandy explore the systems and how each one could provide comfort and support. The *microsystem* is her family, the *mesosystems* are the family and school, the *exosystem* is her church, and the *macrosystem* is the economic area in which she lives, which is very poor. The area provides little in the way of resources for treatment of addiction counseling for families. Having evaluated the four systems, the counselor again tries to engage the parents in counseling with their daughter, which this time is successful. However, only the mother appears for the session. Immediately the counselor notices Sandy's increase in energy and improvement in grades.

Stage of Change

Sandy's stage of change moves from contemplation to action because of her mother's support as well as the school counselor's encouragement. The school counselor, who realized after talking with the mother that the husband's drinking was indeed alcoholic, suggested to the mother to consider attending Al-Anon and Al-a-Tot for Sandy. The mother was provided information on alcoholism and referred to an outpatient counselor in a neighboring county for support and counseling.

From this scenario, the school counselor provided direct services to the student, and as a result, started a self-esteem group for the elementary school. The school counselor also engaged the mother in the process and helped her obtain support, information, and therapy, which ultimately helped Sandy. The identification of the husband's drinking in the dependency end of the continuum helped the counselor realize the trouble at home and how that system was significantly impacting Sandy's attention and grades in school. The counselor also realized the importance of community influence and support, and therefore involved support systems such as the church, Al-Anon, and community counseling. Finally, as a result of this multifaceted approach to Sandy's presenting issue, was the development of support directly in the school with the counselor. Ultimately this systemic approach and model identification helped Sandy refocus, gain support from school, her mother, Al-a-Tot, church, and to reengage with her peers. This resulted in better focus and increased grades the next term in school. In turn, the support for the family and change in behavior with the mother and the daughter could paradoxically intervene on the husband's/father's drinking.

Case of Mike

In this scenario, a 19-year-old African American college student has been caught by the university police urinating in public after consuming large amounts of alcohol at a fraternity party. The student, upon arrest, became belligerent and physical with the apprehending officers. He spent the evening in jail and was released the next morning. He seemed embarrassed the following morning and did not recall the previous evening's events. At that point he recognized how he had blacked out because of his use of alcohol. Mike was referred to the judicial committee the following week; he also met with the local district justice for the violation. In this case, he was dually referred for the alcohol and drug assessment.

Mike met for a preassessment with the alcohol and drug staff member to determine his involvement in the campus program. During their preliminary session, Mike disclosed that his first use of alcohol began at age 16 and his current pattern is to drink only on the weekends, from 8 to 10 beers at a time. He reported that in high school, he drank minimally and experimented some with marijuana. Mike is a 2nd-year student who has a grade point average of 2.85, which has dropped in the past semester. He reported to the evaluator that his last use of marijuana was minimal, "Maybe a few joints every two or three times a month." He denied any other chemical use. He did share that he drank minimally in high school because of his father's alcoholism and his uncle's death from a heroin overdose.

As presented, Mike reported only one other alcohol violation in high school when he was stopped for possession of alcohol and was, therefore, not able to obtain his driver's license until age 18. He presented to the evaluator the following data, which will be important for an appropriate referral. Mike appears to have a pattern of drinking, which has increased, and has a developing tolerance to alcohol. He has presented at least two blackout periods during his drinking. In addition he reported a second alcohol consequence and a significant history of alcoholism and drug addiction within the family regarding his father and uncle.

Continuum
The client appears to be in the area of abusing alcohol with concerns for future progression into dependency.

Ecological Approach
In this case the client is most significantly influenced by his peer group and secondarily by his family. His *microsystem* has switched from his family to his university setting, where

most of his peers drink and use drugs. His family and fraternity brothers have become his *mesoystem*. The *exosystem* includes the university and the surrounding community, which is primarily White and is in a rural setting. Mike reports that he grew up in the city and feels uncomfortable being the minority fraternity brother in a predominantly White town. His feelings of fear and discomfort are eased when he drinks alcohol and smokes pot. The *macrosystem* impacting his life is the minimal money his family has because of his father's alcoholism. The client reports to working a part-time job in addition to his full compliment of undergraduate courses. Racism is also an aspect of the *macrosystem*, which impacts Mike both at school and at home.

Stage of Change

Mike appears to be between precontemplation and contemplation. During the assessment he realized how an incident had happened again, and it seemed to scare him about his inability to recall the previous evening because of the blackout.

Mike states that he has had no prior drug or alcohol education or treatment for his alcohol use. On the basis of the presenting data, the following recommendations could be suggested. Mike could attend an education group, which presents basic information about healthy choices and alcohol and drug use. Mike could also attend the EIG because of the addiction in his family, two blackouts, and a previous alcohol violation. Additionally, Mike would be referred to financial aid to discuss financial support for college and encouraged to speak with his advisor about grades.

Case of Bree

In this case, the client is a 42-year-old White woman referred by her primary physician for counseling. The physician is concerned for Bree's condition, her inability to sleep, and her use of alcohol and prescription medication to manage stress. The physician has taken Bree off of the drug Xanax and has started her on Zoloft for what he has diagnosed as depression. It is not clear in the first session the extent of the stress in her life. She is referred for counseling in order to examine her coping strategies and stress levels.

Bree arrives and presents the problem as her marriage and her husband's lack of affection toward her. Bree reports over the past 3 years her husband has been increasingly distant, angry, and concerned about her drinking. She reports her drinking is in response to his distancing and started using Xanax PRN (as needed) 1 year ago at the urging of a friend who also takes it for stress. Bree describes her pattern of alcohol use as minimal, "Maybe a couple of glasses of wine once or twice a week." Her physician is concerned about her elevated liver enzyme test, which indicates heavier drinking. Her physician is also concerned that she may be obtaining a prescription for Xanax from another physician.

Bree shares with the counselor that she was stopped for speeding and then was arrested for drunk driving. She had a blood alcohol content of .17, which she later said was dropped because the officer did not appear in court. During the interview she appears disheveled and distracted at times, changing her story. When the suggestion of future couples therapy is discussed, Bree becomes very defensive.

The counselor finds gaps in Bree's history along with minimization. Although Bree does not see her use as problematic, clues to her developing problem are presented by the referring physician, and a self-admitted drunk-driving incident (in her mind it didn't happen since she wasn't convicted). She does not see how the problem of her husband's distancing from her could be because of her alcohol use. It seems that the client does not see her alcohol use as a problem in the way her husband does.

Continuum

As we examine this case, the husband's and physician's concern for Bree's use, her defensiveness in the session, blaming the husband for her drinking, the physician's suspicion of an additional Xanax prescription, and her inconsistent stories during the session place her behavior in the dependency side of the continuum.

Bree would need to be continually evaluated for her compulsion and continued use despite negative consequences.

Ecological Approach

The *microsystem* immediately surrounding Bree is her husband. She stays at home each day and has not worked for a number of years (by her choice). Bree discusses during the session her feelings of worthlessness and boredom at home each day. The *mesosystem* in her life is the church she belongs to and the circle of friends she is in contact with each day. Many of her friends also stay at home and share a similar boredom. She finds support from them and tries to eat lunch or initiate outings at least once a week. The town in which she lives is her *exosystem*. She was born and raised in the town and knows everyone and most of the families in town. Bree reports to subtle pressure to be the town socialite and welcome wagon to all new residents. The *macrosystem* in her life relates to the financial success of her husband. His wealth allows them to travel and associate with government and political figures in the area. Again, she reports this pressure to be the perfect wife, host, and conversationalist as contributing to her anxiety. The issue of stereotypical gender roles is an aspect counselors need to take into consideration when working with Bree.

Stage of Change

Bree appears to be in contemplation and has only taken action to seek counseling and stop drinking wine out of compliance because of the pressure from her doctor and husband.

At this point the counselor would be encouraged to obtain a release of information to the doctor in order to establish a treatment protocol. The counselor recommends to the client that she come in for individual counseling sessions each week. She also voluntarily agrees to stop drinking wine at the request of her physician but not because she has a problem. She says that she does not really want to start taking Zoloft but agrees to for the next 2 months. She will not sign a release of information to her husband but will to the doctor.

The plan at this point is for Bree to maintain her abstinence from wine, take the Zoloft as prescribed, follow her doctor's recommendations, and attend weekly, individual sessions to further explore the nature of the relationship with her husband and her drinking and Xanax history. The counselor will monitor how successful she is in maintaining abstinence and following the physician's recommendations.

Summary

This chapter provided readers with a continuum model in order to approach clients with alcohol and drug issues. Along the continuum were ecological considerations and multicultural awareness, stages of change, symptomatology, and systemic interventions used in the process. In addition to the continuum, this chapter provided information on early intervention groups and presented three case scenarios where counselors created a counseling plan through the application of the stages of change and ecological considerations. This multiple approach took into consideration the cultural context and progression of the client's usage.

Exploration Questions From Chapter 5

1. What are your thoughts and beliefs on the disease model of treating addiction? Are you in support? Why or why not?
2. How do clients change? What do you think motivates addicted clients to change? How will you be part of that change process?

3. Spirituality is discussed periodically throughout this text. What are your thoughts as they relate to counseling an addicted client? Do you feel it is important and if so, why? If not, why not?
4. Why do you think people use drugs in the first place? What is your opinion?
5. What are your thoughts on Brofenbrenner's model? How might you use it in your work?

Suggested Activities

1. At your workplace or intern site, ask about the history of the agency and how it has treated addicted clients? What is the treatment philosophy?
2. On the basis of Brofenbrenner's model, create an approach when working with substance abusers in your school or agency.

Treatment and Treatment Settings

Counselors working in various settings (e.g., community agencies, colleges, and school settings) should understand the unique focus found in treatment for alcohol- and drug-addicted clients. Beyond this, they should also have knowledge of the many aspects associated with treatment. This chapter informs counselors on what alcohol and drug treatment entails, the functions and goals of treatment, how counselors can motivate clients for treatment services, who can benefit from addiction treatment, and the levels of treatment and medical care (i.e., outpatient, partial hospitalization program [PHP], detoxification, inpatient, halfway house) that exist. The chapter provides three case scenarios and an application of the information presented.

What Is Treatment?

Treatment is the external therapeutic process that clients are exposed to through education on addiction including group, individual, and family modalities. White (1998) defined treatment as "the delivery of professionally directed services to the alcoholic or addict, with the primary goal of altering his or her problematic relationship with alcohol and/or drugs" (p. 334). Alcohol and drug treatment, whether conducted through outpatient or inpatient settings, is designed for clients who meet the criteria for alcohol and/or drug dependency as articulated in the *Diagnostic and Statistical Manual of Mental Disorders* (4th ed., text rev., *DSM-IV-TR*; American Psychiatric Association, 2000). These clients may also be abusing other substances.

Addiction involves the compulsive and excessive use of drugs and alcohol with subsequent negative consequences. As a result of the well-formed defense system (i.e., denial, minimizing, rationalizing), clients are not always aware of how out-of-control their behaviors are and the resulting impact on others. Treatment provides a setting for addicted clients to identify their defense system. Treatment also provides a means to increase the client's understanding of emotional problems (both current and historic). These insights connect clients with the consequences of their use, which can have a significant impact on the denial system. Treatment also allows for personal examination of thoughts and behaviors that contribute to the continued use of drugs and alcohol. The power of addiction convinces its victims that alcohol and drugs are not a problem. To address this irrational thinking, the therapeutic modality of group counseling is used in most addiction treatment programs. Through the process of group interaction, clients provide one another feedback and support to draw out painful emotions associated with their drug and alcohol use. As a result of such support, along with education on various aspects of addiction, clients are able to understand the realness of their addiction. This culminates in an increased commitment to a recovery program coupling abstinence with new behaviors and management strategies.

Function and Goals of Treatment

The function of alcohol and drug treatment is to provide structure, feedback (peer and staff), education, counseling (group, individual, family/couples), and coping skills to clients. These entities merge as the client internalizes and creates an abstinent lifestyle. Treatment decreases isolation, encourages useful social connections, and instills hope in a seemingly hopeless situation. Ultimately, the goal for most alcohol and drug treatment programs is to help clients cognitively and emotionally assess their relationship with drugs and alcohol. This new awareness results in the development of a personal recovery program.

It is common for clients to attempt abstinence on their own prior to entering treatment. The problem for many individuals is not discontinuing (at least for a while) the drug but rather remaining abstinent on a continuous basis without the proper coping skills and support. For some, medical intervention and inpatient detoxification are needed in order to assist in the process of withdrawal from their drug of addiction (N. S. Miller & Gold, 1998).

This, however, is not the case in methadone treatment where the treatment goal is for clients addicted to narcotics to take their methadone (a narcotic substitute) on a regular basis in order to avoid withdrawal symptoms from heroin or other narcotic drugs. In this type of treatment the client is maintained on methadone. While in the methadone program, clients agree to three key therapeutic rules: (a) to remain abstinent from all other drugs and alcohol except for methadone, (b) to attend counseling sessions, and (c) to take their prescribed dose of methadone at the clinic. Some clients remain in a methadone program for years, while others use it as a means to wean off narcotics and into a drug- and alcohol-free lifestyle.

How Do Counselors Help Motivate Clients to Enter Drug and Alcohol Treatment?

One of the significant challenges counselors have when working with addicted clients is motivating them to consider alcohol and drug treatment. Just because clients discuss their drug and alcohol use in session does not necessarily mean they are ready to make a meaningful, substantial lifestyle change. The more informed counselors are regarding the treatment structure, location, cost, and time commitment for clients, the better able they are to work with client ambivalence.

Referring a client to alcohol and drug treatment can represent a substantial commitment of time and energy on the part of both the client and the counselor. For example, clients who are ambivalent about treatment may need to discuss their fears and anxieties concerning treatment, where the facility is located, and how much it might cost before they entertain the thought of entering treatment. In this process, counselors want to work with clients to sign a release of information to the receiving facility in order to help coordinate the admissions process. This usually entails providing the diagnosis, overall counselor impressions, concerns, and recommendations. The more roadblocks to treatment that are addressed by counselors, the greater the likelihood clients will comply with the treatment referral.

For instance, imagine sitting with your client (Dale) who is presenting symptoms of cocaine and alcohol dependency, yet is resistant to the idea of discontinuing his alcohol and drug use. You feel strongly that he could significantly benefit from entering a drug and alcohol treatment program. As you work with him in individual counseling you realize that most of his problems are intertwined with his alcohol and drug use. He does not agree with this perspective. How do you address drug and alcohol treatment with Dale without him discontinuing counseling altogether?

Motivational interviewing can be an effective method of working with client ambivalence whereby the counseling relationship itself creates the groundwork for a potential referral. Just because treatment resources in the community exist does not mean Dale is prepared to go. What this strongly suggests of counselors is to work on client *preparation.* Failing to do this will probably result in the client *not* showing for the referral appointments and possibly discontinuing counseling.

Picture another scenario: You just received a phone call from parents who want their 32-year-old daughter (who lives at home with them) to enter addiction treatment. How do you help these parents motivate their daughter for treatment?

As in the previous case, counselors need to understand the nature of their clients' motivation and existing therapeutic leverage. An example of therapeutic leverage is found in the court system where judges, in lieu of incarceration, refer clients for assessment and addiction treatment. In these cases, the use of therapeutic leverage suggests counselors might respond to a client in the following manner:

> I understand your hesitation to go for an assessment; however, your probation officer is looking for you to comply with treatment recommendations. He may return you back to court if you don't comply, and based on your excitement about this new job, I suspect that is not what you want.

The intention of the previous statement is to help the client recognize there are choices: to comply with treatment recommendations or risk losing a good job and being sent back to court for noncompliance. It is the counselor's responsibility to remain objective, outline the choices, and explore the consequences of each possible decision. In so doing, the counselor will be practicing in accordance with the *ACA Code of Ethics* regarding freedom of choice in counseling while emphasizing client responsibility (American Counseling Association, 2005).

Similarly, the mother who is calling for suggestions to motivate her daughter into addiction treatment will need to explore what leverage she could employ to assist in the process. She might say to her daughter that unless she attends an addiction treatment program, she will be unable to live in the house, which is a very personal and difficult decision.

Who Can Benefit From Treatment?

Numerous individuals can benefit from alcohol and drug treatment; however, the primary benefactor initially is the addicted client. Others who receive positive impacts from the treatment process include family members, friends, and employers. As a result of treatment, the addicted client can stop using drugs and alcohol, develop a personal recovery plan, and begin the process of healing family relationships. Some clients may enter treatment ambivalent about their drug and alcohol use. For these individuals, complete abstinence may not be a primary goal of the initial treatment. However, they can still benefit greatly from treatment by learning about their addiction, defenses, and the turmoil they have put themselves and others through when using drugs and alcohol. Treatment may plant the seeds for both current and future growth.

There are also those who discontinue drug and alcohol use on their own, without treatment. The literature suggests rates of 80% to 90% abstinence if patients participate in weekly continuing care or Alcoholics Anonymous (AA) or Narcotics Anonymous (NA) meetings following discharge from an inpatient treatment program (N. S. Miller & Gold, 1998).

Clinical Example

When I (Ford) started as a counselor in the field of addiction in 1984, I interned in a detoxification unit where most of the patients were in the later stages of addiction, and their use of drugs and alcohol had significantly devastated their bodies. Most of the clients entered a 28-day inpatient treatment facility following detoxification. There were very few outpatient programs at the time, and the popular mode of treatment was inpatient. The advent of managed care initiated a reexamination of this length and type of treatment, and as a result, outpatient and PHP increased as quickly as inpatient programs closed down.

When Clients Are Ready for Treatment

Let's say you know where the best alcohol and drug treatment program is located, you have helped the client understand and coordinate the financial issues, you have met two of the staff in the treatment program and were impressed, and most important, your client is willing to attend an initial screening appointment. The next step is determining which level of treatment your client needs.

Continuum of Treatment Care

This segment outlines the suggested criteria for admission into a variety of treatment settings: outpatient treatment, intensive outpatient treatment, partial hospitalization treatment, and inpatient alcohol and drug treatment, and how treatment impacts clients. The continuum of treatment care suggests clients are in varying points in the progression of their addiction, and therefore multiple treatment options are necessary.

The American Society of Addiction Medicine (ASAM, 1996; Magura et al., 2003) created criteria that allow for a broader continuum of care and make differentiations between adult and adolescent care. A common set of criteria has been developed to help determine a client's severity and was designed to place alcoholics in the appropriate level of care. Critics argue that the emphasis on medical aspects of treatment may place clients in a higher level of care than appropriate. Indeed, some patients with severe alcoholism may work better in a lesser level of care rather than inpatient treatment (ASAM, 1996).

ASAM has four separate levels of care, as listed below, which are evaluated on six other measures of severity in order to assess and refer a client for appropriate treatment.

ASAM Levels of Care

Level 1: Outpatient treatment
Level 2: Intensive outpatient (IOP) and partial hospitalization program (PHP)
Level 3: Medically monitored inpatient (residential) treatment
Level 4: Medically managed inpatient treatment

Dimensions of Severity

Dimension 1: Acute intoxication and/or withdrawal potential
Dimension 2: Biomedical conditions or complications
Dimension 3: Emotional and behavioral conditions and complications
Dimension 4: Treatment acceptance resistance
Dimension 5: Relapse potential
Dimension 6: Recovery environment

Outpatient Treatment

Outpatient treatment allows clients to attend sessions while residing in their own homes. Clients attend sessions either during the day or in the evening, and thereby are able to maintain regular working hours. A study by Friedmann, Lemon, Stein, and D'Aunno (2003) suggested that outreach programs in the community should liaison with criminal justice and workplace programs in order to attract clients earlier on in their addiction progression and thus are more likely to respond successfully to treatment.

Let's suppose you refer a client to outpatient treatment. What happens once they begin? Following the initial outpatient assessments and treatment planning, they are provided a schedule of treatment groups, which meet every week. N. S. Miller and Gold (1998) reported that the abstinence-based method is commonly used to treat addiction in 95% of the programs surveyed. Control or cutting down is not the goal in treatment, only total, complete abstinence. This model subscribes to the disease concept of addiction, the process of progression, and the chronic nature associated with it. Both education and group therapy are the primary modes of counseling applied in treatment. Additionally, the 12 steps of AA are integrated into the treatment process, and outside attendance is required while in treatment.

Clients entering alcohol and drug treatment may feel scared, apprehensive, and uncertain about the decision to engage in the process. Many clients initially believe that they are the only ones who are suffering from this problem and feel uniquely isolated and alone. This is expressly why most treatment is in the form of group counseling, which addresses the isolation and helps clients recognize the universality of the problem (Yalom, 2005). In outpatient settings, the client is assigned an individual counselor (although most of the therapeutic work is done in a group format).

As clients observe others at various stages of recovery in the group, combined with gaining a sense of trust in the treatment process, they are able to start sharing the pain and consequences of drug or alcohol use in their lives. Through such sharing and self-disclosure arrives, maybe for the first time, a sense of connection with others without the use of chemicals. Patients can experience a profound awareness of the potential for healing in a group. These new therapeutic underpinnings provide clients the courage to open up and allow others to hear their painful journies. In turn, these stories help others who are new to treatment.

Outpatient treatment typically consists of weekly individual sessions and multiple group sessions per week. Outpatient programs regularly require family involvement, either through education groups or family counseling sessions. A sample outpatient schedule might include group counseling on Monday and Wednesday (90 minutes each), attendance at AA and/or NA meetings on Tuesday and Thursday, and individual counseling on Wednesday (60 minutes). Saturday and Sunday are for leisure activities, family interaction, and support meetings.

Outpatient treatment staff usually consists of an addiction counselor, a psychiatrist, and a consulting psychologist to provide psychological testing. One of the primary factors for outpatient admission is the limited or nonrisk of clients for severe physical withdrawal. It is also noted that clients should be able to respond positively to emotional support.

Intensive Outpatient Treatment

Intensive outpatient (IOP) treatment differs from outpatient treatment in a number of ways. One place they overlap is that clients are able to attend treatment sessions and maintain employment while living at home. IOP typically consists of three groups per week, 3 hours per session, as well as weekly individual and family sessions. The primary modality in IOP treatment is group counseling.

The increase in treatment contact is in relation to the need for structure given the client's addictive process. Some clients are able to effectively use outpatient services, successfully meet their treatment goals, and remain abstinent. Other clients may continue to relapse and need significantly greater structure provided through IOP protocol. When counselors are evaluating clients for IOP, the following suggested criteria should be considered in determining the appropriateness for this level of care.

Partial Hospitalization Program

PHP differs from IOP in that it requires increased hours of treatment contact per week. The PHP is for clients requiring regular medical and psychiatric monitoring. PHP clients also do not meet the requirements for outpatient treatment because of their increasing severity of symptoms. At the same time, they are not exhibiting severe enough symptoms for admission into inpatient treatment. Clients typically attend partial treatment activities three to four times per week. Schedules for partial programs may range from 9:00 a.m. to 3:00 p.m. During this time clients are provided education and skills-based programming in a group format, individual and group counseling, case management, and psychiatric assessment. Staff in these programs may include psychiatrists, nurses, recreational therapists, psychologists, social workers, and addiction counselors.

Detoxification

This medical component of treatment is generally associated with a medical facility. However, within the past 15 years, outpatient ambulatory detoxification has also become a viable alternative to inpatient detoxification for some patients. Appropriate clients, as evaluated by a physician, are those with low risk for seizures and those who have minimal medical complications. In some cases, there are clients who attempt abstinence without medical supervision. In other cases, clients realize the challenge of self-detoxification (and all the associated physical, emotional, and cognitive difficulties) and choose to enter a detoxification program. The process of admission to a detoxification unit is similar to checking into a hospital; however, at the time of admission, patients may be under the influence and less than cooperative. While working in the detoxification unit, there were many times that I (Ford) witnessed patients arriving intoxicated and unable to negotiate the short walk down the hall. Within minutes they would pass out in their beds, then awaken later that night disoriented and nauseated, ushering in the detoxification process.

Detoxification provides structure for patients as they are monitored (e.g., blood pressure, pulse, respiration) by the medical staff while their bodies expel the chemicals through various means (urine, breath, sweat). Physicians create a detoxification protocol depending on the chemicals ingested by the patient. Such interventions may include prescribing continuous fluids, aspirin, phenobarbital, Buprenix, or Librium (Caldiero, Parran, Adelman, & Piche, 2006; N. S. Miller & Gold, 1998).

When patients experience withdrawal, physiological issues such as nausea, fever, or muscle cramps emerge. It is during this time when clients (if they were not in detoxification) would potentially begin using drugs and alcohol to alleviate withdrawal symptoms. Instead, during detoxification, the medications prescribed aid in the management of withdrawal symptoms. While patients are detoxifying, the medications enter the patient's body, preventing seizures and delirium tremens (DTs). Throughout detoxification, nurses monitor patients' vital signs and observe for signs of potential seizure activity or respiratory issues. As withdrawal symptoms subside, patients are usually tapered off the prescribed medication before being discharged from the medical unit.

While patients are in detoxification, they are evaluated by nurses, physicians, and counselors. A full biopsychosocial assessment is completed for purposes of referral following detoxification. Although patients may experience physical sickness in detoxification, it is important that they participate in group therapy with other patients during their stay because of the natural tendency to isolate. While these interventions are occurring, the staff counselors (setting the stage for the next step in the process) provide ongoing assessment of clients and involve family, employers, and partners (with appropriate releases signed) in the process. Detoxification, for many, is the first step on the road to recovery.

Inpatient Alcohol and Drug Treatment

In the mid-1930s, when AA was cofounded, few inpatient treatment centers existed. Physicians willing to work with this population found many of their patients in a useless cycle of addiction. Clients engaged in a "revolving door" process where they would be detoxified, leave the hospital, only to get drunk again, and then reappear for help (White, 1998). Throughout the years as Bill Wilson, the cofounder of AA, worked toward his own sobriety, he had a personal physician, Dr. William Silkworth. In his lifetime Dr. Silkworth worked with over 50,000 alcoholics, and as a result believed two things. The first was that alcoholism was not just a vice or bad habit, but rather a disease. The second was that alcoholism was an obsession of the mind that condemns one to drink (Kurtz, 1979). As a result of the development of AA and people like Dr. Silkworth, structured inpatient treatment was introduced (White, 1998). Inpatient treatment staff consists of physicians/psychiatrists, nurses, leisure activities counselors, addiction counselors, social workers and/or psychologists, intake counselors, mental health counselors, and family counselors. A typical inpatient daily schedule consists of group therapy twice a day, lecture education, leisure activity, and employer and family meetings, along with time to complete assignments, meet with counselors, and attend AA and NA meetings. Treatment days usually begin around 6:30 a.m. and end with lights out around 10:00 p.m. The unique feature of inpatient treatment in comparison to partial and outpatient treatment is that patients stay in the facility while they are receiving treatment. Patients' lengths of stay vary depending on their treatment goals. Patients referred to inpatient treatment many times have failed to meet their goals in outpatient programs and are in need of an intensive structure to intervene on the addiction. Patients admitted to inpatient treatment are first evaluated by physicians for a detoxification protocol, and following that evaluation they may or may not enter detoxification. Although treatment programs are structured in different ways, most programs are anchored to the 12 steps of AA as a foundation for a recovery philosophy (N. S. Miller & Gold, 1998).

Halfway House

Following treatment (outpatient, IOP, PHP, or inpatient) clients may continue with structured support through placement in a halfway house. Within the context of a halfway house, individuals live with other recovering clients in a house or residence operated by professional staff. Staff can include a house manager, counselors, a facility director, and food preparation specialists. Clients may enter a recovery house for housing needs following treatment and/or the need for continuing structure. Clients may live in a recovery house for up to a year, usually with the expectation of completing required work. In these settings, clients have weekly individual sessions with their counselors as well as group sessions. Clients are expected to focus on recovery, first and foremost (White, 1998).

Good candidates for admission into a halfway house are typically clients in the later stages of their addiction, who have had multiple attempts at recovery. These clients typically benefit from structure and ongoing support in the recovery process. Living in a recovery house offers clients the opportunity to attend treatment sessions while living in a recovering milieu. The overarching goal, of course, is for clients to eventually successfully transition back into the community.

There are also recovery houses that have no professional staff, relying instead on resident-determined guidelines. There is an expectation in these recovery houses for residents to attend 12-step support meetings on a regular basis and to keep current with their financial responsibilities to the house. They may have weekly house meetings or informal discussions but have no clinical staff to work with residents in individual or group therapy.

Clients in the Continuum of Treatment Care

The following are client examples that help the reader understand the continuum of treatment care shown in Figure 6.1. Counselors need to understand how a client proceeds through the continuum and how they can best help clients through the process.

Mental Health Counselor Treatment Scenario

As a mental health counselor you see 25 to 30 clients per week in your office, many of whom are diagnosed with clinical depression. However, on this occasion, you meet with Jeff, a 32-year-old who presents with marital discord as his initial issue. Upon further communication with Jeff, you realize the precipitating event for his visit to your office was related directly to his use of alcohol. Jeff reports he drank 10 beers last Saturday evening then blacked out. He adds that he learned later from his friends and family that he yelled obscenities at his wife and the other couple having dinner at their house. These actions were followed by Jeff taking off all his clothes and jumping into the pool. The following morning he had no recollection of what had happened but realized he must have been out of control because he woke up naked in the bushes.

Jeff presents to you that his wife was very upset but indicates that this was a very rare occasion and that he typically only drinks one or two beers. However, he also states that he drinks "heavily" once or twice a month with his old college friends. He reluctantly admits that he came in for counseling because his wife was at her "wit's end" and moved out of the house two nights ago. Although he appears remorseful, he doesn't seem to be connecting his drinking with her moving out of the house. He admits that he has cut down on his drinking in the past because of his wife's concerns, only to return to his usual pattern. Jeff also reports that he has promised his wife multiple times that he was going to stop altogether, but ended up drinking anyway.

What Are the Strategies a Counselor Can Employ at This Point?

- Do you refer him immediately to outpatient treatment, or do you refer him to detoxification services?
- Is he a candidate for inpatient treatment, or are you going to see him individually?
- Will you refer him to an alcohol and drug specialist, or will you focus on his depression due to his wife's moving out?

These are the questions counselors need to consider when clients like Jeff present for counseling. Let's begin to review what a counselor could do at this point.

Precipitating Issue and Insight Into Problem

At this point, Jeff's understanding of *why* he is in your office is more related to his wife moving out and his potential relationship loss rather than his drinking. He has not yet

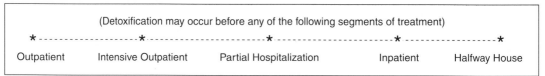

Figure 6.1. Continuum of Treatment Care

begun to connect his drinking with her leaving. His insight into his drinking behavior is minimal at best. However, he admits to tremendous sadness as a result of his wife leaving. Let us review what information Jeff has presented us: He has developed a tolerance to alcohol (by his report), and he has one recorded blackout (by his report). There is patterned drinking and a significant consequence (his wife leaving) of a drunken evening with friends (by his report). He denies experiencing any type of withdrawal symptoms when he stopped in the past.

On the basis of your assessment and using the *DSM-IV-TR* criteria, you see Jeff's drinking as alcohol dependent. In terms of the stages of change (Prochaska et al., 1992), he appears to be in the contemplation stage in that he has some understanding of how his drinking has impacted others, and his wife's absence is motivating him to initiate action, "whatever it takes to get her back."

Creating the Therapeutic Bind

By its very nature, generally speaking, addiction is predictable and progressive. Understanding this construct equips counselors to *work with* clients. As W. R. Miller and Rollnick (2002) described, the therapeutic bind helps to motivate and work with the resistance rather than against it. In Jeff's case, you might consider the fact that he will probably drink again. Additionally, he may do so without control during the course of individual counseling with you. Up until this point Jeff is trying to convince himself and you that he can control his drinking. Addicted individuals think they can control their use, which is described fully in the next chapter. You, on the other hand, realize it is probably only a matter of time before his drinking creates more consequences. As a result, you help Jeff create a contract that stipulates, "Just in case you can't control or stop your drinking, will you go to treatment?" Jeff is now in a bind. If he refuses, he is admitting right there that he is not in control. If he says yes, you can work with Jeff by creating a plan for him to enter treatment.

What Level of Treatment?

Now that you have determined alcohol is the primary problem and that Jeff has some insight into the problem, the question emerges regarding what direction is best as he proceeds. Jeff might be a good candidate and appropriate for outpatient treatment. This assessment is based on his reported absence of withdrawal symptoms, his motivation to do "whatever it takes" to remain abstinent, and his diagnosis of alcohol dependence. However, he may not be willing at this point to enter an outpatient treatment program. If he is willing to enter outpatient treatment though, you can provide him resources in the local area, obtain a release of information signed by Jeff to relay the information to the intake counselor, and then encourage Jeff to take full advantage of the treatment process. You could let him know you would be willing to see him for follow-up care after the treatment program.

The other option, if Jeff is not interested in starting outpatient treatment, is to continue working with him in counseling. The primary goal may include helping him make changes so that his wife may return home. Working with this goal you can ask Jeff, "In order for your wife to return home, what do you think she would need to see from you?" More than likely Jeff will say something like "Not drink or get out of control with my drinking." Maybe he will say "Not go out as much with my old college buddies and drink." Jeff has now identified a pragmatic action-oriented behavior that aligns with the parameters of the primary goal (which will still involve him examining his drinking, the impact it has on others, and the current consequences related to it). Jeff may promise to you that he won't drink or that he will control his drinking. He may be both convincing and sincere in doing so because he believes he has complete control over his drinking. You, however, understand the predictability of loss of control with addiction. Jeff will discover on his own that he cannot control his use and may experience other consequences while he is in counseling with you. You can also introduce early on the following proposition: If Jeff finds that he is unable to control his drinking and suffers more consequences, would he be willing to enter an outpatient treatment program?

After the fourth session Jeff discloses how he got drunk on Saturday night in a local bar and obtained a driving under the influence (DUI) charge while driving home, then spent all day Sunday in jail. In addition to being angry, he also realizes for the first time how alcohol is ruining his life.

Working With Client Consequences in Individual Counseling

At this point you have more therapeutic leverage to help Jeff accept a treatment referral. You could intervene with "Jeff, this must be very difficult for you. I've watched you over the past month and all the feelings you have had related to being alone after your wife moved out. And now again it appears that alcohol is creating more problems. This would be a perfect time to consider outpatient treatment. Not only do the courts typically favor individuals who are taking responsibility for their drinking when there is a DUI, but your wife, based on what you have shared with me, would also be in favor of you receiving structured outpatient treatment." Jeff can now decide to again refuse your referral to treatment, which would go against the promise he made to himself that if he couldn't control his drinking, he would become willing to accept alternate intervention strategies and follow through with the referral. On the other hand, he could discontinue counseling with you rather than accept your referral, which places the importance of the therapeutic relationship and the development of trust in jeopardy. If the relationship has been built, it places Jeff in a therapeutic bind.

Confrontation or *Carefrontation*?

Bernie Siegel, M.D. (1986), who coined the word "carefrontation," believed that for helpers or clinicians to confront clients, they needed to do so in a genuine and caring manner in order for their clients to receive the feedback. Empathic statements help Jeff realize that both his wife and the court system would be supportive of treatment, should he choose to enter it. You are also gently "carefronting" in reminding him of his agreement to enter treatment, should his way not work. There is always the possibility Jeff will attempt a renegotiation of his initial agreement and once again try to control or abstain. Should the court order him into treatment, it would give him a significant message to move forward in the therapeutic process. Should the court referral occur, it is important that you prepare Jeff for treatment, educate him on what will occur, and offer ideas on how he can gain the most from it.

School Counselor Scenario

An 18-year-old student comes into your office to discuss her father's alcohol use. Tiffany reports her father drinks at least a 12-pack every night, verbally fights with her mom, and then falls asleep by the television. She states that this has been the pattern for the past 7 years, after her father lost a job because of his drinking. He has been unemployed for more time than he has been employed over the past 7 years. Tiffany says that her home life is affecting her ability to concentrate in school and that on the weekends she sometimes "smokes weed" to "mellow out." She says it is not a regular thing, but she does it because it makes her feel relaxed and less tense at home. She also said that if her father ever found out she smoked pot, he would kick her out of the house.

As the school counselor you've known of Tiffany from her involvement in school plays and the track team. Since this is her senior year, you inquire about her postgraduation plans, at which point she tells you she is not going to college but will move in with her 25-year-old boyfriend, who also drinks a lot.

Presenting Event and Insight Into Problem

Tiffany came to counseling reporting a lack of sleep, poor attention in class, and feelings of depression. She is aware of how her father's drinking is impacting her life and the rest of the family and realizes how, in turn, this issue impacts her involvement with other activities. Given this information, what might you conclude? Does she have a substance abuse or dependency problem? Would she benefit from addiction treatment?

On the basis of the information Tiffany gave you, you conclude that she is aware of how tired and run down she is related to her father's drinking. However, it does not sound as if she is as aware of the relationship dynamics that are playing out with her boyfriend. Her use of marijuana at this point would need to be explored. Of particular concern might be the feelings she avoids or copes with by smoking pot.

What Level of Treatment Is Warranted?

In this case, it does not appear that structured, formalized treatment is warranted at this point. However, because of the high risk centered around her family and her father's alcoholism, it would be recommended that you continue to see her individually and explore how alcoholism impacts her life, as well as how it may affect the choices she makes with her partners. Continued evaluation and exploration of her marijuana use would also be important. Further, preparing Tiffany for referral to the alcohol and drug specialist might be warranted. It would benefit both Tiffany and the therapeutic bond to acknowledge her honesty with you in the session about her feelings and drug use. For her to share about her marijuana use is a big step in trust, which is the cornerstone to counseling and to any referrals you might make in the future. An Adult Children of Alcoholics (ACOA) group may be appropriate, should it be offered in the school. A referral could be made to the community for ACOA support groups. Should she continue to use marijuana, questions such as "What does marijuana do for you that you cannot do when clean?" "What can you do on marijuana that you cannot do when not using?" or "What does marijuana help you avoid or escape from?" would be appropriate to explore.

Preparing Clients to Accept Referrals and Help

It is important for the counselor to be familiar with treatment program resources. It is just as critical to work with clients to help them accept the referral. For instance, let's say Tiffany mentions marijuana use and immediately you refer her to the alcohol and drug education group. Although it may be helpful for Tiffany to receive the information, she may not yet be prepared for the referral. Quite possibly she will either discontinue counseling or simply not follow through on the referral to group. This failure to prepare Tiffany may also mitigate her reaching out for counseling services in the future. In essence, along with not helping her move toward treatment, you may actually cause harm by setting up conditions that may signal that counseling is deceptive, hurtful, uninformed, uncaring, and so on. Working with her and teaching her how to accept help and the benefits of work in counseling is a goal in itself. Many times with self-referred clients the referral to treatment by the counselor is too quick from the client's perspective. Often, the client is simply not prepared or ready to move on the referral.

College Counselor Case Scenario

The 2005 National Survey of Counseling Center Directors (366 centers surveyed) indicated that 90.3% of the directors observed an increase in the number of clients with severe psychological problems. Ninety-six percent of directors believed that the increase of students with more serious problems is a growing concern in their centers, and 78% believed it was a growing concern for the administration (Gallagher, 2005).

As a college counselor you see a variety of clients each day with varied presenting issues. Patti is no exception. Her initial paperwork suggests she is depressed and has contemplated suicide within the past 2 months (though she has no current suicidal thoughts and has no plan). Her precipitating event, or her reason for seeking counseling, is the breakup of a 6-month relationship. Initially she says he was seeing other women and that is why they broke up. She continues to disclose details of her use pattern, including amount and consequences (she experiences periods of lost memory when she drinks). Patti tells you how she would go to a party with her boyfriend, only to "wake up" in someone's house early the next morning not knowing how she got there or where she actually was. Her boyfriend would get drunk too and "mess around with other women when I was drunk." Patti recollects how, for years, she watched her mother take pills, which would make her drowsy and incoherent. Patti says she really "got drunk" this past weekend and it scared her because some of the people she was now associating with also use drugs.

As with Tiffany in the preceding scenario, we have multiple issues to address: Patti's depression, her significant alcohol abuse, the recent loss of a relationship, the significant consequences (both experienced and possible) related to her blackouts, and the impact her mother's drug use had on her during her developing years. Should Patti be referred to outpatient treatment? Do you feel she has an alcohol problem? To what degree is there a relationship between her depression and her alcohol use, and does one lead to the other?

These are some of the questions most clinicians ask as they begin to work with a substance abuser. Patti's depression appears significant and will need to be continually monitored with referral to the staff psychiatrist. Additionally, further assessment of depression in her family and current depression following abstinence is needed. Patti's report of her alcohol use is of concern, particularly related to the previous weekend.

Might she benefit from outpatient treatment at this point? Yes. Because she is self-referred, she may be at a place where a referral will be accepted. However, it might take you time and effort to facilitate that step in the process. In the meantime, Patti has presented significant information to begin addressing her feelings, her blackouts, her relationship loss, and the previous weekend. All of these issues plus the ongoing assessment of her depression are critical.

Summary

This chapter discussed the various types of treatment sites in the continuum of treatment care and familiarized the reader with criteria for admission into detoxification, outpatient and inpatient treatment, and partial hospitalization. Additionally, scenarios were provided to help readers understand how a client might engage in the treatment process as well as how clinicians can work with them during this journey.

Exploration Questions From Chapter 6

1. What aspect of the continuum might you like to work in?
2. Have you ever worked with a client who has been in withdrawal? If so, how did you approach it?
3. If you haven't worked with a client in withdrawal, how might you know the person needed detoxification?
4. What counseling skills do you feel would be important in helping clients obtain treatment?
5. Do you believe treatment (outpatient, inpatient, etc.) works or is effective? If so, why? If not, why not?
6. What happens when you have clients who cannot afford treatment but are in dire need?

7. How might you work in developing trust with clients of color who you are trying to refer to treatment but who are very wary of going?
8. If you are facilitating a group of clients, of whom only 3 out of the 10 are minorities, how will you bring this up as an area for exploration?

Suggested Activities

1. Visit various sites of treatment care in your region and become acquainted with the treatment program and staff. Ask questions of the staff about their specific duties and determine how you might refer a client to their facility.
2. Talk with patients about their experience in treatment and what was most helpful and least helpful.

Developmental Approaches
in Treating Addiction

From our professional view, clients are multidimensional and complex. We believe each client possesses both the ability to grow and the ability to self-destruct. As counselors, we are privileged to be a part of this therapeutic journey. Along the way we use tools such as an empathic heart, an inquisitive mind, and an archeological and environmental perspective to human development. Our clients' lives are like complex tapestries. Collectively, they represent blended families, wellsprings of culture, and unique genetic creations. Depending on where we meet our clients in their unique stories, we have the opportunity to explore the rich variety of bachgrounds from which they have come and to help them generate the missing patches of fabric in their experiences so they may achieve wholeness. For some clients, such missing patches, or gaps, have been filled with drugs and alcohol. When these chemicals are removed (which occurs in the treatment process and subsequent recovery), the developmental deficits still remain.

This is a unique chapter because of its specific attention to human development and its interaction with the recovery process. The combination of these major tenets informs effective treatment planning and direction for counseling. Within the structure of this chapter are case scenarios and pragmatic considerations for counselors to use in their clinical work.

Why Are Developmental Stages and Models Important for Understanding Recovery?

We have noticed a significant relationship that exists between the recovery process and our work with clients with addiction. Of course, the potential for relapse in recovery is ever present. Therefore, a thorough understanding of potential developmental gaps, which can affect the clinical process, helps identify specific client needs in counseling (Wallen, 1993). An understanding of client developmental needs individualizes counseling, providing increased treatment efforts. For instance, clients who have experienced significant trauma within the first 5 years of life, may have difficulty in developing healthy, supportive, and trusting relationships. As the therapeutic relationship develops, reparenting (e.g., using transference and countertransference) can occur within the counseling relationship, allowing for growth through the potential developmental impasse.

The two broad areas of development we examine in this chapter are life span development through the stages described by Erikson (1963), Piaget (1954), and Kohlberg (1968) and recovery development through the stages described by Brown (1985), Gorski (1989), and Gideon (1975). A combined review of these models along with assessment information outlined in chapter 4 provide the basis for comprehensive counseling and ultimately increased recovery options.

How to Use This Chapter

Chapter after chapter, you are building a multifaceted and multilayered understanding of how to work with alcohol- and drug-abusing and addicted clients. Readers should visualize their alcohol and drug clients, the symptoms, their readiness for change, the types and amounts of ingested drugs, the cultural backgrounds, and the diversity of referral options. This chapter calls attention to the significance of fully examining life span development. Focused attention is on the interplay between initial unresolved stages and drug or alcohol use or abuse. Counselors are provided the central tenets to working with the ways through which the cycle of unresolved developmental issues repeat and contribute to the relapse process. Essentially, counselors are encouraged to help clients identify developmental gaps and develop effective coping strategies for emotions and relationships.

Erikson's Theory of Psychosocial Development

Erik Erikson's stage development theory provides an outline of normal healthy human development (C. S. Hall & Lindsey, 1978). As an ego psychologist, Erikson redirected Freud's view of human development along sexual stages, focusing primarily on social stages. He believed that early relationships with parents or parental figures played a significant role in the development of the child. Kohut (1977), an object relations theorist, agreed with Erikson that the relationship between the parent and the child was of critical importance in the developmental process. Kohut contributed the notion that dysfunction in relationships as an adult stemmed from poor bonding and attachment in childhood. Erikson's stages and related cases follow.

Trust Versus Mistrust

Of primary importance in this stage, which occurs from birth to 2 years, is the development of basic trust with the parental figures. Normal dependency with a parent develops at this stage in which the child can depend on the parental figure(s) to be consistent and present, thereby developing trust. As long as the parent(s) can be consistent, a feeling of trust will develop. However, if a child is unable to develop a felt bond or connection, a strong core message of unworthiness or not being enough can develop. At this stage when a child is yelling and screaming, the parent comforts the child, and eventually the child learns to self-soothe, whereby learning to not only trust the parent but also to begin trusting his/her own innate ability to self-soothe. Additionally, during this stage children learn to trust that they can actually effect movement in their environment. The screaming child (above) may also learn that he or she can trust self in being able to move things (in this case parents) in his or her environment. This is a critical lesson for many tasks in life. Failing to learn to trust self in having some control in the environment can lead to self-defeating talk later in life and a sense of being controlled by the world. Clients who have not developed a sense of trust may fear being abandoned or feel unloved. They also learn not to trust their own feelings.

Case With Trust Versus Mistrust

Gary was a handsome 48-year-old male who, in addition to being addicted to alcohol and cocaine, was also addicted to sex. As Gary attempted sobriety, it was clear how the early relationships in his life with his parents played a significant role in getting sober. He reported that his father was cold, aloof, and worked a lot. He said his mother was very nurturing and was present throughout his life to support and care for him when he got into trouble. When he came in for treatment he was referred to participate in a men's group. Through the group process he began to develop trust with male figures as well as the male facilitator. In contrast to depending on women to meet all of his nurturing needs, he discovered that a group of men could provide a very supportive environment; this helped him begin the process of healing from the core message he received that he was not enough, brought on by his father's neglect. He also learned that he could use his own resources (e.g., open discussion, sharing of reactions and feelings) to get his needs met, thereby developing a stronger internalized sense of trust of self.

Autonomy Versus Shame and Doubt

This stage is typically thought to range from 2 to 4 years old. There are parallels between Erikson's stage and Freud's anal stage. In this stage the child learns to differentiate right from wrong as well as good from bad. During this time of life, the child is working toward the development of a sense of autonomy and separateness. These lessons build to an internal sense of control. Of course, all of this new development learning is hypothesized as being built on the previous stage. Also during this stage, children are setting boundaries by saying "no" and are challenging their environment (specifically considered by Erikson to consist of parents, siblings, and other key immediate family members). Striking out on one's own can occur when a child successfully meets the needs of basic trust. Support of the child creating a healthy sense of boundaries is substantially important for the development of a positive self-esteem. Without that trust the child may feel shame, doubt, insecurity, and may have low self-esteem.

Case With Autonomy Versus Shame and Doubt

Cindy grew up in an alcoholic family; her father was an abusive alcoholic. Cindy was the youngest of three children. She grew up in fear of her father. Currently she is in counseling because of her drinking and her dysfunctional relationships with men. You determine that, as a child, she was verbally abused and did not develop a sense of trust or safety within the family. Early in her life, relationships with boys became very important. The major messages from boys included telling her she looked pretty. These comments merged with her developmental issues, leading to her initiation of sexual relationships as a way of being loved. To quell her feelings of low self-esteem and shame (associated with self-perception and perception of her own behaviors), she started drinking at age 13.

In recovery, Cindy will benefit from attending both women's support and group counseling meetings to develop trust with other women (which she reports she never has had). It would be important for Cindy to abstain not only from alcohol but also from intimate, romantic relationships with men until she more fully develops a sense of self-trust and boundaries in recovery.

Initiative Versus Guilt

This stage occurs typically between the ages of 4 and 6 years old and parallels Freud's phallic stage. Healthy development associated with this stage is facilitated primarily by the parental figures setting reasonable limits. These boundaries, in turn, encourage the child to engage in new initiatives. The initial role identification with adults for both boys and girls occurs in this stage. If the child experiences little or no support in their initiatives, a feeling of guilt may preside. This guilt exceeds normal guilt as it surges through the individual continuously. Successful completion of this stage is promoted by positive, supportive, and limit-setting behavior on behalf of the parent(s) (Erikson, 1963; C. S. Hall & Lindsey, 1978).

Case With Initiative Versus Guilt

In recovery, Tim is discovering he is a lot like his father. Tim has identified two areas that continue to plague his recovery efforts. He watched his father gamble away most of the household's savings while engaging in multiple extramarital affairs. Tim recognizes, in recalling his youth, that he was never allowed to try new things. He further recollects that his father ran the household with an "iron fist" and did not allow for creativity or initiative. Tim realizes he started testing his father's patience in early adolescence. He realizes his drinking and gambling, along with many girlfriends, were ways of both rebelling and making himself feel good. In recovery he realizes the need to effect positive movement, typified by remaining sober. He also recognizes the importance of avoiding casinos and extramarital affairs. Tim learns to recognize how his cycle of relapse leads to feelings of enormous guilt and shame. It can be seen with this example how mistrust, shame and doubt, and guilt all play as factors in relapse. Additionally, the case exemplifies the importance of creating a treatment plan that addresses developmental issues along with the use or abuse of chemicals.

Industry Versus Inferiority

This stage typically runs from age 6 to puberty. Freud described it as the latency stage of psychosexual development. According to Erikson, in this stage the child is observing socially acceptable activities (as demonstrated by both parents and peer groups). Peer groups, in fact, tend to have a stronger influence than the family. As individuals transit through this stage, they need to experience an internalized sense of success. Failing to achieve such internal positive belief leads individuals to feel discouraged. One group particularly at risk during this stage of development is children who have learning disabilities or who have been affected physically by their mothers' chemical use (i.e., fetal alcohol syndrome). As an example, children with learning disabilities associated with fetal alcohol syndrome may not feel as though they are successful in school and self-identify as being "dumb."

Case With Industry Versus Inferiority

Stan, a 23-year-old college student, was a successful swimmer in high school. However, he always struggled with reading and comprehension. He was diagnosed with attention deficit disorder in high school and was prescribed Ritalin, a psychopharmacological stimulant for attention problems. Unfortunately, Stan began taking the drug more often than prescribed. Additionally, he started stealing it from his brother and buying it from friends in college. When he entered treatment for alcoholism, he realized he was also addicted to stimulant drugs (i.e., Ritalin). He struggled throughout his childhood and early adulthood with feeling inferior to others, especially in learning (e.g., school). The primary focus of his therapy was supportive and interactive. These tenets anchored new growth by developing a support network and by providing a place to discuss his feelings of inferiority. While in recovery he remained abstinent, typically attending two support meetings per week and meeting with his counselor weekly. Also during the process, he was evaluated and placed on a nonstimulant medication. The combination of the medication, support, and addressing the inferiority feelings helped him make new choices for his life and career.

Identity Versus Role Confusion

This stage occurs beyond puberty and is highlighted by the individual's struggle for identity and finding an individual place in the world. The initial stage of trust versus mistrust is revisited, with the additional element of the trust portion (in this stage) being developed outside of the parental influence, within the community and environment. Therefore, the role of peers and peer groups in this stage is tremendously important. Freud's genital sexuality would also be found in this stage of Erikson's development. For many parents this is a time of great consternation because of the adolescent's exploratory behaviors, pushing limits, and exploring one's own identity. Such pushes and pulls accompanied by parental support and nurturing helps refine the budding sense of identity in the world. Failure to acquire this sense of self leaves the adolescent with a diffuse and scattered self-understanding. Many times this exploration is in conflict with the parental figures. A healthy sense of identity is fostered as a result of each stage, resulting in the ability and willingness to experiment and explore new behaviors (Erikson, 1963; C. S. Hall & Lindsey, 1978).

Case With Identity Versus Role Confusion

Laura was afraid of her own shadow growing up. She felt insecure and guilty most of her life until she went to a party with one of her friends. With her first shot of alcohol, Laura felt connected, a part of the crowd, and less fearful. After three shots, all of her worries went away. She learned quickly how alcohol and the group of friends she was associating with were providing her with something she had never had—a connection with others (albeit chemically induced). While in recovery, Laura realized quickly that she was revisiting the old fear and distrusts. Her need to develop positive new messages, connect with support people in recovery, and explore her identity as a recovering person are each key ingredients in her sobriety.

Intimacy Versus Isolation

During this stage of life, romantic relationships as well as significant friendships begin to develop. What occurs is a recapitulation of family dynamics with intimate relationships. If a person witnessed two parents fighting constantly, and the interaction between her parents was adversarial at best, the relationships that the person will be involved with will more than likely parallel her parents' relationship.

Case With Intimacy Versus Isolation

The previous case of Laura could include an enmeshed relationship with her father as she grew up. In adulthood Laura has poor boundaries and continually wants to please other men at the expense of her self-esteem. When this begins to occur, she becomes quietly resentful and acts out by either cutting on herself or drinking excessive amounts of alcohol. With either behavior, she is taking her anger and pain out on her body. In recovery, she will benefit from examination of her needs and relationship with feelings. Additionally, she will want to examine her boundaries and the need to please others at the personal cost of feeling resentful. Her resentment, in turn, leads to self-destructive behaviors. Part of this cycle may include statements such as "I know he is not good for me, but I don't want to be alone, so he is better than nothing."

Generativity Versus Stagnation

This stage of life involves the altruistic behavior of humans, either by raising a family or going beyond one's own ego and helping others. Parenthood is one means through which individuals feel as though they are contributing to and helping create a new tomorrow. Others feel compelled to give back to the community through other venues, such as volunteerism. If the sense of giving of self for the next generation does not occur, a feeling of stagnation can surface. Once an individual discontinues drinking, he or she may realize that the *altruistic* sense needs to be addressed. If this sense is left unaddressed, the individual will probably develop feelings of stagnation and boredom. This, of course, can lead right back to drinking.

Case With Generativity Versus Stagnation

Dale just got sober and realizes his job does not provide the altruistic outlets and opportunities he needs. Therefore, he decides that after 2 years of sobriety he wants to become a counselor. He realizes if he stays in his current administrative position he will become bored and drink. Therefore, he begins the process of applying to schools and volunteering at a local shelter, thus addressing this developmental need.

Integrity Versus Despair

This is the final, culminating stage of development in Erikson's model. During this stage, a life review occurs to determine whether life is and has been worthwhile. If the major emphasis is on failures and things not done or achieved, despair can emerge. A sense of despair can have a substantial effect on the recovery process. Many addicted clients (once they sober up) reflect on the fact that their use may have cost them to lose relationships, opportunities, and significant pieces of self. Because of such pain and loss, these clients are at risk for relapse. For those in recovery after retirement, this is most definitely an issue.

Case With Integrity Versus Despair

Don has worked for 30 years as a teacher, drinking alcoholically for half that time. With the onset of retirement, he spends much of his time at home drinking throughout the day. During the first year of his retirement, his wife continues to work. She decides to leave him unless he discontinues his drinking and goes to treatment. He enters treatment, sobers up, and realizes all the missed opportunities because of his priority to drink. He also feels as though his life is over, "Why not continue to drink and die that way?" Don appears to have much despair in his voice. In recovery, Don will probably need to develop a support group. He will benefit from recognizing how his life experience can help others either through regular attendance at support meetings or by contributing to areas he feels were neglected in his drinking (i.e., community projects). It is imperative that Don acquires a sense of integrity in his sobriety and that his life is worthwhile.

Summation of Erikson's Stages

Each mini-case has provided an idea of how developmental issues are important in the recovery process. Clients are typically not aware of these critical life tasks. It is incumbent on the clinician to help clients find peace with the major tasks in each stage. Each case presented an individual who felt either alone, not trusted, isolated, or not worthy. Alcohol and drugs initially anesthetizes the pain of such feelings. It is vital, therefore, to address possible developmental deficits. The next section reviews Jean Piaget's stages of cognitive development.

Piaget's (1954) Cognitive Development

Sensorimotor Period

This period ranges from birth to 1 or 2 years, during which time the child learns primary circular reaction. During this stage, young children experience the world primarily from their sense and motor capabilities. In essence, children must be able to see or touch something for it to really exist. This stage is also recognized by the phrase "thinking by doing," which implies linear, causal, direct interaction with the world on the part of the child.

Preoperational Period

This stage ranges from 1 to 7 years when the child begins to learn language skills and incorporates an egocentric view of the world. The child is unable to see from a perspective outside of self. During this period of time, the child is truly fixated on him- or herself (Brown, 1985; Wallen, 1993).

Concrete Operational Period

This is a period when children can begin to carry out increasingly complex cognitive operations, albeit nonabstract. For example, a client comes in for counseling and is asked, "Could you tell me what brought you in today for counseling?" and the response from the client is "a taxi cab," which is a concrete response rather than an abstract one (Brown, 1985; Wallen, 1993).

Formal Operations

This is when an individual can think and respond in an abstract manner. Taking the above question, a formal operations thinker might say, "I have had difficulty with my relationships and, in particular, their concern with my pot use." This can develop between the ages of 12 and 18 years; however, not all adults are able to develop abstract reasoning or thinking (Brown, 1985; Wallen, 1993).

Application of Piaget to Clinical Work With Addicted Clients

We could speculate the following about clients who are "stuck" in the preoperational period: They would look strikingly similar to active addicts or alcoholics, being self-centered and ill-equipped to see the impact of their behavior from other perspectives. When working with a client it will be helpful to explore the client's family and relationship life from 2 to 7 years. In recovery there could be movement from "me" and "I" to an understanding of others' feelings and viewpoints. Part of the treatment planning would be to help the client see how using or drinking impacts others. In time it would be important to help clients recognize their own self-centeredness.

Determining whether a client is a concrete thinker or a formal operations thinker is important. Every morning for 2 years I (Ford) worked in a partial hospital setting with dually diagnosed patients, many of whom were lower functioning. Much of what I talked about in the education component and the group segment was concrete and straightforward. In the afternoons, in my private practice, I counseled clients who were able to think and understand abstract concepts. Both sets of clients were addicted; however, it was important for me to understand that if I approached the morning group with abstract questions and information, it would be difficult for them to comprehend. If I spoke concretely to the formalized thinkers, it would not meet their capabilities for growth and may set the stage for increased frustration on the part of these clients.

Kohlberg's Moral Development Stages

The work of Lawrence Kohlberg expanded on Piaget's stages of cognitive development from a moral perspective. Kohlberg's model is broken down into three distinct stages: the preconventional period, the conventional period, and the postconventional period (Kohlberg, 1968). Within each of these stages are two areas of exploration.

Preconventional Period

This period includes *punishment and obedience orientation* where the child understands that certain rules regulate behavior and that the child will abide by them in order to avoid punishment. The second orientation, *instrumental–relativist*, examines the child's thought process of whether breaking the rules outweighs the possible consequences of breaking the rules. Essentially, in this phase the individual evaluates the pain they may experience from the decision versus the pleasure they may receive (Kohlberg, 1968).

The first orientation is best understood by the following example: Picture a first-year college student who rigorously follows *the rules*. He has the opportunity to try alcohol for the first time during the initial months of the school year. He debates the potential consequences (e.g., getting caught, being underage, feelings of guilt) and the potential pleasures associated with drinking (e.g., excitement, intoxication, peer acceptance). This is a clear example of how one might weigh out the decision according to Kohlberg.

Conventional Period

Kohlberg found this to be more of an altruistic stage in which the child wants to be helpful. *Good boy and nice girl orientation* is when the individual conforms to family or environmental rules despite personal discomfort. An example of the good boy, nice girl is when a child wants to help at home to compensate for the active alcoholism that is occurring. Despite the personal discomfort (i.e., sadness, fear, and guilt), the child desires to contribute to the needs of the family. This case represents a clear example of how one would conform despite the discomfort. The *law and order orientation* is the individual's adherence to rules and order of the society. This is the particular stage in which the individual begins autonomous judgment (Kohlberg, 1968). For instance, a client, raised in an addicted family, turns a sibling into the police for drug possession. Although a family member, the client is acting autonomously and following the rules of the society.

Postconventional Period

In this period the individual arrives at moral judgments from internal principles rather than the rules of the society. This may start in early adulthood or later adolescence. As with Piaget's formal stage of development, which involves abstract thinking, this period outlined by Kohlberg necessitates an ability to think abstractly.

The *social contract/legalistic orientation* is where individuals have both rights and responsibilities. The *universal ethical principal orientation* is where a person's moral beliefs and attitudes are also in agreement with one's own ethical principles. Those who are in this stage of moral development will also disagree with unjust laws and regulations despite the potential consequences (Kohlberg, 1968).

Although intoxicated, clients may exhibit immoral behavior but not necessarily be immoral themselves. Over the course of addiction, clients behave in ways that are in direct conflict with their internalized value system. Someone who is addicted to drugs may become a liar, a thief, and/or a manipulator in order to obtain drugs. In essence, the drugs or alcohol overpowers their sense of moral judgment. In recovery, clients need to examine their values and what has been compromised as a result of their addiction.

Developmental Models of Recovery

This chapter has outlined several major developmental theories with respect to psychosocial development (Erikson, 1963), cognitive development (Piaget), and moral development (Kohlberg, 1968) and the impact of alcohol and drugs on human growth. In this next segment the focus shifts to models that outline the recovery process and the developmental stages that addicted clients move through in sobriety (Brown, 1985; Gorski, 1989).

Recovery is an internal change process that initially begins when addicted clients contemplate their alcohol and drug use as problematic. As clients move from active addiction into recovery, they discontinue their use of drugs and alcohol and begin to examine their thoughts, emotions, and behaviors in relation to their chemical use.

A suggested equation for recovery is the following: A + T + E + B + S. Recovery is composed of *abstinence* A + an examination of *thoughts* T + an exploration and expression of *emotions*

E + a change in *behavioral* choices B + (for some) an examination of their *spiritual* existence S. The temporal, situational, and logistics through which clients enter the recovery process is both unique and idiosyncratic. Clients initiating a personal recovery process have done so with great personal and familial cost. In point of fact, however, by the time clients are ready to take action, their lives are out of control and unmanageable. For many, the tremendous emotional pain is a primary motivating factor to enter treatment and initiate the recovery process. The emotional pain that motivates clients to act typically stems from a severe conflict between life goals and values and their drug and alcohol consequences (W. R. Miller & Rollnick, 2002).

Three developmental models of recovery are outlined. These models provide counselors with an understanding of the internal process many clients experience when beginning a recovery program. Stephanie Brown's developmental model of recovery focuses on the recovery of the alcoholic. Terence Gorski expanded Brown's model by adding utility with both alcohol- and drug-addicted clients. Finally, William Gideon's model of recovery is described from the standpoint of isolation in addiction to connectedness with others.

Brown's Developmental Model of Recovery

Brown (1985) suggested four stages of recovery: drinking, transition, early recovery, and ongoing recovery. Each of these stages contains three components that interact simultaneously: the alcohol axis, environmental interactions, and the interpretation of self with others. In other words, during each stage all three of these factors merge in a variety of ways (Brown, 1985). The focus on alcohol throughout the first three stages is significant, only to fade in ongoing recovery. The focus on alcohol during the drinking stage is obvious because the individual is both obtaining and drinking alcohol. However, in the transition stage, the person is discontinuing the drinking. As the individual discontinues drinking, the focus turns to *not drinking* alcohol. The focus is still on alcohol except it is on abstinence from alcohol. The preoccupation continues even though the person has discontinued use (Brown, 1985).

Drinking Stage

During this stage, clients spend energy trying to control their consumption of alcohol. This, according to Brown, is when the alcohol axis focuses on control. The environmental interactions with family and friends can be stressed because of the alcohol use. The interpretation of self is that of denial, where the person may not recognize (or may not want to see) his or her consumption as problematic. Significant in the movement toward the transitional stage is the moment when clients begin to recognize their use as out of control (V. Lewis & Allen-Byrd, 2007). Typically this results from the mounting negative consequences of their use (Kurtz, 1979). Referring back to the stages of change (Prochaska & DiClemente, 1986) and the process of motivational interviewing (W. R. Miller & Rollnick, 2002), it is necessary to recognize how both models can be used effectively for clients in the drinking stage. For instance, a client in counseling for marital discord reveals he drinks "a lot" on the weekends, which is of great concern to his wife. The counselor at this point works with the client, using motivational interviewing to help the client examine and explore the impact alcohol has on his relationship with his wife and children. This exploration, in relation to the stages of change, may further equip the client in moving from contemplation to preparation. If this movement happens, he might begin preparing for behavioral changes (e.g., treatment, support group attendance, including wife in counseling).

Transition Stage

This stage indicates a significant change in thinking (of both self and the addiction) from "I am not an alcoholic and I can control my drinking" to "I am an alcoholic and I cannot control my drinking" (Brown, 1985). According to Brown, "The individual who has not truly surrendered or accepted the belief in loss of control may periodically shift back and forth from drinking to nondrinking. The abstinence is not a surrender to loss of control but a temporary compliance" (Brown, 1985, p. 34).

A poignant and significant alcohol axis shift in the client's thinking has moved from preoccupation with the next drink to preoccupation with not drinking. At this point, the client is thinking about times when drinking could possibly occur and the potential consequences of further use. The transition for clients is from a drinking lifestyle to a nondrinking lifestyle, which can present a challenge. Many times clients return to drinking, so it is important for counselors working with clients in this stage to help develop a sober support network for clients. Discussion of both support groups and treatment options is also critical during this stage of the process. The sense of identity is in transition; it moves from control and not alcoholic to not being in control and alcoholic (V. Lewis & Allen-Byrd, 2007). This internal angst is a significant aspect for counselors to recognize, which is the insanity of addiction.

Early Recovery Stage

In this stage clients not only identify themselves as recovering alcoholics but also begin to establish significant relationships with others in which alcohol is not present. The alcohol axis is focused on recovery and sober living. Environmentally, clients are supported by 12-step meetings, treatment, and support from significant others (i.e., family, friends, and work). For many, 12-step meetings are the primary source of support where the continuous focus on recovery is crucial. Brown (1985) suggested a developmental metaphor where clients in early recovery resemble toddlers requiring tremendous reassurance and support. According to Brown, the fellowship of Alcoholics Anonymous or Narcotics Anonymous provides structure, support, and tools for early and ongoing recovery efforts. The alcohol axis focuses on the core of a new identity: a sober person (V. Lewis & Allen-Byrd, 2007). Later in ongoing recovery, the alcohol focus decreases and attention to relationships increases. In early recovery, the person is acquiring a stronger sense of autonomy while continuing to attend support meetings.

Ongoing Recovery Stage

Ongoing recovery incorporates the exploration of spiritual beliefs as well as provides support to others. This altruistic behavior is best exemplified through community work, sponsorship, or the family. New ideas and behaviors, intertwined with the exploration of being a person in recovery within the family, community, and workplace, are created. Brown (1985) and V. Lewis and Allen-Byrd (2007) related this stage of recovery to that of the movement from adolescence to adulthood. In recovery, like in adolescence, individuals develop strong peer groups and lifelong relationships. Significant here is that clients choose meaningful relationships that further enhance their sobriety and new way of living.

Although individuals continue attendance at 12-step meetings, over time, the focus morphs from I/me thinking to helping others in their recovery efforts. This is also a time when problems other than alcohol may emerge. The new sobriety allows clients to attend to issues as life problems (e.g., career, physical, personal relationships) instead of viewing them as being an alcohol problem.

The metamorphosis from drinking to ongoing recovery moves clients from self to focusing on others. Bateson (1971) saw individuals moving from a view of self to that of viewing self within the context of others and the environment. Transition and early recovery are self-focused to promote the individual's attention on abstinence. This stance further enhances the development of support as a recovering individual. As the person becomes more comfortable in sobriety, the focus shifts to helping others and the development of new socially interested activities.

Application of Brown's Developmental Recovery Stages With a Client

For approximately 3 months you have been working in counseling with Jeb, who was initially self-referred because of his concern with depression. For the first month you met weekly with Jeb, actively exploring his level of overall functioning and his symptoms of depression. During this month, a strong therapeutic relationship and basic trust developed. After 1 month, Jeb disclosed that he was a daily pot smoker. He had been hiding this from you because he did not want to stop smoking and he did not want to disappoint you. He felt his low energy may be linked to his pot use and felt compelled to disclose it because he trusts you. You discover Jeb smokes approximately two joints per day and smokes continuously throughout the weekend. With this new understanding of the case, you process his rationale for disclosure and what he wants to do, if anything, about his use. Jeb reports he has tried to cut down, yet found it did not work for more than a month or two, at which time he was back smoking every day again. You explore what he is motivated to do at this point (i.e., continue using, cut down, or stop). He says he wants to stop and commits that between this current session and next week's session he will stop.

At the next session Jeb reports he stopped for 2 days. After the brief hiatus he smoked even more over the weekend. In turn, his increased weekend use caused him to be late for work on Monday (which has never happened before). Jeb appears nervous over the possibility of having to submit to a random urine test at work. Therefore, he was much more amenable to trying other alternatives such as outpatient treatment. He agrees to attend an outpatient appointment that week to try and engage in treatment. During treatment, you maintain regular monthly contact with his counselor (until he has completed outpatient treatment). At that point, he states his desire to return to you for continued individual counseling.

Commentary

Jeb has indicated his initial reluctance to abstinence; however, he was amenable to stopping. Jeb is in the drinking or using stage at this point where his thinking is "I am not addicted; I can control my using." Within a week he came to recognize some vital information: What he thought he could do alone, he could not. Along the way, the potential job jeopardy shifted him into the transitional stage of recovery, allowing another alternative to be explored. Jeb indicates fear and the need for structure and support that, at this time, he is unable to provide for himself. At the session following his tardiness to work he appears motivated and is transitioning to "I am addicted and I am not in control!" Thus, he is both motivated and ready to enter outpatient treatment.

Gorski's Developmental Model of Recovery

Similar to Brown's model of recovery is Terence Gorski's (1989) developmental model of recovery (DMR). This model begins with transition as the first stage; then stabilization; followed by early, middle, and late recovery; and ending with the maintenance stage. Known for his work with relapse prevention, Gorski developed the DMR to provide clients and counselors with a comprehensive model to use with associated stage goals to address in the recovery process. The DMR identifies recovery issues for both alcohol- and drug-addicted persons.

Transition Stage

This stage is similar to Brown's drinking stage of recovery in that denial and attempts to control usage are considered main elements. In Gorski's model, transition occurs when individuals attempt to control their usage. Examples of these attempts include changing either the time of day they drink or the type of drugs they ingest. During this stage they still have not connected life problems with alcohol or drug use. From this perspective, even though they may have three or four significant problems, they still believe none of the issues are directly related to their use of substances. The necessary cognitive shift does start to emerge when they recognize that their using is becoming out of control. This insight is driven primarily through experiencing negative consequences or recognizing excessive use. As a result, they will try and cut down or control their use to prove (to others and self) that their using is really not a problem.

The attempted control is characteristic of an individual who is ironically out of control. The logic that can be worked with clients at this point is as follows: "If you were in control, I wonder why you would need to cut back? If you don't feel it is a problem, why would you want to make any pattern changes in your drinking or drug use?" At this point addicted individuals find their attempts to control short lived, returning to use.

Counselors assist clients in the transition stage to connect consequences to their use of drugs and alcohol. When this shift occurs, the denial system breaks down, allowing clients to acknowledge the powerlessness and unmanageability. The end result is the client becoming increasingly willing to accept help.

Stabilization

Gorski (1989) outlined four specific goals during the stabilization stage. The first goal is the clients' recuperation from the use of the drug. This means discontinuation of their drugs and alcohol use, including, if necessary, using detoxification service. The second goal is the reduction in drug and alcohol preoccupation and increased focus on recovery and supportive relationships. The third goal is to better cope with stress without using chemicals. Finally, the fourth goal denotes developing hope and motivation to continue in recovery.

Post-Acute Withdrawal

When clients discontinue their use of chemicals, as we have discussed in chapter 3, an individual may go through detoxification and physical discomfort. Variables to be considered include the type of drug and the amount being abused. An acute detoxification is relatively short term. However, Gorski (1989) identified post-acute withdrawal (PAW) essentially as withdrawal that occurs long after the initial physical withdrawal symptoms. Not every client in stabilization will need (or benefit from) detoxification, nor will they experience PAW. PAW starts with the emergence of feeling overwhelmed by daily tasks, having difficulty making simple decisions, and managing stress ineffectively. Clients experiencing PAW may also become forgetful. PAW may occur during times of increased stress in the first 6 months to a year of recovery. Of importance in this stage is the need for clients to maintain contact with support groups, develop a healthy and balanced intake of food (minimizing caffeine and sugar intake), and increasing exercise. A structured daily plan reduces idle time and provides the needed support while the body stabilizes and heals. At this point, the cognitive recognition of the consequences related to drug and alcohol use come into awareness. This new insight surfaces stress and possibly triggers PAW symptoms. The importance of helping clients with stress identification and methods of management are critical. The challenge for most clients is managing the stressors without the use of chemicals. Counselors are in the position to aid in stress identification and help clients develop skills in managing anxiety and fear.

The initial process of abstinence in stabilization and early recovery also includes grief for the loss of the drug. Observing chemical use as a significant relationship in itself helps frame this response. The relationship has ended, thereby stress and grief from the loss would be quite normal. Talking about this process with clients who have feelings of sadness or anger is important. The clients' recognition and honoring of this loss is the beginning of early recovery; these are major factors to discuss when they are moving beyond the past relationship and moving on with new behaviors, thinking, and exploration.

Another task at this point for clients is to maintain motivation and energy toward a recovery program. Counselors may hear clients discuss feelings of boredom or anxiety in stabilization or early recovery periods. The zest and initial commitment may wane as clients experience the enormity of their addiction, the daily maintenance of a recovery program, and the work involved. Having clients involved in support groups in conjunction with treatment helps maintain their motivation.

Early Recovery Stage

The goals in this stage, according to Gorski (1989), identify the signs of possible relapse and break recovery down into two parts: (a) the drinking and drugging problem and (b) the thinking problem (the irrational thinking). From our professional experience, we've observed numerous clients relapsing between stabilization and early recovery. This is due to their lack of skills and resources in managing stress and cravings, limited supports, and being unwilling (or unable) to ask for help. Many clients hold the false belief that they can handle it on their own in recovery and control their use.

Counselors help clients explore their new role as a sober and clean person. They also explore clients' strengths and shortcomings, which helps to alleviate emotions of guilt and shame related to their use. Counselors identify the benefits of drugs and alcohol in the lives of their clients. The questions "What does alcohol or drugs allow you to do or become?" and "What does alcohol or drugs allow you to avoid or escape from?" help clients and counselors recognize the purpose for their use of chemicals. These questions further identify areas of needed development. For instance, if clients respond to the first question with "I feel more confident and able to express my feelings when I am using," it provides counselors with information to help their clients work on expressing feelings and developing trust and self-confidence. A response to the second question of "I use drugs to avoid dealing with my past" informs counselors on the areas that need to be explored in the counseling sessions. Without understanding these two questions, clients potentially will repeat the using patterns unless alternative behaviors or strategies are developed. Counselors strive to help clients on accepting their addiction and promoting new choices, freedom, and hope.

Middle Recovery Stage

According to Gorski (1989), this stage occurs when clients begin repairing their lives. This stage is additionally recognized by the client coming to grips with how he or she was impacted by addiction and working to develop a well-balanced lifestyle. Gorski used the analogy of getting injured in a car accident. First the paramedics stop the bleeding (transition), then the person goes to the hospital to be stabilized (stabilization), and then the process of early recovery begins. Middle recovery continues with lifestyle changes conducive to recovery and using recovery principles. This is also a time when clients make amends to those they have harmed because of their addiction. Making a list and eventually making amends represents a significant step in the healing process.

This stage involves holistic self-examination of the client, from emotional and physical growth to spiritual growth. With new behaviors come opportunities to enhance growth and create new choices.

Late Recovery

Clients in this stage have been sober and clean and feel better (mentally, emotionally, physically, and spiritually), yet may ask themselves "Is this all there is to recovery?" Gorski

(1989) recognized that this unhappiness in recovery stems from unresolved childhood issues merged with self-defeating thoughts and behaviors. Clients begin to explore childhood patterns of communication and behaviors that still play out in their adult lives. His suggestion to clients is to keep the chemical dependency focus for the first year of sobriety and not move directly into family issues until clients have a stable recovery and support system.

Gorski (1989) identified a number of challenges in this stage. The initial challenge is the inability of clients to engage in problem-solving thoughts and behaviors. Problems can grow and if left unattended, will result in major life stressors. A second issue is the unrefined skills of clients in managing emotion. A third issue is rigidity in behavior and the subsequent lack of flexibility with lifestyle changes. Taking care of others constantly is another issue that may surface along with people pleasing. Being a placater or entertainer also causes concern during this stage of development. Finally, blaming others or acting out in recovery are areas of challenge in the late recovery stage. Counselors can provide feedback on problem solving, a therapeutic environment for emotional exploration, and a sounding board for resentments and control issues.

Maintenance Stage

This is a lifelong stage, which has no end. Encapsulated in this stage is the primary focus on growing as a human being and developing a high quality of life. Individuals are maintaining what works for them in recovery and are able to address changes and problems as they occur. Should a significant problem arise, individuals are able to garner resources to effectively deal with the problem efficiently. This is done with little danger to their recovery process. Counselors at this stage may help clients focus on issues in life beyond alcohol- or drug-related problems. A client who enters counseling in the maintenance stage may delve into relationship issues as opposed to focusing primarily on alcohol or drug problems.

Application of Gorski's Developmental Model of Recovery With a Client

Carlos was in a horrible car accident that almost took his life. He was returning home late one night from a local bar, misjudged a turn, and collided into a tree. He was taken to the local hospital where he was treated for multiple contusions. While at the hospital he was charged with drunk driving (due to a .35 blood alcohol level). Carlos was recommended to stay in the hospital for 3 days to address his injuries and to detoxify from alcohol. Carlos is a daily drinker, consuming up to 12 beers per day. He continually has a small amount of alcohol in his bloodstream and has attempted to discontinue drinking alcohol once, which resulted in physical shakes and stomach pains.

Carlos is recommended to stay for 1 week in treatment and to attend group meetings in the inpatient unit for alcohol and drug addiction. He is recommended to follow up with outpatient treatment once he is discharged successfully from treatment.

At this point Carlos is willing to address his alcoholism. He has moved from transition, where he was drinking daily and was in denial, to stabilization, where he admits his drinking is alcoholic and is willing to take action in recovery. Carlos is being stabilized in inpatient treatment, where he will be referred to outpatient treatment and will receive help in his early recovery.

For the next year, Carlos attends outpatient treatment and Alcoholics Anonymous meetings. He manages his cravings for alcohol and develops a strong support network in recovery. He also begins working with his sponsor on making amends to those he has harmed in his addiction. Over the next few years he continues with 12- step meetings. Additionally, he initiates exploration into family communication issues, which are impacting his current relationships. He works at developing a healthier life, discontinues smoking cigarettes, and adds exercise to his daily routine. Additionally, Carlos reconnects with his Cuban heritage and embarks on a long-time passion: salsa dancing lessons.

The steps and processes that have helped Carlos maintain his sobriety are evident: He developed a support system, made amends, and worked on family issues and communication patterns in his life. As he continues to develop, he maintains his recovery, continues his spiritual journey, and reconnects with his cultural heritage (which was almost lost as a result of his drinking).

Gideon's Model of Recovery

We've included this model because we believe it outlines the internal process of addicted clients succinctly. Gideon (1975) described the *isolation* of the addict and alcoholic and the free-floating anxiety and tension that surround the individual in this stage. Feelings of guilt, loneliness, and irrational fears abound as the drinking and drugging increase. At the core of the addicted person are emotions of insecurity, inadequacy, and unworthiness. Gideon described how addiction creates both external and internal isolation for clients. He suggested that recovery occurs in *relation* to others. As a result of this interpersonal connection, anxiety and fear are reduced. Freedom, joy, and security are fostered in concert with openness and the ability to love both self and others. At the core are the development of self-worth and an eradication of irrational fears. The third stage, according to Gideon, is the *transformation stage* in which awareness and self-responsibility are present. A new identity as a recovering person focuses on the here and now, recognizing and facilitating connections between self, others, and the surrounding environment. This integration, in turn, leads to *self-actualization*, the final stage in the recovery process.

Application of Gideon's Model of Recovery

Gideon (1975) attended predominantly to the emotional disconnection of clients in addiction. Addiction is isolative by nature, leaving afflicted individuals feeling disconnected from their emotional makeup, as well as those around them. In recovery, clients embark on a difficult personal internal journey. This life transit results, for some, in meaningful connections with others. This is also why group counseling and support meetings are suggested as a means of helping the transitional process and connections with others.

Summary

This chapter provided readers with three human growth and development theories. It offered suggestions on how these models can be applied to work with addicted clients. In addition, three developmental models of recovery (Brown, Gorski, and Gideon) provided a conceptual understanding for assessment purposes as well as treatment planning. The similarity with each model provides counselors with an understanding of the internal recovery process and the options for use with clients, along with application to relapse prevention. Figure 7.1 presents each of these developmental models and how they can complement one another and provide a better understanding for both the clinician and the client in their work together.

Exploration Questions From Chapter 7

1. Discuss with a small group how you might use developmental ideology in working with your substance-abusing or addicted clients.
2. Looking at the clients you have been working with, which stage of development, according to Erikson, do you see most of your clients having difficulty with?
3. What gaps do you see in your own development and how have they impacted your adult life?

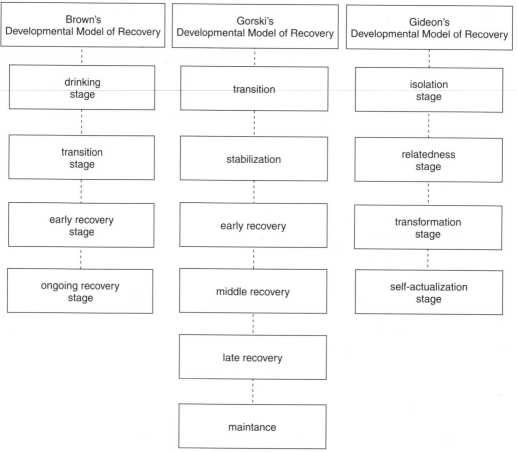

Figure 7.1. Summary of Developmental Models of Recovery

4. How do you see using the developmental approach with clients?
5. How might you work with an addicted client using a combination of the developmental approach and the medical model?

Suggested Activities

1. Talk with a sibling, parent, or relative about your upbringing. Ask them about any observations they made of you as a child that are present today?
2. Observe a young child and try to determine his or her age and developmental level.

Family and Addiction

So far this text has focused predominantly on multiculturalism, drugs, assessment, biopsychosocial underpinnings, treatment, developmental issues, and the internal changes of the individual addict and alcoholic. In this chapter the focus shifts to the family system, where addiction impacts each person in the family in one way or another (Crnkovic & DelCampo, 1998; V. Lewis & Allen-Byrd, 2007; Wegscheider, 1981). Alcohol and drug addiction is recognized as a significant contributor to family stress (Csiernik, 2002) and a demonstrable risk for child psychopathology (Bijttebier, Goethals, & Ansoms, 2006). Because of the power and presence of the addiction in the family system, we have also incorporated general systems theory into the chapter in order to provide the reader with a systemic approach.

In order for any problem, including addiction, to truly flourish within a system, the family system must have developed rules and guidelines to support the behavior (Goldenberg & Goldenberg, 2008). When counselors work with families, whether addiction exists or not, they are looking at the family as an organism (Brock & Barnard, 2009; Minuchin, 1974) and the relationships between each of its family members (Goldenberg & Goldenberg, 2008; Haly, 1986; Wells, 1998). This is referred to as a general systems approach. From this theoretical perspective, the interrelationships and communication patterns are explored within the family (Bertalanffy, 1968; Brock & Barnard, 2009).

Bepko and Krestan Stage Theory

Counselors working with family members assess the degree and magnitude with which addiction exists in the system. It is understood by systems theorists that change is inevitable in the family life cycle and therefore impacts the equilibrium of the family (Ansbacher & Ansbacher, 1956; DeJong & Kim Berg, 2008). Addiction in families significantly disrupts the system. The following stages developed by Bepko and Krestan (1985) help counselors understand the dynamics of working with families impacted by addiction.

The first stage, *establishing boundaries and identity,* involves working with families to unbalance family systems that occur when the addict/alcoholic stops using. Structural family therapy can be used to work with families in examining the family's rules that support the symptomatic behavior and to reconfigure the family's boundaries (Minuchin, 1974). In structural family therapy the family is viewed as a system with subsystems, a hierarchical structure, and boundaries. The structural counselor builds relationships with each member of the family and helps them to enact or act out in the therapy session. As the family develops rapport with the counselor, unbalancing can occur to restructure rules and boundaries within the family (Minuchin, 1974). Family members attending individual counseling or 12-step support groups also unbalance the system through subtle changes in attitude and behavior.

A balanced system is considered to have a prescribed set of behaviors for each member. These "guiding rules" have been handed down from one generation to another, are typically unspoken, and help the members of the system know what to expect from one another. Critical to understand here is that a system can be dysfunctional, chalked full of pain, and might be hurtful to members, yet still be balanced. Once someone or something interjects in a way that causes significant change in roles to occur, the system is considered unbalanced (Minuchin & Fishman, 1981).

During this stage the family is unbalanced, and overt attention is paid to identifying the imbalance within the system. The newly sober/clean person in the family, by nature of being abstinent, unbalances the system. Counselors help to create safety, facilitate clear communication, and develop healthier boundaries within the family.

Bepko and Krestan (1985) described the second stage, *commitment and stability*, as adjustment to sobriety while the family is restabilizing, regrouping, and authoring new roles in the system. The primary family focus is on alcohol or drugs. The major distinction here though is the focus on hoping he or she will not use again. In this stage the counselor redirects attention back onto each family member. Family members are encouraged to share and discuss their individual needs that have been neglected as a result of the active addiction in the family.

The final stage, *clarification and legacy*, involves rebalancing the system in order to support the goal of abstinence. Each family member identifies and explores new behaviors within the family in order to support the addict's recovery as well as the recovery of the family. This stage is an opportunity for tremendous movement and growth of individual members. For example, the 18-year-old sister of a client (older brother who has been stealing from the parents) may have decided (under the old rules) that college was out of the question because she had to "defend" the family home from the addict. With the new-found sobriety of the older brother, she may now reinvest in her future (including enrolling in college).

In addition to the stages, Bepko and Krestan (1985) developed 12 questions that can guide counselors when working with families in which addiction exists. In an effort to include drug addiction, the word *addiction* has been used.

1. "Where is the addiction in the family?" Through assessment with family members, determine who in the family drinks and/or drugs addictively.
2. "Who is most affected by the addiction?" Because addiction impacts the entire family in innumerable ways, this question is difficult to ascertain.
3. "Is it really addiction?" Some addicts and/or alcoholics may use heavily or excessively; however, their use may not be considered addictive.
4. "In what phase is the drinking/drugging behavior?" This question helps to determine if the addiction is early onset (e.g., feelings of guilt, increasing tolerance) or chronic, late-stage using (e.g., morning usage, shakes after using).
5. "What phase is the family in?" Is the family in early phase (establishing boundaries and identity), middle phase (commitment and stability), or late phase (clarification and legacy)?
6. "What phase of the life cycle is the addict and/or alcoholic in?" What issues and impacts is the addict/alcoholic having on the family?
7. "What does the family think about the addiction?" Find out from members their thoughts or viewpoints on the addiction. Not everyone will agree the drinking or drugging is addictive; some members may see it as stress relief.

8. "What solutions have the family already attempted?" This question explores how the family has tried to deal with the addiction.
9. "What does the secrecy map look like?" In working with families where addiction exists, counselors understand that family secrets are prevalent (e.g., sexual abuse, extramarital affairs).
10. "What is the family history of addiction?" Determining who and where the alcoholics or addicts are in the extended family can help counselors understand patterns to best help the family.
11. "What patterns of over- and underresponsibility exist?" Who in the family is overcompensating for the addiction, and who in the family is not taking responsibility?
12. "How is the power structure perceived in the family?" Who has the perceived power versus who really has the power in the family?

These questions help counselors determine the structure of the family, including who has the power, who is aligned with whom, and where the addiction exists, both currently and by history. The collected data will guide effective family counseling and treatment recommendations. In addition to using these questions, identifying where the family is in relation to the family life cycle can also aid with effective family planning.

Family Life Cycle

Carter and McGoldrick (1999) outlined expected stages in the family life cycle, providing counselors with an understanding of how addiction could impact each stage of family development. Although these stages are traditional, we believe they can be useful in conceptualizing the impact, role, and essence of addiction within a family system.

The first stage in the life cycle is the *beginning family.* In this stage, the associated developmental tasks are for the couple to differentiate from the family of origin, develop boundaries between family members, resolve conflicts between them, and identify needs within the couple. The second stage describes the family with *infants and preschoolers.* Resulting from the onset of children, the family renegotiates responsibilities and tasks and provides safety and authority to encourage growth. The third stage, identified as the *school age family*, renegotiates responsibilities within the household. This is accomplished by encouraging discussion of feelings when children are not able to handle school and deciding who will help with the schoolwork. The *adolescent family* addresses the balance between adolescent autonomy and parental control. Also significant during this stage is the changing role of the parent(s). These negotiations prepare the adolescent to leave home. The *launching family* is the fifth stage when the adolescent separates from the family and leaves in a healthy manner to enter college, a career, trade school, the military, or the world of work. The *postparental family* discusses how the couple's relationship will change and how to best use time.

Family Roles in Addicted Families

Counselors working with families impacted by addiction recognize the effects on children and adults (Csiernik, 2002). Vanderlip (2007) described how addiction can impact the children in the family. Children living with a parent who is not in a recovery process for his or her addiction experience significantly impacted stress levels within the family. Even potential future grandchildren may be hampered in their ability to grow developmentally (Moe, Johnson, & Wade, 2007). Further, communication within the addicted family is reported as distant and noncommunicative. Children of alcoholics (COAs) are four times more likely than non-COAs to develop alcoholism and are more likely to be the focus of physical abuse. Research indicates that one in four children in the United States has been exposed to alcohol abuse or dependence in the family (Grant, 2000). COAs are at risk for behavioral problems and tend to be aggressive, impulsive, and sensation seeking. In the United States, currently there are 8.3 million children who live with at least one parent who is in need of treatment for alcohol or drug dependency. One in four children under the age of 18 is living in a home where alcoholism or alcohol abuse is a fact of daily life. In addition, countless others are exposed to illegal drug use in their families (U.S. Department of Health and Human Services, n.d.). Vanderlip continued by stating that COAs appear to have lower self-esteem than non-COAs (in childhood, adolescence, and young adulthood). Research has indicated higher levels of self-reported stress, difficulty initiating the use of mediating factors in response to life events, and increased symptoms of personal dysfunction for the ACOA than for peers who did not experience either trauma or alcoholism during childhood (C. W. Hall & Webster, 2002; C. W. Hall, Webster, & Powell, 2003). Young children of alcoholics many times show symptoms of depression, anxiety, bedwetting, few friends, or are fearful of attending school. Teens may show depressive symptoms through perfectionism, isolating, hoarding, or developing phobias, which can impact school abilities. COAs tend to score lower on tests that measure cognitive and verbal skills and are more likely to drop out of school or be referred to a school counselor. According to Ruben (2001), COAs also tend to follow a number of rules: Don't talk about family problems or emotions, limit communication about what occurs at home, nothing is ever good enough, don't be selfish, do as I say and not as I do, avoid play and conflict.

COAs also benefit from awareness of the characteristics and the roles in the addicted system. The 1980s brought a great deal of attention to family treatment and ACOA approaches to wellness. Therapists and researchers (Ackerman, 1983; Black, 1981; Crnkovic & DelCampo, 1998; Gravitz & Bowden, 1985; Wegscheider, 1981; Woititz, 1983) highlighted the importance of addressing ACOA issues for prevention and intervention purposes and to aid in the recovery of the family. Sharon Wegscheider-Cruise expanded on family roles after having trained with Virginia Satir, a well-known family therapist who first described similar family roles. The family roles Wegscheider (1981) created were specific to the addicted family. She found that as children from addicted families grew to adults, their adherence to these survival roles solidified, impacting life choices. These roles, useful in childhood when active addiction existed, served as coping mechanisms (Rice, Dandreaux, Handley, & Chassin, 2006). In adulthood, the roles that once protected no longer served a significant purpose. In opposition, they interfered with the development of healthy relationships. In a research study conducted by Devine and Braithwaite (1993), an early attempt was made to operationalize and measure the profiles of COAs that Black (1981) and Wegscheider (1981) compiled through clinical observations. The results indicated that there is no reason to assume that the roles described and measured in their studies are solely related to COAs. Devine and Braithwaite suggest that practitioners should regard the roles as coping responses of children who are threatened by the family situation they are living in. Table 8.1 outlines each role with a description of characteristics and subsequent negative impacts of the role if left unaddressed.

The Hero

The hero of the family is typically the oldest child or an only child. The hero tends to be a rescuer and assumes the responsibilities of both the addicted person and other members of the family. The hero rarely gets into trouble. Typically, the hero internalizes negative emotions. Although the hero many times is an overachiever with sports, grades, or abilities, internally the hero feels inadequate and/or guilty. In addition to "looking good" the hero attempts to keep the addiction a family secret from others. The hero rarely discusses the family secret. The hero serves as the family confidant, thus setting up boundary problems. The hero may also help raise the other children in the family. If the hero receives counseling, he or she can learn to accept failures and see imperfections (Black, 1981; Devine & Braithwaite, 1993; Wegscheider, 1981).

Table 8.1. Roles in the Addicted Family

Role	Characteristic of Role	Negative Aspect of Role	With Changes to
Hero	Responsible Successful High achiever	Guilty Inadequate Anxious	Self-acceptance Setting limits Verbalizes emotions
Scapegoat	Legal system Rule breaker Authority issues	Incarceration Addiction Unhappy	Expresses emotions appropriately Becomes effective counselor Respects rules
Lost Child	Isolated Lonely Invisible	Depressed Suicidal Disconnected	Connected to others Creative Good listeners
Mascot	Immature Joker Poor work history	Relationship problems Financial problems Inadequate	Resilient Humor is appropriate Responsible
Addict/Alcoholic	Intoxicated Irresponsible Emotionally unstable	Death Many losses Isolated from feelings	Recovery Family reconnection Helps others
Coaddict/Coalcoholic	Resentful Overresponsible Enabling behavior	Depressed Loss of self Lonely	Serene Sets limits Connected to others

The Scapegoat

The scapegoat tends to appear defiant, angry, and may be the one to act out behaviorally. School counselors may observe these students as loud, aggressive, and rule breaking, with little consideration of the consequences. Inwardly, however, scapegoats may feel hurt and rejected from a tumultuous home life. Their role at home may include being blamed for the problems of the family. This blame results from an agreement to focus on the scapegoat's problematic behaviors as opposed to the addiction. As a result, the negative behavior diverts the attention away from the real problem, which is the addiction. Scapegoats are typically second children, and at some point in their development they realize they cannot compete with the hero. The scapegoat is at high risk for developing addiction problems and getting negatively involved with the legal system. With counseling, however, the scapegoat can learn to take responsibility, be realistic, and express feelings appropriately (Black, 1981; Devine & Braithwaite, 1993; Wegscheider, 1981).

The Lost Child

The lost child tends to feel isolated and unimportant. He or she provides relief to the family through invisibility. Depending on the birth order, lost children typically are middle or youngest children. They tend to be shy, have few friends, and have difficulty making decisions. As they develop they become more withdrawn, may become depressed and suicidal, or sexually act out. With counseling and support they can develop talents and ask for support and help by learning to trust others (Black, 1981; Devine & Braithwaite, 1993; Wegscheider, 1981).

The Mascot

The mascot brings levity to the home and provides a distraction. Mascots tend to be internally fragile and immature in behavior. Their fear is suppressed internally, while externally their hyperactivity, learning disabilities, and short attention spans are manifest. Over time the mascot may develop physical problems such as ulcers from stress. They sometimes seek out heroes to take care of them in adulthood. With counseling and support, the mascot can be taken more seriously, continue to have a good sense of humor, and take responsibility for his or her behavior (Black, 1981; Devine & Braithwaite, 1993; Wegscheider, 1981).

The Alcoholic or Addict

This role is identified by the chemical use of the family member. Internally the addict may feel a deep sense of shame and inadequacy, and externally appears irresponsible and uncaring. This role seeks pleasure from drugs and alcohol and, because of this, impacts the lives of family and friends. With help, this person can begin a recovery process and play a significant role in the recovery of the family through role modeling and support.

The Coalcoholic or Coaddict

The coalcoholic's or coaddict's primary focus is on the addict's use and the consequences related to such use. These individuals take responsibility, thereby providing a levy between the consequences and the addict. Enablers are typically quite responsible. An example of this is that they may obtain a second job in order to offset the money spent on drugs and consequences and the alcoholic's or addict's behavior. Although they voice a sense of powerlessness, enablers tend to be outwardly in control. Internally they may feel frustrated and resentful for having to assume so much responsibility. As a result of taking such responsibility, enablers may be isolated from support. This can lead to the internalization of their feelings, creating stress-induced illnesses (such as depression and ulcers). With support and help in counseling, the enabler can discontinue enabling behaviors and focus on his or her own growth.

A counselor's professional role dictates in what ways he or she might interact with an ACOA client. School counselors will find many of these characteristics present in their students. Whether elementary or secondary, students referred for counseling may be acting out in response to the active addiction at home. The impact of familial alcoholism and drug addiction on children is significant (Black, 1981). For counselors working with children and adolescents, understanding developmental models of recovery helps identify and therapeutically effect change with this particular population (V. Lewis & Allen-Byrd, 2007). Counselors in mental health settings may counsel adult children from addicted families. These clients may present with relationship problems, depression, or anxiety disorders. College counselors may discover that clients enter counseling with relationship issues, developmental challenges, and experimental alcohol and drug use (Jones & Kinnick, 1995).

In our experience, family work with addiction as a primary issue is far messier and more complex than work with a family not struggling with addiction issues. For example, I (Bill) worked with a family who presented to counseling with a concern about the 12-year-old son. There was no mention initially of any addiction issues within the system.

While working with the family, it became apparent that there was a large unexplored and unspoken concern that was being "protected." From a systems perspective, I was aware that the system had created some rules about who can know what about the issue. I also knew that the 12-year-old was the "scapegoat," or as referred to in family systems work, the identified patient (IP). The family wanted me to "buy" the story that the IP was the thing that needed to be fixed.

Over several sessions, I joined the dance of the system by using their sense of humor, openness (to other issues), and care for others. Having successfully joined the system, I began to suggest "reframes" for the roles of the addicted family members.

For the IP (who was suggested by the family to have the problems of not listening, defying them, and becoming increasingly problematic in school) I reframed his role as being really important to the family to remind them of how much love and care they have for one another—that even when facing tough times, the family does not "ditch" one another. This message was also meant to suggest to the addicted family member (the father) that he could move in another direction and that the family would not abandon him (a suspected concern). I also suggested how the 12-year-old's behavior was developmentally appropriate, as he *was* becoming an adolescent and that somehow he had learned to resist the status quo and find his way toward the right direction. This reframe suggested to the family that *they* could go in a different direction as a system as well. I reframed the intentions of the 6-year-old daughter as being important for the family to see the joy and hope in life, even though she was rarely the center of attention. As the "lost child" she was also a beacon of hope to the father that, as the message was intended to suggest, hope and joy *could* return to his life. The "hero," the mother, had a powerful mix of feelings like she needed to maintain order in the insanity of the system while feeling immense guilt over her "mistakes." I offered the reframe that she was the engine of the family. This metaphor was intended to reflect her power in maintaining the problem or finding a solution.

The reframes in themselves were not intended to "fix" the problem but merely to introduce (through the members' current roles) potential new directions. By honoring their current positions in life, I met them where they were.

Several sessions later, as I had suspected, the father's addiction was disclosed (by him). No one in the family appeared shocked or surprised. Rather, there seemed to be a sense of relief that the powerful hidden source of energy had been revealed to someone outside the system.

Some important concepts from this case include the initial suggestion from the family that the 12-year-old boy was the IP. This served two purposes for them: It could start the helping process without breaking the family rule of sharing the secret, and it could (if the addiction issue had not been disclosed) have had the counselor "fixing" the 12-year-old. In essence, the "fix" would have been to quiet the 12-year-old who, according to general systems theory, was probably behaving in "loud" ways to alert someone outside the system to the problem (addiction).

Regardless of your specialty (e.g., school, college, mental health), understanding the roles and possible directions of counseling with families with addiction issues is critical to both recognition and successful work. Important in the work with those impacted by addiction are the support groups. The following groups are available for families and friends of those addicted to alcohol and drugs.

Al-Anon, Nar-Anon, Al-a-Teen, Al-a-Tot, Families Anonymous, and ACOA Support Meetings

Counselors incorporate support groups in an effort to provide something they as counselors cannot facilitate, a true understanding of what it is like to be in relationship with an alcoholic or addict. Al-Anon was established shortly after Alcoholics Anonymous by Lois Wilson (Haaken, 1993). She believed, as did her husband Bill Wilson (cofounder of Alcoholics Anonymous), that fellowship and unity offered hope to those feeling hopeless. Al-Anon is open to family members or friends of an alcoholic looking for support. Nar-Anon is for families and friends of those addicted to drugs. Al-a-Teen is for teenagers living with a parent who is addicted, and Al-a-Tot is for young children living with addiction. Families Anonymous supports parents with a child or adolescent who is abusing or is addicted to drugs or alcohol. ACOA is a support group for adults who have been raised or are living with alcoholism or addiction. Each of these meetings follows the 12 steps of Alcoholics Anonymous, which will be explored later in the text.

Because addiction is isolating, these focused and supportive groups break the cycle of isolation and provide clients with a nurturing environment. Counselors recognize that family members attending meetings are able to make changes in their behavior. Further, these individuals are supported in maintaining the changes, in part, because of the support they receive at the meetings. For families interested in conducting an intervention, attendance can offer support and pragmatic information during the difficult preparation period as well as the actual intervention event.

Intervention Strategies for Both Family and Addicted Member

Counselors often find family members engage in counseling not necessarily for themselves but rather to help those identified as the alcoholic or addict. The first contact by family members usually pertains to methods and means of intervening on the addicted person. We have provided a typical initial phone call to walk readers through the process of engaging family members in the counseling process.

Case Example: Tawny

I (Bill) respond to a call on my voicemail. Tawny says she is concerned about her mother's use of alcohol and wants to "get her help." As I talk with Tawny, it is apparent that she is not interested in getting help for herself but rather just for her mother. Interestingly enough, however, is that Tawny is married to a "problem drinker" but "he doesn't drink like my mom does." Although Tawny ultimately wants help for her mother, I first discuss the possible need for Tawny to come in for the first session to determine potential steps to help her mother. Once Tawny arrives for her session, I can more fully assess how progressed her mother's drinking has become. I will also be able to better determine the impact it has (and has had) on Tawny. Exploring the alcoholism, while validating Tawny's feelings, is the first step in helping her mother. Paradoxically, in order to help her mother, Tawny needs to intervene on her own enabling behaviors. In family systems theory, this is called *joining the system*. In this case, the joining takes place through the relationship with Tawny. Providing a trusting, therapeutic relationship and suggesting outside support meetings (ACOA or COA 12-step meetings) might be an effective start. This is just one example of a family member coming in for help. However, there are four basic methods to intervention, which are described below.

Intervention Approaches

As counselors provide individual therapy for family members, one goal is to examine the ways their behaviors may contribute to the enabling patterns. If successful, the possibilities for family intervention increase. There are a variety of intervention approaches. The choice to use one instead of another depends primarily on who is willing to be involved in the process. The varieties of intervention are the systemic family intervention, the instant intervention, the professional intervention, and the Johnson model of intervention.

The *systemic family intervention* involves family therapy focused on combining family behavioral change with individual recovery within a family context. A counselor who understands enabling behaviors, and the dynamics and roles that occur in the family, can help facilitate the family toward growth. The identified chemically dependent person in the family is invited to each family session. For example, Tawny meets individually with her counselor and begins to identify her personal characteristics, the roles she plays, and her enabling behaviors that contribute to the family dysfunction. In counseling she learns to set limits and boundaries and to detach with compassion from the alcoholism. Because of her own growth, she is able to invite family members into the counseling process. At this point she is also better equipped to facilitate her mother joining therapy (to participate and ultimately receive treatment and support). Continued below is what occurs in counseling with Tawny.

Tawny's Intervention

Tawny comes in for counseling and decides to focus primarily on her mother's drinking. It is clear, from Tawny's report, that her mother is an alcoholic in the later stages of alcoholism. You contract with Tawny to follow through on a number of counseling goals. The first goal is to become educated and informed about her mother's illness. This includes being willing to obtain support for herself to assist her mother. She agrees to attend one Al-Anon meeting between sessions and to inform her mother that she is going to see a counselor about her mother's drinking. The plan is for Tawny to invite her mother to the next session.

So far you are working with Tawny on her goals and how to best help her mother while negotiating with her to obtain support and learn more about alcoholism. You further contract with Tawny to stay involved in a counseling process for at least the next month.

The following week, Tawny is accompanied by her mother, looking angry and distressed. Once you close the door, her mother, Betsy, berates her daughter and you for talking about her drinking behind her back. She reports she came to this appointment only to hear what kind of lies her daughter is telling you.

The mother is now engaged in the process, albeit angrily. From this point you could facilitate a dialogue between the two and have Tawny express her concerns. A number of possible scenarios could follow the session. Betsy could become emotional, actually be able to hear her daughter's concerns, and be willing to enter treatment. Betsy could also get up during the session and leave, never to return. She could say to Tawny and to you how drinking is not a problem, at which point you could suggest an experiment of abstinence for the next week. You could suggest that they both return and discuss how Tawny's Al-Anon meeting went.

The basic idea is to engage both Tawny and her mother in a therapeutic process. Additionally, a major objective is to help Tawny obtain support and have Betsy begin to explore her drinking. Ultimately, of course, the best outcome would be for Betsy to get sober and for Tawny to discontinue enabling behaviors. Counselors need to be patient and willing to empathize with the struggles, sadness, and hurt.

The *instant intervention* responds directly to the crisis at hand. The intervention is swift and relies primarily on the crisis at the moment to motivate the addict or alcoholic into treatment. For example, a client is released from jail after having been arrested for possession of cocaine. Upon his release he is brought to counseling by his family, at which time he immediately enters treatment, based primarily on the legal crisis. The client enters treatment, understanding that if he fails to comply, his family will evoke the bond they posted and he will be returned to jail.

The *professional intervention* is conducted by a group of colleagues who have some amount of leverage in helping the client enter treatment. For example, a partner in a law firm has been absent from work, has spent a great deal of the firm's money on miscellaneous expenditures (drugs), has significant mood swings, and has been caught with cocaine in his office drawer. The partners in the firm agree to provide him an opportunity to enter treatment or no longer be employed as a partner in the firm. Because this option is presented by his colleagues, it is a significant motivator for obtaining treatment. Many state licensing boards around the country have impaired professional services that help facilitate and monitor professionals who place themselves and others in jeopardy. These boards may place individuals on probationary status or indefinitely suspend their licenses to practice medicine, law, or nursing until sufficient treatment and recovery time are demonstrated.

The *Johnson method of intervention* was developed by Vernon Johnson (1980) and incorporates several of the major constructs found in other popular intervention processes. Johnson proposed that family members become educated on addiction and outside support throughout the intervention process. One major difference is that he believed the primary step should be a systemwide intervention. Subsequent to the family intervention is the intervention with the addicted member. Counselors who work predominantly with interventions help clients identify enabling behaviors in the family and construct individualized plans for family recovery. The family members who avail themselves of these sessions most often desire that their loved one receive treatment. Therefore, these members are willing to engage in self-examination and change.

Counselors who specialize in this mode of therapy are referred to as interventionists. Typically they have specific training and credentials to effectively and professionally intervene and work with the potential fallout of such processes. In the preparation phase, the family prepares individual lists that relate specific, factual incidents when the addicted family member affected them. For instance, Tawny may write down her emotions related to her mother being drunk at her high school graduation. She might highlight her internalized response of feeling embarrassed in front of her peers.

Once compiled, family members practice reciting the lists while role playing the intervention process with the counselor. This all occurs in preparation for the actual intervention. In this model, the addict is unaware of the preparation and is usually surprised when it occurs.

Once the counselor determines that the family is ready, the time, place, and date are set for the intervention. The actual time of the intervention is usually when the addicted person is most vulnerable. This is most often in the morning, after a long evening of using. At the actual intervention, the addicted family member is asked to stay and hear the concerns of the family.

Following the expression and sharing of emotions and specific events, the family asks for this person to enter treatment. Generally, if the family is prepared, the individual will be amenable for help. However, should the person refuse, family members are prepared to share what behaviors they will discontinue if treatment is refused. These behaviors can range from loss of financial support to initiating divorce proceedings. The spirit of this is not punitive but rather a statement by family members to the addict that they can no longer participate or be an active part in the addiction process because it is too emotionally painful.

Summary

Most effective addiction treatment programs have a family component that strongly encourages family participation. Treatment programs recognize addiction as a systemic issue. This awareness causes many programs to require family member attendance in sessions before they are able to visit the loved one. Family programs include education, group and family counseling, and referrals to outside support groups and counseling.

This chapter outlined family stages, pertinent therapeutic questions, family roles, therapeutic approaches, family support groups, and intervention methods. Regardless of the specialization a counselor chooses, he or she will work (directly or indirectly) with children and adults who have been affected by a family member using substances.

Exploration Questions From Chapter 8

1. What are your thoughts on the ACOA characteristics? Explore how you might use this list of characteristics with clients.
2. How might you motivate a family or family member to obtain help or support for themselves?
3. Discuss the pros and cons that you see regarding the use of a developmental perspective.
4. How have you observed secrets to affect families?
5. Describe the coping skills or strengths that could be developed from growing up in an addicted family.

Suggested Activities

1. Talk with the family counselor or coordinator at a local treatment center and explore his or her challenges in the position of working with families of addicts or alcoholics.
2. In a small group, discuss which role you might have played in your family, even though addiction may not have been present. Continue to discuss how client roles in the family might impact treatment progress.

Grief and Loss in Addiction

A s professional counselors, we have come to recognize the power and weight of grief and loss issues in all forms of counseling. No lives are lived without the impact of such heavy issues. Clients cope with grief and loss in various ways. Among these mechanisms of dealing with pain, anger, and regret is the use (and in some cases increased use) of drugs and/or alcohol. Beyond the increase or changed pattern in the ingestion of substances as a form of coping with loss is a second paramount issue for counselors working with this population to consider: the loss and associated grief of the substance itself when working through the recovery process (Streifel & Servanty-Seib, 2006). Because grief and loss are so clearly integrated into the patterns of addiction, we felt it imperative to call out the relationship between substance abuse/addiction and issues of grief and loss. This chapter highlights the substantial overlap of the two.

Counselors should recognize that there are patterns and stages that describe the potential emergence of grief and loss as a core issue for a client (Worden, 2002). We will use two primary theories to help counselors better recognize and understand the potential relationship between substance issues and grief and loss concerns.

Before we start, however, we would like to offer our perception of an operating definition and description of grief and loss. We have found that many counselors recognize the typical (major) losses in life (e.g., death, loss of a job, divorce). However, we use an expanded definition for our work that includes loss of any and all aspects of behavior, attitude, understanding, worldview, and/or sense of self that is recognized by the client (consciously or unconsciously). This expanded definition, of course, includes the loss of the substance itself in persons in recovery (Rando, 1995). Additional examples might include significant physical changes (e.g., a 53-year-old woman entering menopause, a 17-year-old high school wrestler finishing his last competitive sporting event), changes in relationships (e.g., coworkers who have worked in an office for the past 10 years being sent to two different departments within the company), or changes in the world order (e.g., a 13-year-old girl discovering through a news broadcast that genocide is occurring in another country). We could go on, but you get the point that grief and loss encompass many aspects of clients' experiences both within self and their understanding of the world around them (Stroebe & Schut, 1999).

Grief and loss describe two separate yet interconnected concepts. Loss connotes the idea that some thing has been removed. Grief identifies the overall affective response to the loss. In other words, grief associates with feelings whereas loss is a cognitive-oriented structure. This is an important distinction because when working with clients who abuse or are addicted to substances, counselors must work to help these clients reorganize their core thoughts and feelings around the loss and associated grief.

Kübler-Ross (1969) demonstrated the stages associated with the actual loss and subsequent grief response by the client. Her work has identified stages that are normal along the route to successfully working through the stages of grief and loss. Worden (2002), who used the frame of "the mourning process," recognized an additional process that included tasks as a means of helping counselors identify direction with clients. The following discussion uses both theories as guides to understanding how clients with substance abuse issues may present in each stage or task.

Kübler-Ross

In her seminal work, Dr. Elisabeth Kübler-Ross (1969) recognized, identified, and described five core stages of grief and loss with terminally ill patients. Though these stages have been identified as being linear in fashion by some, we believe there is no clear pattern or fashion in which all clients progress through the stages; in fact, in many cases we have found clients emerging from one stage only to reenter shortly thereafter. Her general categorizations are denial, anger, bartering, depression, and acceptance.

Denial

Clients in this stage either dramatically minimize or completely ignore the truth that they had a significant loss. For example, a client who is starting the recovery process for the first time may state, "I really don't miss alcohol." Of course, in this stage they really do believe that they really don't and will not miss alcohol. In point of fact, as they continue recovery they will need to address those parts of alcohol that they really will miss (e.g., the sense of connection they felt with others while under the influence).

Another example of denial is a client who recently lost her husband. Perhaps she has always had a glass or two of wine for dinner. Now, 3 months after the death of her husband, she is drinking nearly a bottle of wine. While under the influence of alcohol, she can avoid the reality of the death and loss. If left unchecked and unnoticed, this ineffective coping mechanism of drinking to repress the loss may result in addiction.

In general we have found this type of client to be cheerful, resistant, and/or hard to pin down when discussing use patterns and loss issues.

Anger

Clients in this stage experience and express anger as a means to cope with the loss. For example, a client confronted with excess use patterns may become extremely angry with the counselor, friend, or family member. Such a response can be seen in the following client: A client who has been sober for 6 months (this is the first time in recovery) may, upon the reality of living life clean, have some significant losses (e.g., financial, career, relational). Each loss may be met by the client's frame that "the world has hurt and pained me, and I am angry." The ferocity of such a strong reaction to the perceived negative factors, if left unchecked, may result in subsequent use to "dull the anger."

Another example of the anger stage is the client who starts using substances with increased regularity to alter her or his mood from angry and upset (over the loss) to joyful and happy. In the event that such a behavior pattern is left unchecked, the client may continue to use in increasing amounts and, as with the previous case, result in significant additional losses that then must be medicated away.

We have found these clients to present as angry with us, the referring counselor/agency, and/or their families for placing them in counseling. In some cases, the anger is directed inward and other self-destructive behaviors surface (e.g., self-injurious behavior).

Bartering

Clients in this stage tend to have thoughts and actions that mirror the following statement: "If I stop drinking, then the loss will be reversed." For example, a client who is contemplating starting recovery may think "If I quit using drugs, then my wife will return to me and we will get along joyfully." Though we have seen the power of recovery heal deep wounds, in this case the client may be building too much hope on the outcome of the behavior. In essence, the client is thinking that abstinence will equate to a joyful relationship. The relationship falling short will probably result in rapid relapse. There is too much weight on the external force (the relationship) and far too little on the internal force (personal responsibility and personal growth).

Another example of bartering may be the client who uses substances to ward off the overwhelming guilt associated with the loss. For example, the client who has the repeated self-statement of "If only I had been a better son, my mom would have loved me more" may find solace and refuge in substances that alter or change that particular story.

In general, we have found this type of client to be sorrowful, have a diminished self-esteem, and express unrealistic guilt and regret related to many matters out of his or her control.

Depression

Clients may intertwine addictive substances with the depression in this stage of loss to "feel again" or to attain the fictional feeling of control and increased self-esteem. Though clients typically spend time in this stage after a significant loss, it is clear that increased use of substances typically results in a prolonged stay in the stage along with an increase in the severity of the depressed feelings.

Consider an 18-year-old woman who spent much of her life practicing to become the best soccer player she could. She involved herself in every possible way with the sport. She had posters on the wall of soccer players, class notes interspersed with drawings of soccer fields (with associated players and plays), and all she seemed to talk about with friends and family was her passion for soccer.

Having played so much soccer (every league she could join) and being skilled, she was typically in the middle of the action. It was not uncommon for her to sustain a concussion every now and again. In her last game she was concussed, and the doctor told her she could no longer play soccer as she had developed "concussion syndrome." Another concussion might result in significant damage to her brain and the possibility of a stroke. Devastated, she obviously had been dealt a powerful and unexpected loss. The diagnosis marked the end of her "current" competitive athletic career. Dreams of playing in college, the Olympics, and professionally were crushed.

She sinks into a deep depression. Where soccer used to fill her life with joy, bliss, and a sense of self, she now has a hole to fill, along with a very depressed mood. Entering college not long after the diagnosis, she has new time on her hands, limited social skills, and the right atmosphere to explore the use of drugs and alcohol. After finding a reinvigorated sense of self through the parties she attends (not noticing she is using increasing amounts of alcohol), she moves out of the depressed stage. However, behaviorally she has built a high tolerance and finds alcohol useful (in small amounts initially) in starting her day and socializing with others (in classes and around the dorm area).

Flash forward 12 years. Though still using alcohol in high amounts, she has learned to manage and function in life fairly well, until she received her third driving under the influence (DUI) charge (while driving her 7-year-old daughter to soccer practice). Fined and ordered by the court to attend counseling, she begins the recovery process.

After she moves through the recovery process, she starts to exhibit signs of depression. Here we want to recall the multiple layers of client issues and concerns. If the counselor fails to address the loss of the substance (alcohol), loss of sense of self (when under the influence), and previous loss of soccer, the client might be left to continue to battle the contributing factors to her depressed mood. We suggest that not addressing each of the significant losses will probably increase the chance of a significant relapse by the client. On the other hand, addressing and helping her find ways to cope more effectively with the loss of an athletic career may be a significant part of her personal plan of recovery. For example, choosing a healthier lifestyle might be both beneficial in helping her body heal from the effects of years of alcohol abuse and might help ward off negative thoughts that lean her toward depressed feelings. Suggestions we might have in this case include yoga, running, hiking, biking, or the like as a part of her overall recovery plan. A goal might be for her to compete with herself to increase the likelihood that she will be able to replace the loss of competitive sports. Additionally, she might be encouraged to join a group or class to reinstill the team experience she lost with soccer. Finally, the behavioral replacement of a healthy liquid (water) when working out instead of the unhealthy liquid (alcohol) might be an important distinction to draw for her cognitive awareness of the replacement process.

Yet another route with this client might be to have her become active with youth soccer. The guilt and regret that may be fueling her depressed thoughts related to use (especially with her daughter) might be countered by becoming more active and engaged and helping her daughter learn to play soccer. Giving back to the community, along with using previous skills (her knowledge of soccer), might greatly benefit her self-esteem and sense of self in relation to others. Such experiences could lead to a new understanding of herself and reauthoring of the soccer chapter of her life.

Acceptance

Clients in this stage have come to terms with the loss and made meaning, to some degree, of the grief over the loss. Of course, this does not denote full acceptance or recognition of life as being better after the loss. One example of this is the loss of a child. The parents may never fully recover and accept the loss as being a transition point after which their lives are better. They will, however, in this stage, have made meaning out of the death and have accepted the "new" world in which they find themselves.

Of critical and special note here is that with many other stage models, most clients do not progress in a linear or direct fashion. In fact, for many, they will recycle through and have to readdress issues in each of the stages described above. We have found also that many of our clients exhibit more than one stage concurrently. In this regard, counselors must be fully aware that real clients are never as neat and orderly as they might expect from reading this model. Kübler-Ross (1969) and Worden (2002) identified the concern of beginning counselors trying to move clients in a regimented way through the stages. We have found that most clients must visit each stage and that only when they have successfully resolved the concerns and addressed their particular issues in each stage can they move more fully toward acceptance. For us the core question, once we have identified a possible stage the client is in, is to ask ourselves, "What do they need to get from anger, denial, bartering, etc.?" We find this to be the best therapeutic direction.

Worden

Worden (2002) identified tasks as a way of focusing the clinical work on action-oriented and goal-derived aspects to move through the mourning process. People mourn in their unique ways. Worden has supplied five general tasks that need to be addressed along the way to healthy coping and adjustment to loss. Because there is considerable overlap of concepts with the Kübler-Ross model (although not in the same order), we will use the Worden model to provide specific, pragmatic ways to work toward successful resolution of each task. Our focus is on the purposefulness of the counselor in addressing each task.

Task 1: Accepting the Reality of the Loss

Counselors might consider using specific language that affirms the loss and does not minimize either the fact that there has been a loss or what was lost. For example, the following are two possible approaches a counselor might take in commenting on the fact that the client cannot use the substance any longer.

Counselor 1: It must have been a tough decision to hold off on drinking.

This counselor is making a somewhat empathic statement but is avoiding the truth that the client either has or has not made the decision to never again drink. Counselor 2 uses a more direct approach in making the loss real and tangible for the client.

Counselor 2: You said that you are swearing off drinking. Let's take some time to talk about what you will lose by ending your drinking.

Here we can see that Counselor 2 is introducing the loss and using definitive language, "ending," in relation to the use. Embedded, yet unspoken, is the counselor's empathy for how difficult this might be to say good-bye forever to a friend (drinking).

Another way in which counselors can help make real the loss related to substance use is by addressing the loss that may have been a part of the initial decision to use (or self-medicate). In our experience counselors sometimes fail to surface such losses for fear of "opening old wounds," whereas, in point of fact, we have found clients to be relieved by having the space to heal the old wound.

Counselor 1: You said it was around the time that your marriage fell apart that you started using more and more tranquilizers. Maybe you just needed them to get you through the rough spot, and now that you are getting more control of your life, you don't need them as much.

Here we see a typical (and not harmful) counselor statement. The counselor offers a re-frame of the purpose and need for the substance use. However, the counselor also glosses over the initial loss and associated thoughts and pain. Though the counselor can reopen the door later, this statement sends the signal to the client that he or she doesn't need to talk about that old wound.

Counselor 2: I want to spend some time talking about the loss of your marriage and all the dreams and hopes that must have been destroyed when the relationship died. I know you said that that was when you started using more. So it makes sense that we spend some time addressing the pain, thoughts, and grief over that loss.

Again, Counselor 2 uses a much more purposeful approach to address the true loss, pain from the past, and open the door to discuss what the client experienced then (and may still be thinking or feeling).

Task 2: Working Through the Pain of the Loss

If Freud was correct, we move toward pleasure and away from pain. It seems only natural for us to remove our hand from a hot surface or find a source of relief when we get a headache. However, compared with the previous two examples, a burned hand or headache are minor and temporary pains. In the process of loss, the associated pain cannot simply be avoided, medicated, or ignored. We have found that clients who ignore the pain of the loss usually develop curious somatic and psychosomatic illnesses. In these cases, we suspect the pain of the loss is looking for a place to emerge and be heard. Counselors need to become comfortable with creating and maintaining the space needed by clients to express and work through their pain. Such pain may come in a variety of emotions and thoughts (manifestations include anger, joy, uncontrollable crying, hopelessness, etc.). The space needed for completion of this task varies from client to client. In general, we have found counselors who have difficulty with emotions usually attempt to "cap" the client's pain by moving them from affective responses to cognitive responses.

> *Counselor 1:* I can see that you are really upset about the fact that your drug use has hurt your relationship with your mother. What do you think you can do to make things better between you two?

Here the counselor has both minimized the loss (acting as if it can simply be healed by the client) and stopped the flow of emotion while trying to shift the client to "think" about the problem.

> *Counselor 2:* I can see how much this hurts to realize the impact your addiction had on your mother. It seems clear that you can never go back to the way it was. Let's talk about the pain your tears represent.

Counselor 2 is both honoring the pain and encouraging deeper reflection on the core pain around the loss. The fear for beginning counselors with the Counselor 2 response is the seemingly final decision on the relationship and fear that they are pushing the client into a more hopeless and pained experience. In fact, however, until the "truth" of the loss is fully recognized and the pain truly honored and understood, the client will struggle to work toward a new relationship with her mother. We have found that only after the true pain and regret of the loss occur can we start working with clients on developing a new, more useful, and positive relationship with others.

Task 3: Adjust to an Environment in Which the Deceased (Substance) Is Missing

Here we added the word *substance* to Worden's original language. For our purposes, these words are interchangeable in the connecting of substance abuse issues with grief and loss. This task is critical for counselors working with clients with substance abuse. This task focuses the counseling on one of the core issues in the relapse prevention process and one of the key pieces to successful recovery. The client must now live in a similar world as before the divorce from chemicals but with the knowledge that the substances are available at all times. In essence, during this task the counselor has to help the client restructure her or his worldview to honor the fact that the previous relationship with the substance is dead. In doing this a new, realistic, and constructive story of nonuse must be developed to take the place of the old story of use.

For example, suppose you are working with a client who became addicted to amphetamines as a result of trying to overachieve to meet his perceived expectations of his mother. Of course, the grief and loss issue of the loss (of the potential deeper relationship with his mother) must be addressed before completion of counseling. Beyond that, however, is the aspect that as he recovers from the addiction and recognizes the death of his relationship with amphetamines, he must also come to understand his behavioral, affective, and cognitive changes in a world that has set expectations and understandings of him. As a result of his high level of production at work, he has come to be seen as the "go-to guy." Reentering this world, he must realign others and his own expectations of his workload. This may be more challenging than it seems.

Both school counselors and community and mental health counselors identify this concept readily. School counselors recognize the challenge of helping a student with an issue only to have the family system at home "change them back." Community and mental health counselors identify this same concept in their work with one partner trying to "fix" the relationship or family system. In both cases, working with the client one-on-one is referred to as *first-order change*. The inclusion of trying to affect the entire system is called *second-order change*. In substance abuse counseling, the attempt is not to change the entire system or world of the client but rather to empower the client to stick to the positive changes made in stopping use, while reinventing and reauthoring the previous relationships.

Task 4: To Emotionally Relocate the Deceased and Move on With Life

This task requires the client to compartmentalize the substance and fully immerse him- or herself into a new and healthy life. As the culminating activity for the client in the mourning process, the role of the counselor in aiding such a transition is to help foster new or refound sources of satisfaction that promote healthy living. We have found that sometimes beginning counselors try to get the client to successfully meet the needs of this task too early in the recovery process. When this occurs, the client attempts to start over without having dealt with the psychological issues that led to the substance abuse or addiction and have yet to identify the loss of the substance, relationships, and so on.

To aid in this task, counselors should direct the focus of the counseling toward current and future plans for the client's new life. "Moving on with life" can denote for some that the client is being asked to deny the substance abuse issue or addiction. This is not the case, however. Clients are encouraged to move from recognizing the world and how their relationships have changed since they became sober, which usually requires a lot of energy, to a sense of a newly emerging identity, with energy for living and fullness of life. Simply put, moving from "I know I'm different because I am a recovering alcoholic/addict" to "I feel like I have a second chance at living a full life." In our work we would roughly estimate that the percentage of psychic energy used in relation to being "recovered" shifts from 90% to 20% during this stage. Though the recovering client can never forget and must always attend to mechanisms that keep him or her from relapsing, the useable energy in this stage becomes much more directed toward the new life.

Multicultural Issues and the Grief, Loss, and Mourning Process

As we have discussed throughout this text, it is not possible to remove multicultural and issues of difference from any aspect of substance abuse or addiction counseling. In this regard, the grief and loss process looks different from one culture to another as well as from one family system to another. Cultural rules guide the individual through the path of recognition of the loss to establishing a new sense of self and the world, with the loss clearly recognized and honored.

For example, I (Bill) had the opportunity to participate in a yearly meeting of Lakota (Sioux) Indians in South Dakota. This meeting, titled "Red Road Days," is a series of storytellings, sweat lodges, and social events geared toward "healing" wounds. One moment that highlighted significant differences between myself and my "dominant White culture" and the Lakota culture of healing was as I listened to a Lakota woman tell her story of loss and healing.

Her story was powerful and riveting. She shared that, despite her best efforts and those of her immediate family (note here that Native American's have a sense of *all* people being relatives), she and her family could not prevent her husband from continuing his alcoholism, which subsequently led to his premature death. What struck me the most as she shared her story was that her mourning process included living for extended periods over the last year at different relative's homes. This was not due to financial concerns but rather was a way of honoring each of those who had reached out to help him (and of course her) during his time of great need.

What I experienced as she told her story were the following emotions and reflections: pain, grief, sorrow, sadness, respect, awareness, circularity of life, energy, calling and direction, hope, and thanks. One might be tempted to apply the models above to ascertain her "stage" or "task" in the grief/loss/mourning process. This would serve to misunderstand the dominant story for her and her culture, which is that "Although his earth time is complete for now, and we will miss him in our world, his beautiful spirit has both moved on from us and is still here with us. We will be reunited in another world-time."

This story serves to remind counselors of the importance of not simply applying stages and tasks as if they are fully accurate and can capture the experience of people from all cultures. The models (described earlier) reflect the predominant theoretical acknowledgment of typical experiences of people from the dominant White culture. Counselors must remember to actively engage in working with each client from a multicultural perspective. In sum, we have found that applying the theories presented in this chapter is quite useful for many clients, but we must always be wary of overapplication, that might dishonor the rules of other cultures.

Summary

This chapter addressed the importance of understanding how integrating grief and loss issues into substance counseling is not only necessary but a pragmatic way of understanding the client. Relapse can be triggered by unresolved grief and loss issues. Helping clients move from useless behaviors intended to mask or deter the effects of the mourning process to healthy activities promotes increased effectiveness throughout the recovery process.

Exploration Questions From Chapter 9

1. What are your family rules about grieving? Loss? Mourning?
2. When you had to give something up that you really liked, how did you honor the loss?

Suggested Activities

1. Identify two or three significant loss issues you have had in your life that others might not see as major losses. In a small group, discuss these issues and what you experience when others "dismiss" your loss as minor.
2. In pairs, discuss the stages and tasks of grief and loss. Identify which stages or tasks might be more difficult based on your personality and your style of grieving.

Group Counseling and Addiction

This chapter highlights group therapy as a significant and viable approach in the successful treatment of alcohol and drug abuse and dependency. Once thought to be a lesser form of therapy than individual counseling, it has emerged as the modality of preference in treating addiction ("Group Therapy Works Well," 1997). An introduction to the stages of group development, the creation and maintenance of a group, and the various skills needed to facilitate a group are covered in this chapter.

Group therapy is used in most drug and alcohol treatment programs (Matano & Yalom, 1991). Most of the work conducted in an inpatient setting occurs in a group. Counselors working with this population need to have training in group work. Although clients benefit from individual counseling as an adjunct to group counseling, group therapy is the preferred modality for most addiction treatment programs (Flores, 1997). A 2001 study suggested that frequent attendance at group counseling increased the likelihood of abstinence from alcohol and drugs, even among participants who did not attend or participate in 12-step meetings. The study concluded that neither the frequency nor duration of individual counseling sessions improved abstinence rates (Fiorentine, 2001).

Isolation plays a significant role in maintaining the individual's beliefs that they are unique and different. When they enter a group and begin to share their stories with others, clients recognize that they are not so unique, alone, or different after all. In fact, many realize they have more of a connection with others than they had ever thought possible. This is a powerful aspect of the healing process found only in group therapy. The results of a study conducted by MacGowan (2006) indicated that building group engagement through a process that is interactive and reciprocal among and between members and the group leader is expected to maximize the benefits of the group experience.

Recovery from addiction can be considered a "we" process, meaning that individuals recover in community and fellowship with others. The first step of Alcoholics Anonymous (AA) states, "We admitted we were powerless over alcohol" where the operative language is *we* as opposed to *I* (AA, 2001). Although much of the work in recovery is internal, support in the group interaction is significant in fostering an individual recovery process (Yalom, 2005). Group therapy offers what individual counseling cannot: feedback and interaction between peers trying to get sober and clean.

Individual counseling is typically not relied upon as the primary modality for the treatment of addiction. As addressed previously, individual counseling can help motivate clients toward group counseling, where behavior change can occur. Individual counseling can be used in preparation for group therapy through motivational enhancement therapy. The combination of individual counseling, 12-step meeting attendance, and group counseling provides an effective, comprehensive treatment protocol (Fiorentine, 2001; Flores, 1997).

On more than one occasion we have witnessed clients becoming more genuine and honest in a group setting than in individual counseling. This phenomenon occurs because groups are able to see through the manipulation, defenses, and deception. The main reason group members see behaviors so clearly is because they have said similar things and can therefore spot it from others (Flores, 1997; Yalom, 2005). The multiple interactive processes cannot occur in individual counseling. A large proportion of a group is presenting constructive feedback to another group member. This feedback process increases the possibility of having a significant impact and therefore experience by other group members. Thus, a group provides a substantially more powerful mechanism to deliver feedback versus an individual counselor presenting virtually the same information.

What Is Group Therapy?

Group therapy addresses individual and interpersonal problems with others who have experienced similar problems, maladjustments, or disorders (Association for Specialists in Group Work, 2009). Group work with a substance-abusing or addicted population is considered homogeneous in nature. It is a group where drug and alcohol use is a main focus of the group discussion and interaction. Although the group members consist of varied cultural and ethnic backgrounds and genders, the common, predominant thread is the use of drugs and alcohol and the impact substances have or have had on their lives and the lives of others.

Support groups such as AA and Narcotics Anonymous (NA), however, are not therapy groups. There are numerous noteworthy differences between support groups and therapy groups. The two groups are differentiated in Table 10.1.

Group therapy is facilitated by a trained group practitioner, and support meetings are chaired by a nonprofessional and a member of the support group. The chair of support meetings generally opens and closes the meeting and organizes the reading of support literature. Beyond that, the chair is a member of the support group.

In group therapy, the counselor works to create a safe environment through modeling and facilitating group interaction among members. In a support group, the interaction

Table 10.1. Group Therapy Versus Support Meetings

Group Therapy	Support Meeting[a]
Facilitated by a trained group practitioner	Chaired by member of the support meeting, which rotates
Focus is on group interaction	Individuals share experiences, strength, and hope; no cross-talk
	Example: a member shares, and then another, then another; generally no questions or confrontation
Commitment to group attendance	Membership is voluntary, no commitment to meeting attendance
Financial cost	No dues or fees; donations only
Facilitator adheres to ethical code	No ethical code; however, anonymity is stressed with all members
Facilitator screens clients for group	No screening is done; whoever attends the meeting and desires to not drink or drug is considered a member
Facilitator keeps group member progress notes	No records are kept
Size limited to 8–13 members	No size limit; if there are 2 people, it is considered a meeting
Typically have a finite date for closure	Members attend same ongoing meeting for years

[a]These are generally called meetings rather than groups.

between members is not facilitated and generally there is no "cross talk," which means members share their own individual experiences without addressing others in the group. Support group members may relate to the stories of others in the group and subsequently might share about their own experience. In a therapy group, there would be direct, person-to-person interaction, questions, and feedback.

Group therapy attendance is very important in order to create a consistent and safe environment for group members to begin working on specific issues. During the group therapy screening process, counselors will attempt to determine the commitment to attendance in the group process. A group contract is generally used for clients to commit to a set number of group meetings and usually make a financial commitment to the groups.

Although support meeting attendance is encouraged, mandatory attendance is not required. A member could go once a month or once every other month; no requirement is set. There are also no dues or fees involved; however, a basket is passed at the end of the meeting for donations to cover coffee and support meeting literature expenses.

Another difference between group therapy and support meetings is a code of ethics that is adhered to by counselors. Counselors facilitating groups should have education and training as outlined in the American Counseling Association's (2005) *ACA Code of Ethics*. Support group chairpersons, on the other hand, do not follow a code of ethics nor do they need training to chair the meeting. However, anonymity is very important for all support group members where only first names are used.

As stated before, group counselors screen their clients for group appropriateness, whereas support meetings only require that a person has a desire to stop drinking or using. As therapy group members attend group sessions, notes are taken; in support meetings, there are no records.

Therapy group sizes, particularly for adults, are recommended to be between 8 and 13 clients. In support meetings, there is no limit and some meetings can be as big as a few hundred or as small as 2.

Finally, therapy groups for addiction generally have a set date of termination, whereas support meetings can be, for many, a lifelong group. A summary is found in Table 10.1.

Comparison of Inpatient Versus Outpatient Addiction Group Counseling

As discussed previously, outpatient treatment groups allow clients to live at home, keep a regular work schedule, and attend treatment activities. Outpatient treatment groups range in time length from 90 minutes to 3 hours, upward to three times per week. Outpatient groups typically consist of 8–10 patients in order to have optimal effect (Gladding, 2003; Yalom, 2005). There are a number of differences between outpatient and inpatient groups. The primary difference is the level of patient acuity. Clients accepted into outpatient treatment generally have fewer medical concerns or withdrawal issues. Many times insurance companies are the primary deciding factor of whether or not a client enters inpatient versus outpatient treatment.

In outpatient treatment, counselors must be sensitive to clients who will be returning home at the end of the group as opposed to returning to their patient rooms, as is the case in inpatient treatment. For example, if the discussion in the outpatient group has been focused on external triggers to using drugs, it would be important for counselors to debrief and explore what each person's feelings were before they went home from group. An inpatient counselor might explore what the group experience has been like for each patient; however, counselors do not need to be quite as concerned that the clients will use after group because they are in a controlled hospital setting and have the structure to continue discussing their experiences after the group. That is not to say, however, that clients do not get high in treatment or have the urge to leave against medical advice.

This brings up the issue of client abstinence in outpatient treatment, which typically is one of the major treatment goals for clients. The use of random urine screens and Breathalyzers is common practice in outpatient treatment. Unfortunately, this can shift a client's perception of the role of the counselor from counselor to that of probation officer. If possible, those clients who are referred by licensing boards, probation officers, or employers should have their urine obtained from the referring sources, thus removing the perceived punitive aspect of treatment. If this is not a possible protocol, counselors need to inform clients upon admission into the program that this is an integral part of what is expected from them while in treatment. Addressing this at the beginning of treatment and discussing it with clients helps minimize distrusting feelings toward the counselor and treatment staff.

Another difference in outpatient versus inpatient groups is how confrontation is used with the client. Confrontation is a technique whereby the counselor points out discrepancies between the client's behavior, affect, and cognition. For example, a group member tells the group that he is grateful to be in the group, that he loves being in recovery, and that his life is wonderful. However, 2 days ago he told the group that he disliked coming to group, that being in recovery was for weak people, and that treatment was just a money scam. This client's discrepancies could be pointed out with support, focusing on his change in attitude, tone, and involvement from one session to the next. Seemingly the best and most effective confrontations come from other group members and not necessarily the group facilitator. The use of effective confrontation skills by the counselor and timing are critical aspects to effective group work, and develop with experience and supervision.

Counselors who confront too frequently and too quickly in the process usually have high group turnover, minimal group participation from members, and increased member defensiveness. Group counselors need to develop rapport and trust with group members before confrontation can be optimally effective. Because of the intensity of inpatient treatment, inpatient counselors tend to take more risks and can be more confrontational than outpatient counselors. This is because their clients are living in a supportive setting that generally requires continuous honesty. In outpatient treatment, clients return home and will not have the immediate support of the group. Therefore, it is important for outpatient counselors to temper confrontation with support and be mindful of what transpires in the group. An article on group therapy and addiction in *Behavioral Health Treatment* ("Group Therapy Works Well," 1997) described Philip Flores's (a significant author in group addiction treatment) approach within a group, "At first you want to give them a lot of support, gratification and containment, so that they don't react to their anxiety or depression by self-medicating" (p. 2). He further said, "But as they continue to get some sobriety underneath their belt, if they don't start confronting and dealing with their emotions, they will likely go back to drug and alcohol use. Somewhere around the middle phase, you start getting them to take a cold, hard look at themselves, and to deal with the feelings they've been avoiding" ("Group Therapy Works Well," 1997, p. 2).

Inpatient groups occur throughout the day. Whatever is discussed in the morning group can be carried on into afternoon groups, offering a powerful continuity not usually found in outpatient groups. Another aspect of inpatient treatment that occurs outside of group is the impact of the therapeutic milieu. The time spent within the therapeutic community has a significant positive impact on clients' spiritual well-being (C. W. Brooks & Matthews, 2000). C. W. Brooks and Matthews's research found the spiritual well-being of clients in an inpatient addiction treatment program significantly improved while in treatment, suggesting the importance of the therapeutic milieu.

Inpatient groups are intense and can be very powerful. Patients admitted to inpatient treatment typically have medical concerns, dual diagnoses, or relapse issues and do not respond well to outpatient treatment. Over the course of treatment, client defenses decrease. This allows real emotions to surface in the group setting. Inpatient stays tend to be short, so counselors have a lot to address with clients in the group settings.

Psychoeducational Groups

This type of group combines counseling and education in one group. For example, a psychoeducational group in an inpatient drug and alcohol treatment unit may focus on relapse prevention. For 2 hours in the morning and 2 hours in the afternoon relapse prevention information and facilitated interaction occurs in the group. Treatment programs typically have an educational component (e.g., lectures or videotapes) that focuses on specific topics. Psychoeducational groups provide information on a specific topic and then explore how the information relates personally and with each other in the group setting (Gladding, 2003).

Early Intervention Motivational Groups

Depending on the counselors' work setting, they may have a plethora of groups already running. Other counselors may have none at all and need to start from the beginning. College counselors, for example, may have multiple groups running with regard to eating or relationship problems, whereas counselors in an outpatient mental health program may have a group focused on developing coping skills. In school settings, college environments, and mental health agencies, the treatment of alcohol and drug issues is usually referred to agencies that deal specifically with addiction.

Velasquez, Maurer, Crouch, and DiClemente (2001) developed an imminently useful stages of change therapy manual for group work and substance abuse. Importantly, this manual is designed to use in a variety of settings before referring the client to formalized addiction treatment. This is an excellent manual for those interested in creating these types of groups. These groups initially do not focus on abstinence but rather on clients being able to connect the emotional consequences of their behaviors with their alcohol and drug use. Urine screens and attendance in AA or NA are not incorporated in this approach. These early intervention motivational groups work with clients who present minimal symptoms of alcohol abuse or dependency, are at risk for movement into addiction, and have a family history of addiction. These clients are not ready or will not meet criteria for treatment yet need more than education. Bridging this gap, the group helps motivate and prepare clients for treatment if and when that time presents itself (Velasquez et al., 2001). As a result, effective screening is critical so the clients are not inappropriately accepted/denied/referred.

Prescreening Clients for Groups

Most if not all treatment groups, regardless of being inpatient or outpatient, are considered "open-ended" groups. Open-ended groups continually add clients to the group membership. Simultaneously, clients terminate from the group, resulting in a continuous change in group membership (Flores, 1997). Closed groups, on the other hand, begin with a set group membership and at no time are new group members added. Closed groups meet for a set period of time until the group has concluded altogether. For open-ended groups it is suggested that no more than two group members be added at a time in order to minimize the change in group interaction and trust levels (Flores, 1997; Yalom, 2005).

The importance of screening clients for a group is an ethical prerequisite for counselors to follow (American Counseling Association, 2005). Counselors meet with clients before their first group in order to assess and prepare clients for the group process. Couch (1995) identified four aspects to pregroup screening:

- *Step 1—Identify client needs, expectations, and commitment:* In this step, counselors begin the preparation process and assess the commitment to the process.
- *Step 2—Challenge myths and misconceptions about group:* In this step, counselors explore with clients what their beliefs and understanding of a group may be in an effort to reduce anxiety and increase safety.

- *Step 3—Convey information:* In this step, counselors share information about the group, how it operates, number of participants, and expectations. This is done in hope of reducing anxiety and outlining the guidelines of the group.
- *Step 4—Screening:* Clients are able to verbalize their reason(s) for entering the group, their hopes, and their desires for change. In this step, counselors provide information on what group therapy consists of, what occurs, and how it can best be used. Counselors ask clients why they are entering group therapy and ask about their hopes for the experience. Overall, the more informed and prepared the group member is, the more willing the group participant may be.

During the prescreening appointment, counselors determine if each of the prospective clients would be a good candidate for group counseling (either at this point or maybe in the future). Most treatment programs already have groups in existence. Yalom (2005) suggested that outpatient counselors should deselect clients for a closed group rather than select group members. He suggested that clients who are actively suicidal, psychotic, or intoxicated may not be appropriate for outpatient group membership until stabilized on medication for depression, psychosis, or detoxification. Those clients remaining will be considered for the group.

Determining which group is appropriate for clients is an additional aspect of the assessment process. Counselors need to consider age, developmental level, motivation, and financial resources of the client when referring to a group. In addition, counselors need to be aware of the types of groups available in the community should treatment not be accessible. For example, a school counselor, after consultation with a substance abuse specialist, determines that their 16-year-old client is not appropriate for outpatient drug and alcohol treatment yet could benefit from a psychoeducational/motivational group. The problem, however, is that no such type of group exists either in the school or in the surrounding area. In this example, the client was appropriate for group therapy, yet no group existed. If there are enough students who would benefit from this type of group, a group could be created to meet the needs of the clients within that school.

Counselors need to consider a client's extraneous variables that would contribute to group attrition. These variables include comments from the client like "I'll give it a try." Or, in some cases, these comments may point toward existing resources such as "Sometimes I like to bowl on Thursday, so I might not be able to make every group." Counselors also want to be aware of transportation issues (e.g., clients who depend on others for transportation to and from group) as well as future changes in living situations (e.g., a potential group member who will be leaving the state in 1 month). Depending on the therapeutic setting, some counselors will need to discuss the client's financial commitment to the group. Although counselors tend to be hesitant with this aspect of the counseling process, it needs to be addressed from the beginning, along with other aspects of the informed consent. Counselors may have clients who want to attend group yet insurance won't reimburse for group therapy, in which case clients need to discuss financial arrangements with the counselor.

Once assessed as being appropriate for group therapy, the client needs to be informed of the nature of the group, what is expected of them, and what they can expect from the counselor. This information is typically disseminated through an informed consent.

Informed Consent

An informed consent "informs" clients about the clinical expertise of the counselor, the theoretical approaches of the counselor, the financial responsibility of the client for counseling, the limitations of confidentiality, after hours crisis procedures, court appearances, insurance filing, the nature of the counseling process, voluntary participation, diagnosis, and consultation and supervision procedures (Corey, Corey, & Callanan, 2007). When providing group services, the nature of the group and the limitations of confidentiality in the group are also included in the consent form (American Counseling Association, 2005).

The informed consent provides the client with information regarding the counseling process and the procedures within the office. This is time well spent to prepare clients for therapy and reduce the possibility for misunderstandings and subsequent ethical issues. In this process, the counselor reviews the informed consent with the client, at which time the consent form is signed and the client receives a copy of it for their records. The original is placed in the client file along with the other clinical data.

Confidentiality in the Group

As part of the screening assessment, clients need to be informed about limits to confidentiality in the group process. Counselors have an ethical and legal obligation to warn authorities and intended victims if clients are verbalizing intent to harm another human being or are in danger of harming themselves. Suspicion or evidence of child and elder abuse also constitute required reporting by the counselor, despite the counselor–client relationship (Ahia & Martin, 1993). During the screening session, counselors need to inform clients of the limitations of confidentiality as it pertains to the counselor's ethical and professional obligations. Counselors also cannot guarantee that other group members will hold confidences or maintain confidentiality. It is imperative that counselors challenge and charge each client to maintain confidentiality with what is said in the group and about who attends the group. This initial discussion of confidentiality between counselor and clients generally leads to discussions of trust and safety, which is a normal and important group focus early in development of the group (Gladding, 2003). In closed groups, for example, the initial group discussion typically includes a decision made by the group not to break the confidentiality of the group. In open groups, this group norm can be brought up each time a new member joins the group.

The Creation and Development of an Outpatient, School, or Community Mental Health Group: What Is Needed?

Initially, the need for a group or justification is most important. Following the epistemology of "form following function," the creation of a group usually follows systemic or community needs. Imagine three college counselors who consistently have clients who are in need of a group that addresses alcohol and drug issues. The clients may not be appropriate for treatment but could benefit from a group experience.

Creating a group from need also allows counselors to consolidate clients, thus allowing for more client contacts. Consolidation is found in school settings where counselor caseloads reach 700–800 students. Of course, counselors with this large of a caseload are not able to see each student for individual counseling. However, in a group, counselors can effect change in more students. Additionally, the group format also maximizes counselor time in providing information and tools to address their problems.

Once the need for the group is determined, obtaining permission to initiate a group is the next step before moving ahead with group planning. Permission from the clinical team, supervisor, and administration garners full support for the group initiative, thereby increasing the potential for the success of the group. Clinical and administrative support is crucial in the creation and development of the group.

Questions a counselor might ask in the preparation process include

1. What type of group will they be facilitating and when will it begin?
2. Will it be an open-ended, psychoeducational substance abuse group? Or will it be a closed-ended, motivational group for at-risk alcohol and drug students?

3. Will the group be structured and if so, what activities will be used during each session?
4. Will the group have cofacilitators, and what will the group be named?

Once the type of group is determined, finding space to hold the group will be the next task. This can be daunting, particularly when room space is limited. A space that is devoid of interruptions and is quiet and sequestered is optimal. Once the space is found, finding enough chairs and making sure the room is available each time the group meets is also critical.

A next step is to advertise the group to necessary stakeholders such as peers, teachers, the community, administration, parents, and other clients. The title of the group, many times, will be enticing to potential group members. Creating a short but intriguing title of the group is recommended. If there is a fee involved, the advertisement should indicate the cost and will need to be discussed with the client during the prescreening session.

To summarize, if counselors have determined a need, obtained permission, developed the group structure, and marketed well, the success of the group is increased. Many times counselors do not put the necessary time into group preparation and end up with clients but no permission from staff or no group room. Preparation is very important to group success.

Attracting Group Members

One of the best methods of creating a group is from in-house or in-center referrals. Not only are the clients already familiar with the counseling process but they also have therapeutic experience. For example, two counselors have decided to create a men's posttreatment recovery group to be held in a university counseling center. The counselors discuss their interest in initiating this type of group with the counseling staff and receive overwhelming support from their supervisor and colleagues. The counselors then determine from the clinical staff meetings that each counselor has two clients who might benefit from this type of group, thus indicating a possible need. Each counselor in the center then talks with their two perspective clients and determines if each of them is interested in the group.

Each interested client is given a referral to the group and the telephone number of the two facilitators. Each potential client calls to set up a screening appointment where the two counselors cointerview each client for 30 minutes. During that session, the counselors provide information such as the group being closed-ended, that it will meet for approximately 12 weeks (one semester), and that the group will be nonstructured and will focus on early recovery issues (i.e., triggers, cravings, environment, and lack of support).

Role of the Facilitator

The facilitator has multiple responsibilities and functions within the group. It is typical for group members to enter the group having the facilitator as the common denominator. An initial task of the facilitator is to focus on creating an environment of safety and trust within the group, thus allowing members to explore feelings and interactions.

Facilitating a group is a dynamic, exciting, powerful, and affective experience. The counselor's use of self in the group process plays a significant factor in group trust and development. A spontaneous, creative counselor who is willing to explore can significantly contribute to the energy in the group setting. Sitting in the group as a facilitator, from our perspective, is electric; there is always something going on in the group, whether it is overt or covert.

Yalom (2005) suggested that student counselors learn the skills associated with facilitating a group through various methods. The first is for the student to participate in a personal growth group in order to understand what it is like to sit in a group as a client. Second, it is important for counselors to observe experienced group counselors as they facilitate the group process. This allows students to observe firsthand what the dynamics and process of a group look and feel like. A third point is the need for supervision as students facilitate their own groups. Yalom suggested that for every hour of group therapy, 1 hour of group supervision should be provided by an experienced group therapist. It is important for new counselors to be supervised and have time to debrief with cofacilitators and colleagues.

A final aspect to group learning is to have a class or training on the basic components of group therapy. Combining these learning opportunities helps student counselors understand the importance of self-knowledge along with group counseling experience and how the two in combination make for an effective client experience.

The development of group norms occurs in the early stages of a group and, once created, is difficult to change. The counselor has an impact in the development of these norms, which allows the therapeutic factors of therapy to occur (Yalom, 2005). According to Yalom, the counselor has two basic roles in the development of norms within the group: technical expert and model-setting participant.

The Technical Expert

The technical expert provides guidelines, structure, and knowledge of the group process. In this role, the group counselor is the authority, using his or her knowledge during the screening process and subsequent group meetings. As a technical expert the counselor will outline guidelines for the group such as confidentiality issues, he or she will keep time (starting and finishing the group), and will maintain awareness of the group process. In essence, the technical expert assumes the role of knowledge deliverer for the group. This is important, especially when the group needs specific information or needs the facilitator to increase the structure of the group.

Model-Setting Participant

The model-setting counselor demonstrates honest and genuine communication between and with group members (important here is that the facilitator is also considered a group member). The counselor has a responsibility to be authentic, spontaneous, and consistent. The counselor models the development of healthy and honest communication among members. Through such meaningful interactions, group members potentially will exhibit similar behaviors. In the role of model-setting participant, the counselor has the opportunity to help develop group norms. This is accomplished through a variety of techniques (e.g., encouragement of affective disclosures and unconditional positive regard; Rogers, 1957). The counselor, through direct and indirect actions, impacts the group norms. In fact, the counselor cannot *not* impact the development of norms in the group. If the counselor remains silent during interactions or if the counselor makes comments following client participation, there is an impact on group norms. With either behavior, the counselor will be a participant in the development of group norms.

Group Counseling Skills for Drug and Alcohol Groups

Group counseling with addicted clients is unique because of a number of factors: the group is considered homogeneous, the group tends to jell and become cohesive more quickly than heterogeneous groups, the group has specific jargon used by members, and the group consists of members either in crisis, denial, and/or emotional pain. Addiction groups are considered homogeneous because of the unifying, consistent factor of addiction shared by each group member. This homogenetic mirroring allows group members to see themselves in others and ultimately helps them work through their own defenses and denial (Flores, 1997). The resulting effect is typically a rapidly established cohesive group. Researchers from Cornell University found that "social contact with people who have gone through the same crisis is highly beneficial" ("Group Therapy Works Well," 1997, p. 1). When group members participate, counselors can reinforce their involvement by encouraging disclosure. For instance, if after a client shares how difficult it is for him to trust in a group there is silence, this could ultimately send the message that it is not acceptable to share within the group. On the other hand, if the response from the counselor is positive and reinforcing, the client is more likely to continue sharing. The reinforcement of the counselor is keenly observed by the other group members, which in turn helps establish the norm that sharing is important, supported, and a part of the group experience.

Rogers (1957) believed that the counselors' ability to be genuine in the counseling relationship and demonstrate unconditional positive regard with their clients was critical in fostering and maintaining the environment for change. He also felt that being accurately empathic with clients was crucial for the development of client trust and the process of change. He believed these three conditions were necessary and sufficient in all therapeutic relationships in order for change to occur. In a group setting, these conditions manifest the development of a safe and supportive environment for personal growth and exploration (Rogers, 1957).

Recognizing Client Defenses

A recognized and very real aspect of addiction is denial. Clients in denial are usually convinced that they do not have a problem with drugs or alcohol. In turn they become exceedingly skilled at convincing others around them (i.e., family, friends, employers, counselors) that there is not a problem. A counselor can work (in individual counseling) with a client in denial on many issues (e.g., relationship, childhood, depression) without ever addressing the denial system. However, take that same client and appropriately refer him or her to a group of addicts and alcoholics, and very quickly the defenses and denial of the client will be addressed by individuals who have verbalized the same things before in their own denial.

As clients in denial enter recovery groups, they hear others talk about their experiences. These life narratives include where they are now in recovery and what needed to occur in order for them to reach out and accept help. Denial in a group setting may emerge in the following ways:

Examples

- "I think I have a problem with drinking, but I am not addicted to it." In this statement, the client is aware of some consequences but is still minimizing and denying the loss of control over the chemical.
- "I hear what each one of you is saying, but my case is different and unique." Some counselors refer to this as a "terminal case of uniqueness," which acts as a way to separate and maintain the idea that "I am not like you drunks, I am stronger than that."
- "Yeah, I agree with you, I am addicted to alcohol, but once in a while, on special occasions, I plan on smoking a joint just to relax." This client is trying to maintain control by switching from one drug to another.
- "My using was not really that out of control. When I went to detox this time I had been drinking for only 4 continuous days rather than 6, so I must be getting better." This client is clearly minimizing and denying the enormity of his or her drinking.
- "I really don't think my drinking affected my children because they never, ever witnessed me actually drinking. Anyway, I drink vodka and you can't smell that." Again, this client is denying the impact his or her drinking has on the family and then believes they did not smell of alcohol.

- "I'm fine. I have stopped using and I am just fine. Everything is okay as long as I don't delve into all those feelings related to the consequences of my using." The defenses in this case are around feelings and the fear of experiencing them.

Counselors need to help clients identify emotions related to the consequences of their use. By facilitating this connection to materialize, counselors help clients to recognize the link between emotional consequences and use. This insight, maybe for the first time, helps clients identify what others around them may have felt when they were using. Helping clients become aware, with the help of other group members, of their defenses is an important aspect of getting well in recovery. As clients identify defenses such as minimizing, rationalizing, and intellectualizing, they are more adept at self-intervention and can observe when they begin to defend their feelings related to the consequences of their using.

Facilitating the Group in the Here-and-Now

Facilitators have multiple tasks during the development of a group. One task is helping group members interact in the here-and-now. This is a daunting task for counselors because of the initial resistance by clients. General social conversations typically do not bring the focus of the interaction into the "now." Being in the moment takes focus, energy, and the willingness to be vulnerable. These attributes are usually uncomfortable because interpersonal interactions between members are explored. For instance, in the initial stages of a group, lack of trust by members can be a normal topic of discussion. A counselor who is focusing on the here-and-now could offer a comment that would highlight the potential silence in the group: "I've noticed for the past 2 minutes that not only is the group quiet but many of you appear to be uncomfortable with the silence. Could we spend some time talking about your feelings as you sit in the group right now?" This comment presents an observation into the here-and-now of the group with hopes of exploration into the silence and the feelings beneath the surface.

Counselors facilitating groups in the here-and-now demonstrate the significance of being in the moment with other group members and with their own feelings. This is a very important aspect of group counseling for clients as they work on their recovery. Most clients agree that when they were using they would think ahead to the next high or the process through which they would get more of their drug. Very little time was spent in the present. In fact, it is the present (i.e., feelings, consequences, stressors) that the addict is trying to avoid or escape from. As the counselor helps focus group members on the present, it is normal and natural for the group to resist. Paradoxically, it is a significant aspect of learning in their recovery.

Group facilitators need to explore how clients are feeling emotionally in the moment. The cliché question "How does that make you feel?" is ironically a very, very important task in the here-and-now. Clients who have spent the past 25 years under the influence of some type of substance are going to have difficulty identifying the various and varied levels of emotional experience. Once an individual sobers up and the group counselor asks "How are you feeling today?" the response many times is "fine." Group counselors are in a position to help clients move beyond this vague and hollow statement of physical being (e.g., fine, okay, all right, good, and/or tired) to the deeper nuances of their emotional makeup. Clients getting sober can usually identify feelings of anxiety, depression, and anger; however, they typically have difficulty initially in identifying and expressing the feelings of hurt, insecurity, shame, or guilt. Usually such feelings are wadded into one general feeling of anxiety, depression, or anger. The task of the counselor in the here-and-now is to help clients peel away at the onion, so to speak, so that a statement of "fine" can move to "I'm feeling anxious" and then to "I am afraid of losing my wife" and ultimately to "I'm so ashamed of myself and what my drinking has done to my family."

Process Versus Content

In addition to focusing on the here-and-now is the use of process statements or comments. This is a most challenging task for counselors because it requires the counselor to look beyond shared client material and search for the "story behind the story." This deeper meaning of the discussion yields significant fruit once successfully presented to the group for exploration (Yalom, 2005). Process comments are used by the counselor to elicit discussion at a deeper and more genuine level. Content in the group can be found in the data presented by clients, such as their histories of using drugs. Content is exactly what it indicates, the presented story or data. A naturally flowing group will have both process and content in its interaction. However, the task of the counselor is to help the group move into the here-and-now through the use of process comments. Yalom described it as a reflective loop. Take as an example the group members sitting in silence. The counselor could say after a prolonged period of time, "Although we have been sitting in here for the past 2 minutes in silence, I suspect each of you has thoughts running around in your head and that in the silence you have been reflecting upon them." Not only is the counselor's comment bringing the focus into the here-and-now but it is also a reflective process comment suggesting that although the group members are silent, significant work is occurring in their minds and hearts. The combination of the two is powerful in unearthing rich material for group exploration.

Counselors facilitating addiction recovery groups need to be cognizant of members who share "drunkalogs," or stories about their using. Mistakenly, these stories can fall under the heading of content disclosure. Although this is important for the client to share (to a point) in order to feel heard, the counselor needs to keep the focus on the feelings the member is having at the moment concerning the stories. A helpful way to look at this is how does the client feel here-and-now about the there-and-then? Counselors can merge the content of the past with the present for discussion between members. The group counselor may say, "I'm hearing how difficult it was for you 5 years ago during the divorce and how your drinking was the main reason for the split. If you would, talk about how you feel now talking about it."

Facilitating Interaction Among Members

Group counseling is not individual counseling. Effective group therapy challenges the counselor to work with the ebb and flow of the group interaction to create individual awareness and personal opportunities for growth. A counselor facilitating a group from an individual counseling focus will be doing individual therapy in group, which is not the goal of group therapy (nor is this procedure effective). Group therapy is a counselor-facilitated social microcosm.

Another important task for group counselors is to help members interact with each other and provide feedback, support, and awareness. We use the analogy of the circus performer spinning plates on thin poles. Group counselors initially act as the energy cell to get discussion moving. This helps clients relate to each other and both support and empathize with clients' feelings. As the group develops, the responsibility of spinning the plates (which started with the counselor) will eventually move to the clients as they help each other in the group process.

Examples

Client: This has been a very difficult group for me. I've shared a lot about my life today, and only a few individuals have shared with me their experiences.

Counselor: I am hearing that because you have been very open in the group that you are feeling pretty vulnerable, and because you have only heard from a few members, you are feeling even more vulnerable. That being said, I am wondering if there is anyone in the group you would like to get feedback from or what they have been experiencing here today in the group.

Or the counselor might say the following:

> I am hearing that because you have been very open in the group, you are feeling pretty vulnerable, and because you have only heard from a few members you are feeling even more vulnerable. That being said, what have the rest of you been experiencing or thinking about as he has been disclosing?

With the first response, the counselor encourages the client to ask others for feedback. The second response has the counselor asking for feedback from other group members. The goal of both of these responses is to foster honest interactions among members to explore what was occurring as the group member shared. Although facilitators recognize and honor the fact that clients bring material to work on in the group, much of what is learned occurs through the interpersonal interactions with other group members (e.g., asking for feedback, perceptions of others, emotional expression).

Opening the Group Session

For addiction groups, we suggest an introductory format of having each client say his or her first name, sobriety date (the client's last use of alcohol or drugs), how the client is feeling emotionally at that moment, and what he or she wants to focus on in the group experience. This entire introductory process for the group should take no more than 10 minutes. It helps the counselor and clients determine possible areas for discussion and exploration. The technique of therapeutically cutting off clients who are going beyond the initial introduction is important; otherwise, some clients will monopolize the group and set an unhealthy group norm. The counselor also needs to remember the issues presented in order to help group members focus on their agendas and connect group experiences with personal recovery agendas.

Example

Counselor: We've gone around the room today and at least three of you are dealing with feelings related to your using and the impact on your children. The rest of you seemed to identify feelings related to the impact your drug use had on intimate relationships. Could we take some time to help each other understand a bit more about what this feels like in here today?

This counselor's comment summarizes what has been said and does not alienate those without children. Further, it is inclusive of how all relationships have been impacted. It also identifies the goal of "Let's explore together in here today this really painful stuff."

Other opening activities can include asking clients to identify a color that represents their emotional state, or select a number from 1 to 10 that describes their feelings (1 being *very depressed* and 10 being *joyous, happy, and excited*). Counselors can also use connective introductory statements that link session topics or unresolved issues from previous group sessions. An example of this might be, "I appreciate what you have outlined for today as an agenda, but before we proceed, I would like to take a few moments to talk about the last 15 minutes of the group last week. Mary seemed quite upset at Carl. Could we take some time to find out where the group is with that?"

Evocative Empathy Statements

Evocative empathy helps group members identify and explore their feelings in a safe context. When presented evocatively, the statement usually elicits a response from group members.

Example

Client: I am really frustrated today. I am so tired from the schedule I am on and feel like I need to take a vacation. I've been working 60 plus hours a week and have found little time for relaxation or time with my family. I am also worried that I might drink because this is most definitely a time when I would drink.

Counselor: You sound very frustrated, overwhelmed, and sad. In what you just said, I also thought I heard some fear that if you don't relax, you will end up drinking.

Client: Exactly, I am afraid that with all that is going on, I will lose what I have worked so hard to gain in sobriety.

Counselor: You seem to have invested a great deal of your heart into getting your family and work situation back on track, and in order to do that you seem to have created a schedule for yourself that is overwhelming. And now you feel as though your sobriety is in jeopardy due to the stress of the schedule you have created.

Client: It's as if I am trying to keep many balloons under the surface of the water, all the time. I can handle one or two, but any more than that, one of them is going to pop out of the water, and the one I feel might this time is my drinking.

Counselor: I wonder if anyone in the group can relate to that feeling of keeping the balloons under the water or keeping everything under control, and knowing something has got to give, and using or drinking in the past has been that escape?

The group facilitator in this case has worked briefly with the client in order to elicit feelings and a description of what is occurring. Following the client–counselor interaction, the counselor then moves it out to the group and asks if anyone can relate to the description, which will elicit a response and potential interaction from group members.

Clarification Probing

As clients share in the group, another task for the counselor is to understand and clarify what has been said while probing for more information and clarification. The combination of clarification and probing helps the group to understand the nature of the information being shared.

Example

Client: You don't really understand what I have been through. In order for me to meet with a group of people, I had to be high or at least drunk. This is a very difficult place to be in and I am not sure how much I will be able to get from the group experience.

Counselor: Being in this group sounds like it takes a lot of courage, that in the past you would have been high in order to do this, and that you have some skepticism whether or not this group is going to help you out at all. You also said that the group might not understand what you have been through. Could you talk a little to the group about what you have been through so we could begin to understand?

Client: I know you all are here to help me help myself, but sometimes I just want to quit treatment and go back to drinking because that is all I know. Anyway, I've been through a lot, two divorces, five jobs, prison, you name it, I've done it.

Counselor: So despite all you have been through you continue to come to treatment anyway. I suspect there are other members here who have felt as you do now. I would ask the rest of you, what has kept you motivated to come to treatment and stay in recovery?

The counselor is trying to clarify feelings as well as explore what the client has been through. The probing question from the counselor begins with "Could you talk a little to the group about what you have been through so we could begin to understand?" and then moves to a general probing question to the group, "What has kept you all motivated to come into treatment and stay in recovery, despite your history?" Again, the group counselor is working toward the group interaction.

First Step Assignment in Group

Group members in most treatment programs are asked to complete a *first step assignment* and eventually present it to their therapy group. The first step assignment helps clients begin to identify how drinking and drug use impacted each faction of their lives, from finances to emotions. Each client writes responses to the questions (below) and the feelings related to each consequence. Along with the assignment is the presentation of a time line, on which clients identify for the group when they started using and the progression of their use.

The following are sample questions asked in the first step assignment:

1. How have alcohol/drugs impacted your mental abilities?
2. How have alcohol/drugs affected your relationships?
3. How have alcohol/drugs impacted your work and leisure life?
4. How have alcohol/drugs affected your spiritual life?
5. How have alcohol/drugs interfered with your education or training?
6. How have alcohol/drugs affected your emotional life?
7. How have alcohol/drugs affected your physical life?

Following the presentation of responses, group members are offered an opportunity to ask questions, provide feedback, and relate to what has been presented. Group members have an opportunity to complete and present a first step assignment to help them become aware of their defense system and identify repressed feelings (both of which are critical in remaining sober). Clients who maintain rigid defenses keep others at a distance and remain both internally and externally isolated. The client presenting an "I'm fine" facade while suppressing feelings is actually creating more and more stress, which contributes to the relapse dynamic.

Group Development

In addition to techniques, norm setting, and modeling, counselors work with the group to help facilitate group development. Tuckman and Jensen (1977) suggested five stages to group development: forming, storming, norming, performing, and adjourning. Closed groups, found mainly in outpatient settings, and open-ended groups, found in both outpatient and inpatient programs, fluctuate through these stages. This is due to consistent membership versus constant change in membership. Closed groups usually successfully resolve the forming stage of the group. Because of this, most of the group's time is invested in the norming and performing stages. On the other hand, open groups will need to spend time addressing new membership, periodically returning to the forming stage of the group.

Stage development and movement through these stages is fluid and continuous. One group session may focus on the here-and-now where the group members are sharing feelings and interacting with each other. The next group may involve disagreements, arguments, and alternative perspectives and be in more of a storming stage. Therefore, the group counselor needs to be cautious about expectations for the group based on the previous group experience. The stages of a group outlined by Tuckman and Jensen (1977) are described next.

Forming

This stage occurs early in the group development, and its main focus is in the discussion of trust, expectations, guidelines, and meeting the new members in the group. The following are comments that might be stated in the forming stages of a group.

Client Comments: I am not a group person and I don't know any of you. Trust is a big issue for me and I am not sure how much I am going to share in front of a group of strangers. My parents always said to keep my business to myself.

Counselor Response: I realize this is your first group and how awkward it may feel for you; however, let's spend some time talking about what inside of you may interfere with your participation.

Or

Counselor Response: There has been a lot of discussion today on what "'should" be talked about in the group and how this group experience will help you when you leave here today. With that in mind, can we talk briefly about how today's session can be useful in the coming week?

The counselor's comments addressed the client's resistance by helping clients name the fear and identify and discuss expectations for the group.

Storming

This stage generally involves conflict with other group members as well as the facilitator. The group at this time becomes more honest with fellow group members and the counselor. The important aspect of storming is for the conflict(s) to be discussed and worked through inside of the group and not outside of the group. The expressions of anger, fear, or distrust are avenues for counselors to help clients develop conflict resolution skills, which are needed skills in recovery. Clients will discuss at length how they tend to mismanage feelings of anger and either rage out at the person they are angry with or stuff their feelings and implode. The group setting can provide a crucible for change where clients can work with each other and experiment with new and healthy behaviors through appropriate expression.

Client Comment: You know, I've been coming here to this group for a month, and you counselors don't share a whole lot about yourselves. In fact, I don't know much about either of you.

Or

Client Comment: Last week in group you said I wasn't serious about being sober, and that really pissed me off. I am committed to sobriety, and what you said hurt.

Counselor Comment: During the first few groups you were quite shy and reserved, and now you are able to share your feelings of distrust as well as curiosity with the group. That's a major change in behavior.

Or

Counselor Comment: It kind of sounds like Joe hurt your feelings. What is it that you would like Joe to know about you that you don't feel he understood?

The client's first comment reflects feelings of distrust with the leader and possibly the group process while the second comment presents conflict and hurt feelings between two group members. In either case, the counselor's task is to help facilitate the discussion between the group members and to deflect the personal affronts while looking for the process behind the comments. In this case the issue is trust.

Norming

During this stage the group is determining what is appropriate behavior in the group, what is acceptable to discuss in the group, and possible goals for the group process

(Tuckman & Jensen, 1977). The norms that are created are typically covert. For example, after a month of outpatient sessions, the group members begin to share more and more feelings within the group. One group member who tends to share a lot of feelings during the group receives a lot of attention from members. Other members notice this and when they share their feelings, they too are given support and attention. The group's reinforcement of members who share feelings creates as a norm the acceptance of emotional disclosure. Although no one directly states this in the group process, it is inferred and has become part of the group culture. Once norms are developed, they are very difficult to change; therefore, it is equally important for counselors to be aware of their unintentional reinforcement of unwanted behavior either through verbal responses or nonverbal gestures (Yalom, 2005).

> *Client Comment:* I really feel comfortable with the group. I would like to talk, if I could today, about what my sobriety has been like for the past few months. It has been exhilarating as well as terrifying, and today I am grateful to have a group like you to talk with [tears].

Or

> *Client Comment:* I am not sure if what I am going to say is okay with the rest of you, but since we have been talking about childhood pain, I feel I can relate and would like to share.
> *Counselor Comment*: You seem to have a lot of emotions rolling around since you have gotten sober. It really is beautiful to watch as in each group you share more and more about how you feel.

Or

> *Counselor Comment*: Many of you have discussed the impact your childhood has had on your current methods of coping as an adult. Although it is important to explore these areas, it is just as important to bring those feelings into the present and determine how those stresses can and have contributed to relapse.

The client comments demonstrate how the group has become a place of comfort to explore issues and feelings. The norm of sharing feelings has been reinforced along with the permission to discuss childhood experiences. The counselor reinforces the sharing of feelings by highlighting the changes made in one group member. The second comment reinforces the group interest in childhood exploration yet encourages members to bring the feelings into the present and discuss how they relate to current recovery issues.

Performing

The group at this stage has worked through many of the initial trust issues, has successfully worked through conflict more than once with other group members, and has established norms. The performing group takes responsibility for the process in the group, for they have observed facilitators modeling healthy behaviors. Group members start with an issue and bring it into the room for interpersonal learning. The facilitator's role is to keep the focus in the present, making fewer and fewer comments as the group continues.

> *Client Comment*: I would like sometime today to discuss my situation at home with my wife since I've gotten sober. I know that a few of you have had some rough roads with relationships since sobriety, so I would like some feedback on my behavior in here. My wife says I am still stubborn and self-centered, which I don't see and need your help.

Or

Client Comment: I've thought a lot about the feedback you gave to me last week on my impatience, and I have realized how unaware I am of my own behavior and feelings. I really need suggestions on how to deal with my impatience.

Counselor Comment: I really hear how open you are to learning and hearing from your group members what they see in you. What a remarkable piece of growth for you to ask for help.

Or

Counselor Comment: You too are making major strides by asking for help, particularly when last week you adamantly defended your position of not being impatient.

In both client comments there is a desire and willingness to learn from other group members and how that experience can translate into the world outside of the group. The performing group helps each other through feedback, honesty, and genuineness. The counselor's comments reinforced their desire to make changes and ask for help within the group for issues they were not aware of previously.

Adjourning

The process of ending a group and coming to closure is very important to group members. In adjourning the counselor helps members make closure with each other, process what the group has been like for them, as well as achieve closure with the facilitators.

Client Comment: This group has allowed me to open up to others like I never thought possible. I have shared with you more than I have ever shared with my family. I am going to miss each and every one of you after this group is over.

Or

Client Comment: I am very sad and angry that this group has to end. I don't like it. It has become a major aspect of my recovery program, and I need to figure out what I will replace it with, although I don't think I can.

Counselor Comment: We have three more group meetings left, and I want each of you to take the opportunity to reflect back on these past few months. What have you learned about yourself in recovery so far?

Or

Counselor Comment: Since this group is ending next week, think about what you are going to do in place of meeting here on Thursday nights.

The clients are beginning to share their emotions (e.g., sad, joyful, grateful) of closure while thinking about what they have learned and what they may do in place of the group. The counselor is making comments to help members with self-reflection and to explore what they will replace the group with once it is over. As the group unfolds and eventually terminates, therapeutic factors occur, which illuminate the changes so critical to group work.

Therapeutic Factors in Group

Irvin Yalom (2005) proposed in his book, *The Theory and Practice of Group Psychotherapy*, a number of therapeutic factors, which he believed occurred in group therapy. He suggested, "Therapeutic change is an enormously complex process and occurs through an intricate interplay of various guided human experiences, which I shall refer to as 'therapeutic factors'" (p. 1). The following is a list of Yalom's proposed therapeutic factors, which will be explained as they relate to drug and alcohol groups:

- Instillation of hope
- Universality
- Development of socializing techniques
- Altruism
- The recapitulation of the primary family group
- Imitative behavior
- Imparting of information
- Interpersonal learning
- Group cohesiveness
- Existential factors
- Catharsis

Instillation of Hope

It is Yalom's belief that hope is a necessary aspect of successful therapy. Clients in group therapy who have improved or grown in recovery can "instill" the hope for change in others. AA uses sponsors as well as the testimonials at speaker meetings to provide hope to those feeling hopeless. Counselors who believe themselves to be catalysts for therapeutic change can also influence clients to believe in the group and their recovery program.

We have observed repeatedly how our belief in the process of recovery and faith in the power of the therapy group combined with clients attending outside support meetings have been significant factors in clients beginning to believe in themselves. At times, clients admitted early on in the process how they depended on other group members and us for the strength to move forward.

Dialogue With Instillation of Hope

Client 1: This past week has been rough. There have been a number of times I wanted to use again but didn't. I really thought through my actions this time and thought about this group. Without this group and the support of AA, I couldn't make it. Coming here to this group means a lot to me and my recovery.

Client 2: I can certainly relate. I too have had a difficult week with the divorce and all. I haven't been able to see my kids in 2 weeks, and I really miss them. I could relate to what John was talking about last week with his custody situation.

Counselor: It really sounds to me that this group is meaningful to a great many of you, almost providing a sense of strength and hope that life can be different in recovery.

Client 3: Absolutely! Most of the time I walk into this group feeling down, and I almost always leave here feeling recharged and ready to work in recovery.

This group is sharing the experience of what it is like to be with each other week-to-week in recovery. They are able to pull strength from each other and, at the same time, relate accountability to each other to stay clean and sober. The facilitator makes a brief statement about how the group is meaningful and provides a sense of hope over the course of the week.

Universality

In heterogeneous groups the group focus may vary from depression to relationship issues. Homogeneous groups, like alcohol and drug groups, connect and jell more quickly because of the universal theme of addiction. Because shame, guilt, and embarrassment accompany clients into the homogeneous group, the rapid realization that they are not alone is therapeutic and healing. For many, this is the first time they have verbalized their feelings of self-hatred and rage. Whereas heterogeneous groups may initially struggle to find universal connections, homogeneous groups quickly begin to understand that each person in the group has experienced similar feelings and consequences from their chemical use.

As inpatient counselors, we witnessed this phenomenon each day as new patients entered the existing group. Many patients arrived tired, depressed, and believing that no one on this planet could possibly relate to their life experiences. As fast as within the first session, group members shared how they could relate to being in treatment and the self-loathing that accompanied the first initial steps in recovery. These realizations, verbalizations, and expressions of connectedness ultimately reduced defenses. Combined with hope, inspired and helped patients progressed forward, armed with the knowledge that they were not alone on their journey and were universally connected through addiction.

Dialogue With Universality

Client 1: I feel so alone here in this group, I don't belong. I am a drinker, not a drug user.

Counselor: What you are saying to the group is that you feel disconnected from this group because the chemical that you use is alcohol and not drugs. I wonder if anyone in the group can relate to what he is feeling?

Client 2: When I first started the group I thought I was the only one with a drinking problem. What I soon found out was that most of the people in this room are alcoholic and addicted to drugs.

Client 3: Yep, I am a hard core alcoholic, have been for 10 years. I just switched to another drug, now I am addicted to both. Be lucky you haven't picked up another chemical.

Client 4: Hey man, we are all in this together. Doesn't matter what you did, it is what you do now that is important.

In this discussion, the group counselor rephrased what was said by the first group member and then opened it up to the group with a general question. The group responded by sharing, and thus a sense of universal "we" was presented and allowed the new group member to hear that he is not alone.

Development of Socializing Techniques

Group counseling provides an experience whereby clients observe and test new behaviors within other interpersonal relationships. Clients vary in their ability to socialize and relate to others. A group can be composed of members who are articulate, socially relaxed, and able to interact with others without too much anxiety, to members who are terrified at the idea of sharing anything in front of others. Group members learn to appreciate the struggles and strengths of each person. Introverted and withdrawn group members can observe how others interact and express empathy, and as a result, they can experiment with new behaviors, transferring newly formed skills to relationships outside of the group. This is particularly important as each member is developing an outside recovery support network.

Dialogue With Development of Socializing Techniques

Client 1: You all seem so comfortable sharing with each other, and I am not sure how to go about talking with the group about what brought me here.

Client 2: Yeah, you seem a little apprehensive about being here.

Counselor: Maybe if you could ask members of the group how they have come to being more comfortable in the group, that might help.

Client 1 seems to have apprehension about sharing in the group. Through observation and direction from the facilitator, the client may begin to learn skills in communication and engage more fully in the group process.

Altruism

Altruism occurs when group members help others in the group. Such behaviors and attitudes are demonstrated through sharing, supporting, and empathizing. Group therapy and AA support meetings function as altruistic settings and are one of the reasons why these therapeutic milieus work well together.

Dialogue With Altruism

Client 1: I'm not sure I can do this recovery 'thing' because I have been through so many treatment programs before. At times I feel I don't have the tools to deal with the reality of life. My life is a total mess, and I don't know where to begin. I lost my job, my wife has filed for divorce, and my kids are not speaking to me.

Client 2: Man, can I relate. This is my fifth rehab and my third marriage. I haven't talked to my kids in 5 years, and I just lost my job. The one thing that I do have is hope. I really feel that this is the time I am going to do it. So, although you feel down, I want to share my hope with you, that our lives can become better. I have had some sobriety in the past and it was wonderful. I want that back. It is possible.

Although Client 2 is not providing the "answers," he is certainly empathic and is trying to share his hope with a group member and help him hear that there are possibilities for the future. The idea of altruism is one person helping another, as was Bill Wilson's (cofounder of AA) understanding of sobriety. In order for him to remain sober, he had to seek out other alcoholics. His sobriety was based on helping others, a main premise of AA (Kurtz, 1979).

The Recapitulation of the Primary Family Group

If you could sit with each client and ask them individually if anyone in the group reminded him or her of a family member (e.g., parent, brother, sister) or evoked a similar feeling as someone in their primary family, you would find the *honest* response to be "yes." Group members transfer their family experiences onto group members as well as onto group counselors. A client raised with an abusive, authoritarian parent might experience strong reactions to members displaying authoritarian behaviors. Those already in positions of authority (i.e., group counselors) act as lightning rods for transference and therefore must continually attend to this dynamic as it plays out in the group. In concert with such awareness is the ability to help clients work through transference.

Dialogue With the Recapitulation of the Primary Family Group

Client 1: You remind me a lot of my father: stubborn, rigid, and funny. Each time you speak I hear his voice in my head. He has been dead for 10 years. He drank himself to death just like you are doing.

Client 2: Stubborn you say, I don't think so [laughs]. Yeah, I've heard that before, particularly from my sponsor. He says I'm hard headed, got to do it my way all the time. That doesn't work so well when you are trying to get sober.

Client 1 presented her feedback concerning a group peer. What resulted was a discussion on how his behavior was not conducive to sobriety. For Client 1, a further exploration by the counselor could help her examine her relationships, how the loss of her father affects her relationships, and how this factors into her recovery.

Imitative Behavior

Social learning occurs throughout the group process (Bandura, 1977). Group members may imitate other group members or the facilitator. This imitative behavior is an important aspect of recovery, allowing the client to practice observed (useful) behaviors by other group members. For instance, a client may observe the positive changes within another group member where the observed behavior is asking for help. Outside of the group, the observing member begins to ask others for help in AA, culminating in the acquisition of a sponsor. Within the group, this member may dress, talk, even act like the observed member. Many times clients have said, "I like what he/she has got in recovery," and because of that they imitate those behaviors.

Example of Imitative Behavior

Client 1 sits next to a group member she finds intriguing and wise. They both arrive early and talk in the parking lot and talk about relationships they have had in the past. Client 1 has begun to dress in a similar fashion as her peer, wearing long, flowing dresses; listens to similar music; and tends to interact with others like her peer.

This particular group member seems to have found someone she can relate to and look up to. She appears to want to be more like her peer, resulting in similar styles and music.

Imparting of Information

This therapeutic factor tends to be present in psychoeducational groups where counselors are imparting or presenting information to clients. The group I (Ford) facilitated every week in a treatment center consisted of information dissemination and client interaction. The information I shared with the group consisted of relapse prevention, which became a topic for discussion in the group.

Information can also be transittted from member to member. Seasoned clients will inform new clients about the process of group therapy, what is expected in the group, and how best to participate in the group to obtain maximum benefit. This peer-level information sharing is powerful because it emanates from the client and helps provide newcomers with structure and meaningful information.

Dialogue With Imparting of Information

Client 1: Well, what I did was to call my EAP (employee assistance program) and discuss my back-to-work plan. What you could do is call your human resources person and find out what your company's policy is on leave. You could also have a back-to-work conference here in treatment before you go back.

This group member is sharing his or her experience with back-to-work issues while providing suggestions to another group member on handling this aspect of recovery.

Interpersonal Learning

An aspect of interpersonal learning that Yalom (2005) described originated from what Henry Stacks Sullivan called *parataxic distortions*. In essence, the client has the "proclivity to distort his or her perception of others" (p. 21). Similar to transference, parataxic distortions are considered to be broader in scope (Yalom, 2005). The patient views and relates to group members with interpersonal distortion. Patients achieve mental health as they become aware of interpersonal dynamics within the group setting.

Important in interpersonal learning, according to Yalom (2005), is the counselor's task in creating and providing an environment for a corrective emotional experience. Such learning occurs when the client has an emotional experience that corrects any previous traumatic or painful events. For example, clients may reexperience sibling rivalry, issues with authority figures (such as the group facilitator), or compete for attention of group members and the leader.

An example of parataxic distortion in a drug and alcohol group is when resistant group members view the facilitators as part of the all-encompassing system that has wrongfully referred them to the group. In this example, members transfer distrust of authority figures, resulting in a distortion of their view of the leaders. Additionally, this mistrust occurs with other group members as well.

When clients begin to trust one another, a corrective emotional experience is more likely to occur. Members having difficulty with other "siblings" in the group are relating to each other in a healthy sibling manner. These challenges can facilitate the emergence of emotions while providing the platform for a corrective experience. In turn, the learning and experimentation involved in the corrective experience can be taken outside of the group and incorporated into behaviors.

Dialogue With Interpersonal Learning

Client 1: I am discovering how difficult it is to open up in this group. I see many of you as not interested and the leaders as judging.

Client 2: Wow, how did you get that? I am very interested and glad each time you participate in the group.

Client 3: Not at all. I really appreciate what you have to say and have learned a great deal from you.

Counselor: It seems as though what you perceived about your peers in the group is not necessarily matching up. Could you talk a bit about where this perception has come from?

As previously discussed, Client 1 is distorting her perception of others in the group. She experiences other members as being disinterested in what she is saying. Parataxic distortion is most probably related to her family of origin where she may not have been validated or listened to, which now transfers to others in the group. Client 1 is learning that her perception of others may not be accurate.

Group Cohesiveness

According to Dickoff and Lakin (1963), former group members found, from a patients' perspective, that group cohesiveness accounts for major therapeutic value. Patients who were able to improve in the group were more likely to have experienced the following: feelings of being accepted by other group members, the ability to perceive some type of similarity with others in the group, and the ability to refer to other group members when asked about the group experience.

Dialogue With Group Cohesiveness

Client 1: I really feel so connected to you all. I feel at times it is us against the world.

Client 2: Yeah, us recovering people among the earth people.

Client 3: I could tell any of you my deepest, darkest secrets, and I would know that you would not judge me and that you would hear me.

Client 4: But boy, we certainly have had some battles getting to this point. Remember those first groups where everyone was defensive. It was like we were just checking each other out and wondering who would break the ice first.

Client 2: And when you two got into it one day, I thought you were going to start throwing punches. And look at us now . . . how awesome.

This conversation demonstrates the struggles this group has experienced along the path of becoming a cohesive group. The group, which started with distrust and fear, has now developed a sense of genuine trust and connection among members.

Existential Factors

Yalom (2005) identified five items relating to existential factors in a group setting. The first factor begins with life at times being unfair and unjust. The second factor addresses the realization that there is no escape from life's pain or, ultimately, death. The third asserts that no matter how close we get to others, life must still be faced alone. Fourth, as a result of realizing the life and death issue, life can and should be lived more honestly. The final component articulates that we are ultimately responsible for the manner in which we live our lives, regardless of the degree of support and guidance we may receive from others.

Addiction can and does lead to death. Inevitably, overdoses, suicide attempts, or being in dangerous situations can surface during the course of group sessions. As a result, members who desire to live life without drugs or alcohol find themselves in a precarious position. While much of their addicted life was spent being dishonest, isolated, and alone, recovery will mean demonstrating honesty on a daily basis, connecting with others emotionally, and living each day fully.

Dialogue With Existential Factors

Client 1: I cannot tell you how many times I have thought of suicide. I ran out of my dope, was on the street, hadn't bathed in a week, and I thought, just end it all.

Client 2: What is it about us addicts? We all have thoughts of killing ourselves at least once. I know I tried once by overdosing on heroin. I just woke up the next day feeling horrible and still had the needle stuck in my arm. And you know what I did? I went out and used again. How insane is that?

Client 3: But you know what? My life has meaning like it never has had before. I know that I am living more honestly, genuinely, and happily, which is a whole lot more freeing.

With death being an ever-present issue in working with addiction, the discussion of death and the new meaning of life take on new meanings in recovery.

Catharsis

Yalom (2005) and colleagues found that catharsis (i.e., intense emotional release), in and of itself, may result in members having a negative group experience. Meaning, in some instances, that when a client has a strong emotional release in group without support or "normalizing of the experience," he or she may experience the release as negative and painful. However, catharsis in combination with other factors was shown to increase group connection and cohesiveness. It is clear that group members do not have to experience a cathartic experience in order to benefit from therapy. Client catharsis without some form of cognitive learning was found to be significantly less effective then when the two were combined.

Drug and alcohol group members have lives filled with intense emotions. Simply allowing them to emote without a cognitive container could lead members to feeling vulnerable. Therefore, when facilitating groups, it is important for counselors to help clients work between emotion and cognition, and allow for personal integration.

Dialogue With Catharsis

Client 1: [Sobbing] Losing my children to child protective services was my bottom. Nothing could be worse than watching your children being taken away in a car because of your using. Now that I am in treatment and detoxed, I feel as though I have hope [still sobbing], but I know it will be tough when I leave this treatment program.

This client is able to share the pain of losing her children, which is directly related to her use. The release found in sharing this with the group is knowing that there is hope for getting her children back.

Closing the Group Session

Group facilitators have a multitude of options for group closure. Closure can denote the end of a session or could signal termination of a closed-ended group. Loss and abandonment are significant issues in the recovery process. Therefore, appropriately closing each session is important. Failing to do so may increase the likelihood of negative results from the group members.

Suggestions for closing each group session include discussing (a) personal awareness and new insights from the group experience, (b) what will be focused on in recovery this week, and/or (c) a significant issue from the group that could be explored in next week's group.

- *Personal awareness:* The group counselor can ask group members to briefly share what they are more aware of now than they were at the beginning of the group. This brings focus to the client and what they have gained in the group for that session. We have found that once introduced to the group, the request manifests into a group norm, with group members doing this without being prompted each week.
- *Recovery focus:* The focus is action oriented to help clients integrate and take action on recovery issues brought up in the group. This process encourages group members to engage in new behaviors and experiment with taking healthy risks in recovery. For example, "On the basis of what you heard in here today, and what you discussed personally, what can you work on this week in recovery?" We have found often that clients return the next week with reports on their newly experimented behaviors.
- *Setting the agenda for the following group:* This process helps clients to not only bring to awareness what they have explored in the group but also helps them create a continuum of what they want to continue to work on in group therapy. Through encouraging continued growth and future plans, we have found that clients are better armed to cope with "down time" between groups. Hope in future plans is a powerful elixir.

Closure With Closed-Ended Groups

Counselors working with groups with a defined ending date should address closure needs 3 to 4 weeks before the final session. During those 3 to 4 weeks, the counselor can ask group members the following questions:

- What will it be like to not be in the group?
- Who has impacted you in the group and why?
- Who in the group has made significant impacts and why?
- What has the group meant for your recovery?
- What was it like at the beginning of the group and what has been learned?
- What meaning have you made from the group?
- How has the group made a significant difference in your life?
- What aspects would you like to continue to work on and how will life be different for you without the group?

The facilitator can also

- Provide group members with feedback on what they did to increase awareness.
- Make space for the members to share feelings related to loss (e.g., fear, sadness, anger).
- Help clients remember what they sounded like when they first came into the group, and help them see that any changes they have made are important.
- Ask members to provide their own feedback on what they have seen in regards to progress and suggest any areas for continuous attention.

- Facilitate the emotions related to the loss of relationships. For many clients, this will mimic the discussion of the loss of their drug and can stimulate feelings related to previous losses in life.

In Appendix 10.A at the end of this chapter is a process I (Ford) have used both in teaching the group class and for clients leaving group.

Summary

This chapter provided the basics of group development and the therapeutic factors involved. The aspects of process versus content were discussed as well as the need for a here-and-now focus in the group discussion. This chapter has built on the previous chapters by preparing readers to understand addiction and the models of recovery. The next chapter reaches further into group by highlighting relapse prevention and the importance of collaborative support and addiction support meetings.

Exploration Questions From Chapter 10

1. What types of groups have you facilitated in the past, if any?
2. In your mind, how does group counseling benefit the addicted client?
3. How might you implement a group in your work or at your internship site? How would you create and market the group?
4. Describe methods in which you already help clients focus on the here-and-now in session.
5. Discuss with a small group the use of individual counseling versus group counseling with an addicted population.

Suggested Activities

1. Observe a counselor facilitating a drug and alcohol group. Notice how the counselor initiates the process and the techniques used during the session. Record your experiences and discuss with the counselor.
2. Develop a group program for your particular work or at your internship site. Develop the topic, how you will obtain clients, how you will market the group, the length of time, cost, and goals/objectives.

Appendix 10.A
Closing Group Activities

Stony Giveaway

This activity is primarily for closed-ended groups and is designed to help provide feedback to each group member while bringing closure to the group process. Before this exercise, a great deal of time has been spent in previous groups talking about loss and the feelings related to loss. The day of the final group is a time of both celebration and saying goodbye.

Some polished stones are set in a bowl and placed in the middle of the group. One at a time, each group member goes to the middle of the circle and selects a stone. The first person who selects a stone (stone owner) passes it to his or her right. The person receiving the stone will provide feedback to the stone owner by filling in the blank: "My hope for you is _____." Following this sentence completion, brief parting comments from that person are made. The stone is then passed to the right and that person goes through the same process. The stone is then passed all the way around the circle until it reaches the stone's owner. At that point each person in the group has provided feedback to the stone's owner. The stone's owner then provides brief parting words to the entire group.

Each group member will go through the same process. This procedure typically requires 60 to 90 minutes to provide feedback for each group member. The group facilitator participates as well. At the end of the group, the facilitator can choose to pick up a stone and pass it around in order to help clients with their closure toward the facilitator.

After all of the stones have been passed around and the feedback provided, each member of the group stands and places his/her arms around the shoulders of the members next to them, if they feel comfortable doing so. The counselor can then choose to say a parting comment or read a particular meaningful passage to the group about closure. I (Ford) have included below the narrative Collective Spirits that I wrote about group experience and continue to read it to my groups when they close. At the end of the group I give them a copy of the reading, plus they take the stone with them.

Collective Spirits

When we examine ourselves through the lenses of others, it is important to recognize that in order for this to happen, we must first be willing to be vulnerable and begin facing our back rooms of darkness and fear. The darkness we are willing to face empowers us to voice that pain and truth with others, so as to make it real and alive in our hearts. As a result, we begin to face the darkness and take action.

This process can allow our demons to be set free within the safety of others and in turn loosen the grip, which stifles the exploration of our individual truth. For some, this process awakens action not thought possible; for others, it is a continuation of connecting with relationships and an enhancement of heart.

You see, this group has had implications far greater than a circle meeting each day or week. I entered this group with some trepidation. I am leaving with an understanding not only of group and individual processes but also, and maybe even more importantly, my own process. I have begun to face the dark and misty edges of my life that I had not explored to the degree I did in here. I found that a great deal of my examination and exploration really came outside of the group, while interacting with others or sitting alone in silence. This group has allowed me to view life through different lenses and look for the teachable moments and individuals who surround me. I can say through this process that I have become much more aware not only of my own thoughts and feelings but also of the environment and the people and conditions that are around me on a regular basis.

What strikes me most is how this process of exploration, both in a group and by myself, has helped me develop insight and awareness. We cannot exist in isolation and need the connection with others, the connection of which has allowed me to see the unity and similarity with others amidst the differences. This to me has global and environmental implications, and this experience can be expanded to the enormity of life: the connection with a group, a community, my culture, and something much greater that I cannot explain. Meeting together as a group is all of this, spiritual yet concrete, terrifying yet comforting, lonely yet connecting. It has represented the paradoxes in life and has opened my eyes to the possibilities that I never knew possible.

As a result of this group, I personally commit to examine the process that occurs in life and how my actions and choices impact others and my environment. I will also continue, day-by-day, to see the importance in connecting with others and how my life will be used as an instrument in the facilitation of helping those in need.

To all of my group members, thank you for your insight and feedback. Your life has helped me grow, which in turn will help others grow. In order for us to keep what we have, we need to learn to pass it on, for the circle truly never ends.

Relapse Prevention and Recovery

A number of years ago I (Ford) worked for Father Martin's Ashley, a renowned inpatient treatment facility located in Havre de Grace, Maryland. I was hired specifically to create an outpatient relapse prevention program in Richmond, Virginia, to address the needs of relapsing clients. Those who entered the program were *veteran* treatment clients who had received treatment services from many of the detoxification units and treatment programs throughout the state. These clients recognized their addiction to drugs and alcohol; the major problem was that they were unable to stay sober for any considerable length of time. Subsequently, I developed a specialty in working with relapsing clients. This chapter outlines the lessons learned at this setting and others in which we have worked. The chapter further extrapolates the relapse (and relapse prevention) cycle and considers ways to address this diverse, challenging population. Throughout this chapter readers are exposed to a process of relapse prevention combined with spiritual dimensions of recovery. This combination highlights pragmatic and practical information for both generalist counselors and addiction-specific counselors.

According to Gorski (1989), clients not actively addressing recovery issues potentially move closer to relapse. We can infer from this postulate that clients need to be vigilant in their recovery efforts. The process of relapse, according to Gorski, can occur over a period of time or may quickly escalate depending on the client's immediate environment, physical cravings, coping skills, and support. It is critical that counselors respect the imperfection of the process, understanding that client relapse is part of the change process. The relapse process culminates with the actual use of chemicals, and therefore it is critical for clients to understand their idiosyncratic relapse patterns, triggers, and warning signs as an outcome of effective counseling and treatment.

Relapse prevention offers clients an increased opportunity to identify their core beliefs, emotions, and behaviors in an effort to self-intervene and choose alternative, healthier behaviors. Left unaware and therefore unchecked, clients repeat the same thoughts, feelings, and behaviors, resulting in chemical use and repetition of the cycle. Recovery begins with a shift in thinking followed by a change in behaviors (abstinence and recovery activities). Relapse, like recovery, also begins internally and culminates in behavioral change (using chemicals). The approach to working with relapsing clients differs from that of working with clients who have never been in treatment before and have never attempted sobriety. Therapeutically, the initial hope with relapse prevention begins with the relationship between the counselor and the client.

Relapsing clients generally have a multitude of issues that can combine to sabotage their recovery efforts. These variables may consist of depression, personality disorders, or other compulsive behaviors (e.g., shopping, gambling, and sex). After clients have been in multiple addiction treatments, 12-step meetings, and are facing the multitude of consequences from their relapses, they usually experience powerful self-messages of feeling hopeless, suicidal, and very depressed. It is incumbent on the counselor to recognize and then avoid the abyss of hopelessness. Useful counselor behaviors here include listening and empathizing with the client's feelings and current felt position in life. By so doing, counselors can forge a therapeutic relationship of honesty, genuineness, and hope. We truly believe, after having worked with many relapsing clients, that it is the hope and spirit of the counselor that can make a significant difference with clients and their belief in recovery. Throughout our careers we have listened attentively during clinical staff meetings to other counselors (as well as ourselves) present case after case of relapsing clients. In many of the clinical presentations we heard value judgments, blame, and overall feelings of hopelessness. When counselors reach such a point, they temporarily lose the helping spirit and are caught in the cycle of our own hopelessness and despair. This is an example of how countertransference unfolds in the counseling relationship, creating a potential therapeutic impasse. Relapsing clients transfer feelings of hopelessness, which, in turn, may evoke unconscious responses from counselors. These responses can evoke overprotection from counselors or evoke emotions of anger, rage, or even hate for clients.

What Are the Unique Aspects of Relapse Treatment?

Clients entering treatment for the first time usually do not have a deep understanding of addiction. Treatment programs educate clients on the disease of addiction, the impact alcohol and drugs have on the body, and the effects on family members, employers, and friends. Additionally, the focus of treatment is on helping clients learn about their disease, identify emotions and defenses, commit to the development of a support system and ongoing recovery program, and involve family members in their recovery.

Relapse treatment, however, focuses primarily on helping clients identify how they moved from a recovery process to a relapse process. A client's relapse does not mean all is lost. On the contrary, clients can learn a great deal from the relapses if they are willing. The operative word, however, is *willing*. As the relapse process unfolds, so does the reinforcement of the denial system, which is ultimately strengthened by chemical use. Outcomes studies indicate that most relapse occurs within the first 90 days of sobriety ("Relapse Prevention Therapy," 1999). In an interview, Terence Gorski suggested that treatment professionals and counselors need to readjust their thinking. He contended that counselors need to work with clients in treatment on relapse issues and not wait until relapse occurs. "Now it is no longer a matter of waiting for a relapse history to develop. We are working more and more toward a set of treatment principles that can be used immediately at the first signs of real or potential relapse problems" ("Relapse Prevention Therapy," 1999, p. 34). Clients may enter treatment multiple times. The goal is for clients to put together more and more abstinent days so that ultimately it will become continuous sobriety. Each time, however, clients will potentially have teachable moments when they can obtain missing pieces to their recovery puzzle. However, some clients lack the ability to be honest and are unable to remain abstinent. "Those who do not recover are people who cannot or will not completely give themselves to this simple program, usually men and women who are constitutionally incapable of being honest with themselves" (Alcoholics Anonymous [AA], 1976, p. 58). Through it all, counselors working with relapsing clients need to be nonjudgmental and supportive of clients reengaging in the recovery process, rather than punishing them for returning to using.

Counselors need to help clients learn from their relapses by asking, "What have you learned from your relapse? What did it teach you about areas in your recovery that needed attention?" Additional information that augments the insight process includes merging the responses to the questions above with previous and current assessment data. It is critical for counselors to codevelop a comprehensive understanding of the current situation in order to formulate an effective plan of action. The following example describes a client who has relapsed and how the counselor has helped bring all the information together in order to create a treatment plan.

Case of Dennis

For years Dennis attempted sobriety. At an early age he witnessed his father slowly medicate himself with alcohol. He eventually died a premature death from cirrhosis of the liver. Dennis was the middle child and married early to get out of the house, to work, to be on his own, and to depend on no one but himself. He said he would never drink like his father or put his family through the hell that he endured.

Unfortunately, his drinking pattern was just like that of his father, and in 1983 Dennis's wife of 10 years threatened to leave him if he didn't stop drinking. Dennis entered detoxification and inpatient treatment and followed through with aftercare for 6 months. He became involved in AA, obtained a sponsor, and was able to remain sober for the next 3 years. In 1986 Dennis's wife was killed in a car accident, decimating his life and leaving him as a single parent of two children. At that point he reduced his AA meetings and focused on raising his children, working extra hours to meet the mounting financial responsibilities. In 1990 both of his children graduated from college, and very quickly they found jobs in their studied professions. Dennis realized he no longer needed to work extra hours, and with that change came idle time. He spent more and more time isolated, feeling alone, and missing his wife and his children. Although he had not returned to AA after his wife died, he was able to remain abstinent. Dennis thought he could drink controllably, which he did for 2 months. He started with two beers, which soon led to a 12-pack, and eventually to half a fifth of vodka each night.

Coworkers, and eventually his supervisor, confronted Dennis over the smell of alcohol on his breath. Dennis was warned, yet he continued to drink. Finally, the supervisor gave him an ultimatum: either go to treatment and sober up or lose his job of 23 years.

Once again Dennis went to detoxification; however, this time he needed less time at the inpatient treatment facility. After inpatient treatment, he attended 2 months of intensive outpatient treatment and regular 12-step meetings. Dennis understood the routine and was familiar with AA, except this time he was ashamed, angry, and less motivated for sobriety. However, he did enjoy his work and did not want to lose his job. He continued with treatment, was successfully discharged, and continued with AA for another 5 months, at which point he again stopped attending.

Dennis remained abstinent but was still very bitter about the death of his wife and his employer's intervention. One night on the way home from work, Dennis decided to stop by a local bar and watch the playoffs. After two sodas he ordered a vodka martini and stayed until closing. On his way home he was pulled over by the police for swerving, was arrested for drunk driving, and spent the rest of the evening in jail. Because of his incarceration he missed work and lied to his supervisor. As a result of the arrest and subsequent conviction, Dennis lost his license for a year.

Commentary

There are a number of significant issues presented by Dennis that would factor into a relapse prevention plan. The warning signs for Dennis began with his belief that he could control his drinking, isolation, resentment, and discontinue his support meetings. In addition to these warning signs is his difficulty in expressing emotion. At an early age, he witnessed his father handle stress and emotions with alcohol. Dennis learned not to talk about his feelings or to depend on anyone but himself (Black, 1981). Dennis also brought unresolved grief into his marriage from childhood, which (just like his father) he self-medicated. Dennis learned to not depend on others, so even though he has been involved in AA, he finds it difficult to develop relationships or reach out for help, which leaves him feeling increasingly isolated and alone. His wife's death only compounded his already present unresolved grief and anger. The multiple relapses, shame, and resentments have all con-tributed to justification for drinking. Additionally, Dennis may be a candidate for medica-tion evaluation concerning his depression, on the basis of his upbringing, loss of wife, and difficulty initiating interests, activities, or relationships.

This vignette offers an example of how the life history and patterns of relapse can pro-vide both the client and the counselor with treatment goal planning information. The fol-lowing pages describe areas to address in relapse prevention: shame, other compulsions and addictions, and other relapse prevention models.

Case of Mandy

Mandy has been using alcohol, marijuana, and cocaine for the past 5 years, producing dev-astating results. She entered counseling at the urging of her friends and after legal charge, which occurred 6 months ago. At that time, Mandy made the decision to discontinue her drug and alcohol use and then chose to enter counseling. She has been concentrating on abstinence and other complicating issues.

Mandy's past includes a significant trauma and instability. At age 8, she was sexually molested over a dozen times by a trusted neighbor. When she disclosed this trauma to her parents, they dismissed it (and her) and accused her of lying. At age 10, Mandy's father was killed in a car accident, leaving her mother to raise two children. Mandy reports that she coped with this loss and earlier molestation by acting out sexually and through disor-dered eating.

Her life has been manifest with problems with weight, depression, and the healthy ex-pression of emotion. As an adult she reports being attracted to intensely controlling and abusive men.

When Mandy was 14 she started smoking pot; at 15 she starting using alcohol; at 17 she started using cocaine with her boyfriend. She found alcohol and drugs to hold pleasurable results: They numbed her emotions and helped her lose weight.

The past 6 months represent the longest period of abstinence since her first use of pot. Now, at age 30, Mandy is trying to negotiate the emotions of the past and the consequences of her chemical use.

Dealing With Shame in Recovery

Shame, for many addicted clients, is at the emotional core of their being (Bradshaw, 1988). Shame may originate from familial upbringing (i.e., abandonment, trauma), their active addiction (behaviors under the influence), or a combination of both. For example, Mandy has the combination of a shame-based upbringing and shame-related consequences stem-ming from her drug use. These are potential pivot points for relapse, if left unaddressed in treatment.

As Mandy remains abstinent in early recovery, a number of possibilities exist. She may remain abstinent and unconsciously repress her feelings and early experiences. This in turn might lead to enacting previous behaviors (preusing) that brought about emotional relief (e.g., compulsive eating, relationships, depression). Conversely, she may become aware of the painful experiences, emotions, and memories that have surfaced as a result of being abstinent and become willing to address these in counseling. Movement in either direction will probably increase the potential to continue using chemicals. However, in the latter scenario, because Mandy is much more cognizant of her emotions, she has an increased possibility of exploring options for managing her chemical use and expressing her emotions.

Shame is a core feeling for many addicts and alcoholics. Because early recovery includes the remission of self-medication with chemicals, shame and other feelings typically surface. As shame is identified, the mind and body act to eliminate pain. This usually occurs through control, developing and maintaining family roles, perfectionism, as well as blame and judgment of others. Bradshaw (1988) suggested that compulsive and addictive behaviors take away the pain associated with shame. Additionally, it is in those behaviors that take much of the life of the addict and alcoholic. Further, Bradshaw stated that shame is an intolerable pain needing immediate relief, either through some thing, person, or behavior, each of which can significantly alter emotions.

Types of Compulsive and Addictive Behaviors

Food

Food (in particular, those with sugar and white flour, which are high carbohydrate, high fat products) can be consumed to medicate painful emotions. Mandy, our client, instead of drinking alcohol may consume three boxes of sugared donuts to medicate her emotions of sadness, shame, and guilt. As she continues this behavior with food, she may experience increasingly more guilt, shame, and anger for consuming large quantities of food. In turn, this behavior initiates an increase in her weight, and thus she may consider using cocaine again, as she did before, to lose weight. Mandy may also binge and purge, so as not to gain weight. This cycle of behaviors may initially repress emotions of self-hatred, yet paradoxically it makes these emotions more pronounced.

Codependent Relationships

Codependent relationships originated from the word, *co-alcoholic–addict*. It was used to identify individuals in a relationship with alcoholics or addicts who defined themselves through those other relationships. In other words, "Who I am is who you want me to be…my world depends totally and completely on you." So as a codependent, the feelings of shame, loss, and guilt are medicated and avoided by involvement in a relationship with someone else of great need (Beattie, 1987).

Work

For many clients early in recovery, working excessive hours at their job is not uncommon. Because of the financial toll their addiction costs, clients may work 70–80 or more hours per week to pay bills, fines, and mortgage companies. Unfortunately, as clients work those long work weeks, they are usually not attending ongoing treatment or support meetings with any regularity because they are too involved in work. Compulsive workers work regardless of potential consequences in their recovery program. For instance, clients who have paid their bills and are now financially stable, still continue to work long hours. This behavior impacts their families because of their absence from home, and, work has now become the primary focus rather than their chemical usage.

Sexual Behavior

An area of recovery from alcohol and drug addiction that is minimally addressed in treatment and recovery is addictive and compulsive sexual behavior (Carnes, Delmonico, & Griffin, 2001). Addiction to drugs or alcohol can readily switch to sexual behaviors through various avenues: Internet compulsive sexual behaviors, frequent use of prostitution and strip clubs, pornographic materials, or affairs that are sexual in nature. These sexual behaviors medicate clients from emotions through an alteration in brain chemistry via sexual stimulation (Carnes et al., 2001).

Clinical Example

A large proportion of male addicts and alcoholics we have worked with who are attempting sobriety and recovery find relief in compulsive sexual behaviors, which ultimately creates a separate set of consequences. For example, a client I (Ford) worked with discontinued using crack cocaine, however, he began online discussions with other women (he was married at the time). The online discussion was followed with subsequent physical meetings and sexual intercourse. Instead of him using cocaine, he was now medicating with sex, lying, being preoccupied, and hiding his behavior with sex just as he had with cocaine. He switched from one to the other, both with considerable consequences. Not only was he lying to his wife and me but he also eventually returned to his cocaine use, which he said medicated his feelings of guilt.

Patrick Carnes has written a great deal on the subject of sexual addiction. Most recently his cowritten book titled *In the Shadows of the Net: Breaking Free of Compulsive Online Sexual Behavior* (Carnes et al., 2001), focuses on equating both the addiction to online sexual behavior to alcohol and drug addiction and recovery. The authors have described the challenge for clients in identifying feelings and cravings or impulses to seek sex as well as modalities of intervention in the process, which include support groups, therapy, and journaling.

Delmonico and Griffin (2002) suggested when screening for problems with sexual compulsivity that clinicians recognize the disorder generally does not stand alone. A comprehensive initial screening is very important for effective treatment planning. The initial interview should include questions that distinguish between sexual concerns and sexual compulsivity. Questions also need to evaluate whether their substance affects their sexual behaviors. The sexual history, frequency, loss of control, obsession, and negative consequences of the sexual behaviors need to be evaluated to determine if treatment is warranted. Formal assessment tools include sexual interview instruments such as the Sexual Addiction Screening Test as well as a thorough medical and psychiatric workup. Clients requiring treatment for sexual compulsivity should be provided referrals to support groups such as Sexaholics Anonymous (SA), Sex Addict Anonymous (SAA), Sexual Recovery Anonymous (SRA), Sexual Compulsives Anonymous (SCA), and Sex and Love Addicts Anonymous (SLAA; Delmonico & Griffin, 2002).

Treatment issues include individual as well as group therapy, celibacy contracts, and psychoeducation. Sexual disorders and substance disorders need to be treated concurrently. Identification and treatment of sexual disorders need to be included as an active part of the recovery plan. Relapse back to either sexual behavior or drug/alcohol use is increased if both are not treated together.

Money, Gambling, and Shopping

This behavior of addiction and compulsion includes any form of gambling, both sanctioned (e.g., casino, poker, horse racing) or unsanctioned (e.g., dice games on the street, flipping coins). The excitement is in the possibility of winning and eternally chasing the intoxication that follows the win. Despite the growing insurmountable debt, loss of family, employment, and so on, the addicted individual presses on. Shopping, although not gambling, uses money to temporarily medicate or soothe emotions.

Nicotine, Caffeine, and Sugar

All three of these substances will alter the mood of the consumer and, in large quantities, develop into an addiction. In thousands of 12-step meetings around the world, on any given day, one can find vast amounts of all three being consumed. Although participants are not using alcohol or drugs, there is a replacement with these substances that can also create physical as well as emotional distress.

Take for instance a person who 8 years ago stopped using heroin and alcohol, only to increase his nicotine use to three packs of cigarettes and two pots of coffee each day. He is no longer using heroin or alcohol, is still with his family, is gainfully employed, and is enjoying the freedom in recovery. However, his addiction to nicotine has created other problems: an increase in blood pressure, which has caused him to take blood pressure medication daily, lack of exercise, and the need to smoke every 30–40 minutes. His consumption of caffeine has created dependence where he must have it in the morning to stave off headaches. Because of his increasing consumption of sugar, he has been warned by his physician that diabetes is a possibility if he does not alter his diet.

The devastation of this combination, if not altered in some manner, will ultimately create increasing medical problems: circulatory, digestive, and respiratory. Of course, on the positive side, he is not incarcerated, nor is he leaving the house at 3 a.m. to buy drugs; however, his "prison" is now with nicotine, caffeine, and sugar. Without these substances he would most certainly experience withdrawal symptoms and an influx of emotions.

What Can Counselors Do to Help?

Counselors need to visualize an individual trying to balance in water on top of many large balloons. The initial balloon the client tries to push down to maintain some amount of balance is alcohol or drug recovery. However, another balloon (e.g., disordered eating) may rise to the surface to which the client needs to attend. Then a third balloon may surface as the second balloon is being balanced under the water (e.g., sex), and now the focus shifts to that balloon. This process may rotate back to using alcohol or drugs. Or the client may begin to achieve a sense of balance in his or her recovery with each balloon and place less and less energy on the surface behaviors and more on his or her internal experience (thoughts, emotions, spirituality).

[handwritten margin note: Balloon analogy]

Once counselors have an understanding of this process, they can help clients explore emotions, urges, and high-risk thoughts that trigger these behaviors. Counselors need to examine this process through the lens of progress rather than perfection with their clients. Clients get scared, and when they do, they many times want to medicate the emotions with chemicals or behaviors that derive instant pleasure, regardless of long-term consequences. Emotions can become overwhelming, and rather than using chemicals, they spend money on gambling or compulsively eat. Helping clients recognize this cycle is a significant step in recovery awareness. The hardest work for clients begins *after* the drug and alcohol use stops. The *Big Book* of AA (1976) states, "Our liquor was but a symptom. So we had to get down to causes and conditions" (p. 64). It could also read, "Our [eating, gambling, sex] was but a symptom." Counselors help clients to recover values, a sense of self, emotions, and dignity. Responses to emotions discussed here keep clients from that process. Therefore, counselors and clients need to identify and address emotions as they surface, which means counselors should be familiar with specific treatment referrals, support groups, or medical practitioners who specialize in each of these unique areas.

What Can a Counselor Do When the Client Relapses?

When clients relapse, doesn't that mean all is lost? On the contrary, clients can learn a great deal from their relapses. As the relapse process unfolds, so does the reinforcement of the denial system, which is ultimately strengthened by chemical use. However, a client could relapse, as suggested by Gorski (1989) and Marlatt (Manisses Communication Group, 1994), to signal use that was prior to compulsive, out-of-control using. In these instances when the client is potentially able to cease the use of chemicals on his or her own without medical or hospital intervention, learning and growth can occur. In such cases, clients may have a moment of clarity or very quickly find themselves in trouble, thus reengaging in a recovery process. However, some clients lack the ability to be honest and are unable to remain abstinent. Through it all, counselors working with relapsing clients need to be nonjudgmental and supportive of clients reengaging in the recovery process, rather than punishing them for returning to use. Asking open questions such as "What have you learned from your relapse this time that you were not aware of before?" or "What were some of the thoughts, feelings, and behaviors you experienced prior to this use?" can help clients learn missing pieces in their recovery plan. As counselors, we need to recognize relapse thinking and behavior in clients and help them discover signs prior to using. When clients relapse, they typically have a set pattern of useless behaviors. Counselors need to have patience and a helping spirit when working with relapsing clients. Many times, clients will call and report to their counselors that they have used again and ask if they can come back in for counseling. The underlying meanings many times sound like this, "Hey, I screwed up again and I am really ashamed, but I am calling you because I trust you. Please don't give up on me." Included in that can also be, "I am willing to exercise new strategies and take action on areas I have been resistant." This is change talk, suggesting that they are willing to initiate new action (W. R. Miller & Rollnick, 2002). Following relapse, clients can reengage in counseling, review their previous plan, add new strategies to the plan, and act on new behavior. In conjunction with treatment and counseling is the importance of outside support meetings and the role spirituality plays in the recovery process, which is discussed in the next chapter.

Below are examples of possible options for postrelapse counseling:

- *Treatment referral:* Eating disorder clinics, gambling and sexual addiction specialists, programs, or support groups.
- *Support group:* Overeaters Anonymous (OA), Gamblers Anonymous (GA), Sex Addicts Anonymous (SAA), which are all faith-based support groups focusing on these issues.
- *Medical practitioner:* Psychiatrists as well as physicians who work with smoking cessation or other medical problems.
- *Nutritionist:* To work with clients on developing and maintaining a healthy regiment of food each day.

As clients follow through with other support and referrals, counselors can work with clients exploring the emotions that are considered to be the causes and conditions that perpetuate these behaviors.

Emotional Identification and Management

The denial and repression of emotions are at the core of these behaviors. They are the causes and conditions. Counselors need to spend time helping clients identify those emotions they experience throughout the day. The use of an emotions chart can help clients select and identify that with which they feel. Counselors also want to explore and encourage emotional growth and maturity.

Essentially, counselors bring all of the chapters in this book into practice by being multi-faceted, ranging from assessment to the actual counseling with clients as they discontinue using drugs and alcohol.

Models of Relapse Prevention

Relapse Prevention: Mackay and Marlatt (1994)

Mackay and Marlatt (1994) believed that relapse is a process that occurs with a host of variables, including negative emotional states, social and environmental peer pressure to use or drink, and physiological factors such as cravings and euphoric recall. They suggest an approach to relapse prevention that identifies problem behavior and situations. Following this awareness is to intervene in hopes of preventing the entire relapse process from unfolding. Relapse prevention is initiated with the assessment of high-risk situations for relapse. Witkiewitz and Marlatt (2004) described high risk as a circumstance when the person attempting relapse is threatened by the situation. High-risk situations can include previous using establishments, people, events, or times of year. Mackay and Marlatt have encouraged counselors to explore and challenge clients and their expectations and perceived results, which ultimately can help clients make a more informed decision. This particular model distinguishes between a relapse and a lapse, where relapse is viewed as a significant step backward and the prediction of future behavior is unknown (Mackay & Marlatt, 1994). This relapse prevention model helps clients identify personal high-risk situations and conditions, then create coping skills to help negotiate those particular conditions.

Relapse is not identified by one particular thing, but rather it often results from a combination of factors including internal factors, environmental factors, and physical or physiological factors (Mackay & Marlatt, 1994). Included in Marlatt's initial work on relapse are concepts that include apparently irrelevant decisions, the distinction between relapse and lapse, the significance of altering one's lifestyle, the relapse process as a teachable experience, engaging in an earnest review of the relapse and what could be learned from it, and finally, the idea of going beyond the disease concept of internal causation to help clients identify external cues and stimuli as part of their relapse prevention efforts.

Washton's Model of Relapse Prevention With Cocaine Addicts

Like most other relapse protocols, Washton and Stone-Washton (1990) suggested abstinence, regular urine testing, relapse prevention education, individual and group sessions, along with therapy for family members and couples. Encapsulated within therapy is client attendance at 12-step support meetings. Creating significant structure early in the recovery process while addressing emotional and environmental triggers is tantamount. Washton and Stone-Washton believe the focus on treatment must be on abstinence first and then on relapse prevention.

Outcome data on relapse prevention efforts with cocaine addicts suggest that they can be treated successfully in outpatient or inpatient programs that are followed by intensive continuing care focusing on relapse prevention (Washton & Stone-Washton, 1990). Washton and Stone-Washton concluded that 68% of outpatients and 64% of inpatients were abstinent at a 6- to 24-month follow-up, according to interviews and urine screen results. Abstinence results for individuals who smoked crack or free-based cocaine (58%) were lower than for those individuals who snorted cocaine (78%; Washton & Stone-Washton, 1990).

Terence Gorski's CENAPS Model of Relapse Prevention

Chapter 7 addressed a developmental model of recovery that suggested stages of recovery. Gorski (1989) stated that as clients transit the stages of recovery, they may experience stuck points. A stuck point might be an issue with a relationship that needs to be worked through. It could also be a financial issue such as the client has difficulty paying bills and is overwhelmed by the lacking funds. The issues that become stuck points can either be early recovery issues (e.g., lack of trust from partner) or everyday issues (e.g., flat tire going to work). Regardless, these moments, experiences, and reactions could be flash points for the beginnings of a stuck point.

For instance, a client in early recovery, who is attending AA meetings, and who is sober has a disagreement with his supervisor. The client becomes angry and overwhelmed and feels unable to talk directly to the supervisor. The client ultimately has two primary directions of action: address the issue with the supervisor or avoid the discomfort associated with talking about the issue with the supervisor. The longer he avoids the situation, the more anxiety and stress he may feel, and potentially the more resentful he may become. As he decides to avoid the issue and the stress increases as a result of the inaction, he begins to feel stuck, frustrated, and/or depressed. Although he is aware of the feelings, he is unwilling to address them, ultimately contributing to stress and feeling immobilized.

Another client, in a similar set of circumstances, could handle the situation in a completely different manner. He could go home that night and talk with his AA group, sponsor, or other AA members about how to handle the frustration. Of importance here is that he is not isolating or suppressing emotions. He is asking for help, which is important in the recovery process. The next day he wakes up, sets up a time to talk with his supervisor, and attempts to resolve the issue with the supervisor. Whether the issue is resolved or not is not the point; that is not nearly as important as the process of dealing with a potential ember of relapse. His willingness to ask for help and follow suggestions made may have a major impact on his remaining sober. Conversely, the person in the first example who decides to handle it alone may be setting himself up for a potential relapse. We see the same situation handled in two very different ways. The first client gets stuck, whereas the second client maintains connection to others in recovery, remains humble, and is open to direction and suggestions.

Gorski (1989) provided a useful acronym for understanding the first client described above: ESCAPE. Using this lens, we can see how the first client responded to the issue at work: *evade* the situation or stuck point; *stress* (which is created by the evasion); *compulsive* behavior (what the client participates in to temporarily salve the emotional stress); *avoid* others such as sponsor, 12-step members, friends, and family; these responses ultimately create new *problems* (lack of trust and communication); and as a result, create more *evasion* from more problems.

The acronym indicating how the second client handled the situation is RADAR: *recognize* that a problem exists (i.e., realize there is an issue with the supervisor and not deny it); *accept* that it is normal and okay to have problems or issues in recovery; *detach* to gain a new perspective and step back from the problem; *ask* others for help and their viewpoint or experience; and *respond* with action when appropriate and when ready (Gorski, 1989).

Clients who do not address stuck points in recovery, according to Gorski (1989), will move into a relapse process where they are internally avoiding and evading uncomfortable feelings. This choice promotes an increase in levels of anxiety and stress. As internal stress increases, the external defenses increase, which in turn increase the stress level even more, creating a stress loop. The initial issue with the supervisor has now become an internal dysfunction where the client begins to have difficulty thinking clearly, managing feelings, or sleeping well. As the internal dysfunction grows, so will the behavioral signs (i.e., avoidance, immobilization, depression, and confusion), which are more visible to friends, family, and coworkers. Those surrounding the individual may begin to express concerns. The denied feelings contribute to stress, which in turn impact behavior and lead to out of control behavior, compulsiveness, and physical or emotional collapse, culminating with the relapse of the drug.

The second client, instead of minimizing or negating feelings, works through and addresses the feeling, maintaining the recovery loop. Stuck points for clients may occur at any point during recovery. The more clients have in the experience of working through these stuck points with the help of others, the more coping skills that are developed, and the more clients feel at ease in asking for help, thus reducing the discomfort.

Gorski's seminal research was interviewing relapsing alcoholics. From these discussions, multiple signs of relapse were identified in Gorski and Miller's (1986) book and workbook, *Staying Sober: A Guide for Relapse Prevention*. The following pages outline the basic themes suggested by this research.

Phases of the Warning Signs

- *Phase I* describes the return of the denial system where clients begin to minimize, rationalize, justify, and distort their feelings. When asked by others how they are feeling, many times the response is "I'm fine" even though internally they may feel a great deal of stress and anxiety. This is the beginning of the separation from the emotional self.

- *Phase II* indicates the presence of denial and avoidant or defensive behaviors. Clients in this phase believe they will never use again and tend to focus on others rather than themselves. Additionally, if confronted about their well-being they become defensive and engage in either impulsive or compulsive behaviors, which result in isolation.

- *Phase III* is when the internal dysfunction grows and clients are avoiding others. The crisis builds, resulting in multiple problems where denial increases. Recovery plans that have been made may unravel, resulting in minor depression. At this point clients may be disconnected from self and others, thus increasing the feelings of being stuck.

- *Phase IV* of the relapse process has clients feeling as though they are going through the motions and wishing life would be different.

- *Phase V* brings confusion, overreaction, and a loss of faith in the recovery process. Family and friends may observe irrational behavior and anger and feelings of being overwhelmed may be apparent. Although clients may be attending therapy, 12-step meetings, and remaining abstinent, they may not be talking about the feelings occurring internally.

- *Phase VI* clients are presenting symptoms of relapse that are very similar to depression: lethargy, irregular sleeping and eating patterns, and feeling very depressed.

- *Phase VII* is when the depression worsens and clients begin to reject help, miss treatment and support meetings, lie, and lose self-confidence. In addition is an "I don't care" attitude, which is the beginning of a justification to drink or use.

- *Phase VIII* is far down the process, and some clients become suicidal rather than picking up and using again. The options are reduced and feelings of being trapped consume clients. Twelve-step meetings and treatment group attendance typically discontinues at this point, and overwhelming loneliness inhabits the soul of clients.

- *Phase IX* is the actual return to use where clients either use and get back into treatment and a recovery process, or use and return to uncontrolled, compulsive, addictive use. Most clients experience feelings of guilt and shame, which are numbed by the continued use of drugs and alcohol, resulting in more consequences.

Gorski (1989) suggested that relapsing clients typically have a pattern that, once understood, is predictable and *can be intervened upon at any point in the relapse process*. The CENAPS model of relapse prevention, developed by Gorski, outlines the process as follows: The counselor should take a comprehensive assessment, which includes a relapse calendar, a developmental history, alcohol and drug history, and a psychiatric history. The relapse calendar highlights for the client and the counselor the previous attempts at sobriety and active using periods. This tool helps clients begin to see patterns in their relapse history. Following the assessment, clients identify relapse warning signs, beginning with their most recent relapse. Counselors help clients review previous relapses in order to help them understand what is missing in their recovery program. Once the warning signs are identified, clients rank each of the warning signs and discuss in group or individual counseling how the process unfolds. Once the relapse process is outlined, clients develop management strategies for each warning sign identified. For example, the warning sign of isolation may be managed through interaction at AA meetings twice per week. Helping clients identify strategies and coping skills is a significant aspect of Gorski's prevention protocol. After strategies have been identified for all the warning signs, a final recovery plan is developed, including activities to address each of the warning signs. For example, it would be important for clients identifying with isolation to attend and discuss feelings of isolation in AA. This is because such a venue is a discussion meeting rather than a speaker meeting where there is typically less group interaction. The more specific the plan in addressing warning signs, the more likely the desired results will follow.

Using Warning Sign Identification Cards

An aspect of Gorski's (1989) model is the use of relapse warning sign cards. This technique consists of clients identifying warning signs along with negative thoughts, feelings, and behaviors. Clients are provided a set of index cards on which they write identified warning signs. Counselors work with clients to arrange a sequential order of relapse cards to outline the progression of relapse.

Additionally, the client arranges the warning signs sequentially in order of previous relapses. This process allows clients to see very clearly, in front of them, how their relapse unfolds. Essentially they are outlining how they become more and more out of control and unconsciously set themselves up. This awareness and insight help demystify how relapse unfolds and provide options for intervention.

Once the client places his or her initial warning sign cards down, other cards may be added after discussion with counselors or group members. For instance, a client identifies his first relapse card as when he started missing AA meetings. However, what he soon discovers is that he was in a relapse pattern long before he started missing meetings. The core feeling he identifies with is fear of abandonment, which has cascaded into multiple behaviors (e.g., isolation, sexual compulsion, and irritability). His core thoughts center on not being enough or worthy. These core thoughts are at the genesis of his relapse cycle, and coupled with his fear of being abandoned, act as a catalyst for future relapse behaviors. With this in mind, Gorski integrated brief cognitive therapy into relapse prevention where the drinking or drugging problem becomes a thinking problem ("Relapse Prevention Therapy," 1999). At the end of this chapter, in Appendix 11.A, there is an outline of how to create a warning sign card and how to work with a client using this activity.

Using Gorski's Model With a Client in Individual Counseling

The following counseling session highlights the counseling process for both generalist counselors as well as addiction-specific counselors and illuminates the process of relapse prevention.

Case of Fred

Fred is a chronic relapsing alcoholic and addict who initially entered counseling for relationship issues. Currently he reports being sober and clean with regular attendance at both AA and Narcotics Anonymous (NA) meetings. The presenting issue is his fear of losing a current relationship and how his sober behavior (i.e., impatient, explosive, and agitated) is pushing his girlfriend away. Fred indicates he successfully completed treatment over 3 months ago and used alcohol once during that time. He is employed as a service manager with a local technology store, which he enjoys a great deal. His girlfriend is not an addict; however, her father was an abusive alcoholic. Fred states he met his girlfriend, Patricia, at a party 3 months ago, about the same time he completed treatment. They have been inseparable ever since and plan on moving in together within the next month. Patricia, however, is concerned about Fred's early recovery and does not want to recreate her family of origin, which brings up distrust and anger in the relationship. Fred has entered counseling to help him deal with her reluctance to live together.

Commentary

The information presents Fred as being in early recovery and, at some level, defocusing his recovery energies on a new relationship. He is no longer engaged in a treatment process, which might provide him with direct group feedback on this situation. His immediate need to move in with Patricia is also of concern. The dynamics that will play out in the relationship over time may also be a major factor to attend to as well. His presentation of

"All is well with my recovery" to the counselor, however, does not fit with his realization of minor "blow ups" when things don't go his way. This client has already identified himself as a chronic relapser, meaning he has practice at his pattern.

Over the Next Month

Fred attends individual counseling each week; however, on the fourth week, at the last minute, he calls and cancels his appointment. At the previous session he seemed a bit more irritable with Patricia and her unwillingness to move in. He also discussed his supervisor at work and how they "got into it" at a regional meeting. Fred shared that he was getting bored again with AA meetings and found his mind wandering at the last meeting over to a new female group member. His discussion in counseling seemed to lack both depth and a desire for change; instead, it focused more on pleasure, either through sex or compulsively spending money on computer equipment.

Fred called the following day to reschedule the appointment and then arrived for the next session looking very tired. He apologized for missing the previous meeting, stating that he had to meet with his regional director. He said that he was terminated from his job because of poor work performance. What Fred neglected to discuss in previous sessions was that he had been oversleeping and missing time from work. The time he did spend at work was on the Internet buying equipment, until one day his supervisor caught him, and that is why he had been angry with the supervisor. Fred also stated that because he lost his job, Patricia would no longer consider moving in until he was gainfully employed. She added a second caveat that he had to remain sober for at least 2 years. Much of the session focused on the supervisor for "turning him in" and how he had "ruined his life." The blame, it appeared, was squarely on someone else and not Fred; he was not taking responsibility for his behavior.

Commentary

Fred developed a number of resentments that could lead to a justification to use. From his perspective, everything was just fine (other than a few "blow ups"). His supervisor turning him in had a major impact on his relationship. His perspective indicates a reactivation of a defense system that says, "I am right, the rest of the world is wrong." Following this line of thinking are a host of feelings expressed by Fred (anger, depression, loneliness, rage) followed by blame. At this point the individual sessions, AA meetings, and his relationship are potentially the only possible sources of external intervention.

Counselors sitting with someone like Fred at this point in the relapse process should help review relapse signs (assuming the counselor has worked with him already on this) and collaboratively identify where he is in the process. If the therapeutic relationship has developed, Fred may be able to respond to counselor feedback. Counselors help clients explore and recognize thoughts and behaviors in relation to recovery. In this case, this intervention may help Fred redirect his energies back to recovery and initiate personal responsibility for his actions, or he may move further down in the relapse cycle.

Next 3 Weeks

After the counselor appropriately provided observation-based feedback to Fred, some significant changes occurred. Fred was able to understand the need to reconnect with AA and talk with his sponsor about the relationship and his recent job loss, both of which he had neglected to share with anyone in AA. He also realized he was not yet ready for a relationship based on his pattern of relapse (previous relationships early in recovery always led him back to using). Finally, he was able to express fears of being alone and abandoned (feelings he has had since childhood). The combination of identifying his feelings, being willing to share them in counseling and in AA and with a sponsor, as well as his willingness to take responsibility for his job loss were all efforts to intervene on his relapse pattern. His pattern of relapse in the past started with isolation, the development of sexual rather than intimate relationships, feelings of guilt, followed by more relationships and then anger and lies. This cycle culminated in the loss of relationships, feeling abandoned, and then depression. On two occasions he considered suicide but instead went back to using. This intervention by the counselor was the first time he was able to redirect his energies back into recovery and avoid using.

Commentary

Fortunately, this counselor was able to address the relapse warning signs being presented by Fred. Fred was also open to the feedback and became honest with his feelings and the difficulties he had been having. As a result, he was able to redirect his energies out of the stuck point and maintain his recovery.

Clinical Example

Using Relapse Prevention Cards in a Group Format

A number of years ago, I (Ford) facilitated a relapse prevention group 1 day a week for 4 hours. During that time I introduced the ideas discussed in this chapter about relapse prevention. In the mornings, the patients would identify at least five signs in their relapse process, which they shared with the group. Before lunch I worked with two people in the group and demonstrated how to organize their relapse warning sign cards. After lunch I broke the group into triads and had them work with each other to organize their relapse warning sign cards. I walked around to each triad and discussed questions or observed each group member as they helped each other.

After they all had created a set of warning sign cards, I asked them to turn the cards over and write down their recovery strategies; then each group member read out loud the actions he would take. Once each member had an opportunity to share, I asked them what the process was like and what they learned about themselves from this exercise. The last part of the group in the afternoon involved a progressive relaxation process and a breathing exercise to help manage stress. This process took 4 hours. Over the course of the day, the participants were provided tools on focusing internally, breathing, identifying warning signs, ordering warning signs, and creating management strategies.

The beauty of a relapse prevention group is that the members of the group are not only all addicts but also most of them have a history of relapse, which helps to remove the embarrassment, shame, and guilt of relapse. Members are typically very supportive of each other because they understand what it feels like to relapse. Those who have not relapsed and are in treatment for the first time learn from the other group members. Group members also tend to confront each other, knowing that it is important to point out relapse behavior and not avoid it.

Making Decisions in Recovery

The combination of having clients involved in a relapse prevention group, individual counseling, and attending 12-step meetings on a regular weekly basis is effective for continued recovery (Fiorentine, 2001; Gorski, 1989).

Included in the cycle of relapse are three significant aspects of recovery that need to be addressed: decision making, structuring time, and developing coping skills. By the nature of addiction, clients' lives are chaotic, crisis oriented, and unstructured. As addiction progresses, the ability to make healthy decisions, structure time, and cope with life becomes increasingly more difficult. The First Step of AA refers to the unmanageability of the addicts' or alcoholics' lives because of their addiction. With sobriety and recovery comes responsibility, and with responsibility comes decision making, which contributes to stress. Helping clients learn effective skills to better manage stress, as well as providing information and discussing decision making, is critical. Clients will often make impulsive or irrational decisions based on little if any information. Their ability to exhibit patience is difficult early in the process of sobriety and, therefore, discussing how to handle daily decisions and structuring time is important. Clients usually have the best intentions as they leave treatment, only to be looking at the bottom of a beer glass within days of discharge. What happens?

For a moment, understand how overwhelming it would feel to realize that every decision you have made for the past 15 years was tainted by your addiction. Decisions regarding relationships, employment, and the manner in which you raised your children or communicated to others have all been impacted by your using. Now, in recovery, you realize the enormity and power your addiction has had over you and all the feelings associated with those decisions. Add to that your commitment to abstain. You realize that if you use a drug or drink (no matter what the consequences may be), all those worries and fears will temporarily go away.

It is important for counselors to understand, if they are not in recovery themselves, how it would feel to be overwhelmed and at the same time discontinue the chemical that created the anxiety and fear in the first place. Therefore, the decision-making process in recovery is important and is outlined below.

1. *Identify the dilemma:* A client who was getting upset about not being able to make his individual sessions wanted to schedule another appointment; however, the family had only one car, and they lived way out in the country. He had been anxious all week, so when he came in for his weekly group session he talked about it with other group members. When he did, six other members had six different ideas of how to get to the individual sessions, which ultimately taught him that soliciting feedback from others was helpful.
2. *Explore all the options:* Once this client talked about the presented choices, he realized he could stay after the group for his individual session or come before the group, meaning that he could come in only once but have two therapeutic contacts per week.
3. *Talk with others about the options and gain perspective:* Exploring with those whom the client trusts is a wonderful way of asking for help and gaining the needed perspective. All too many times decisions are made impulsively, without thought to the outcome or impact on self or others. In this way the options are discussed, resulting in a detached perspective.
4. *Identify and discuss the benefits and the liabilities of each possible choice:* Outlining where the possible choices could lead and how each choice impacts personal recovery plans is an important step.
5. *Follow through on the decision made:* The client develops a plan for each of the viable alternatives being considered for selection.
6. *Make the decision:* Finally the client makes a decision and follows through with the plan.
7. *Follow-up and review:* After the decision has been made it is reviewed for benefits and liabilities. If the individual, after review, feels as though the decision was helpful, he or she will continue with that plan. If, however, the decision was not helpful, the client can review the other choices and implement another option. The important part is for the client to feel as though he or she has choices, even after the initial decision has been made. Clients sometimes believe that if they make a decision, they cannot change their minds.

Structure, Preparation, and Coping Skills

Three areas where counselors can be most helpful include discussing clients' daily structure, how they prepare each day for their responsibilities and recovery functions, and how they cope throughout the day without the use of alcohol or drugs.

Daily Structure

For many clients suffering from addiction, a healthy lifestyle is generally not the norm. Moreover, the consistent aspect in their lives is the regular use of chemicals. Once the drug and alcohol use stops, clients generally are left with a great deal of time that was once filled by the use of drugs and/or alcohol. Questions to be answered include "What will they do with this time? How will it be structured? In what ways might it be structured?"

Clients leaving inpatient treatment without a comprehensive daily plan of action will soon find their prior behaviors and thinking returning. Therefore, it is crucial that clients think ahead and plan recovery activities (i.e., meetings, time with sponsor), time with the family, working time, and leisure time. A structured outline prior to discharge from treatment, however, does not necessarily mean the client will follow the plan of action. Counselors need to help cocreate and craft a viable and realistic approach to recovery based on a structured 24-hour plan.

Daily Preparation

We've asked clients prior to discharge from treatment how much of the structure they have experienced in treatment will transfer into their daily routine? Many times clients pick and choose what they like about treatment structure. As a result, clients create and structure their own recovery based on what they have learned in treatment and ongoing 12-step meetings.

Generally, clients are encouraged to consider waking up earlier in the mornings to create reflection time when recovery readings and meditation occur. Some clients prefer to exercise and stretch in the morning, whereas others enjoy sitting in peaceful surroundings. The important part for counselors is to help clients adjust unhealthy patterns that, when left unattended, contribute to the relapse process. Throughout the day, clients need to have access to recovering support either by telephone, Internet, or through 12-step meetings. These communication vehicles help create a new pattern of living while developing support. The more structure the client can reasonably create, the more occupied his or her mind is on recovery, family, or work tasks.

Coping Skills

Clients need to focus their attention on developing coping skills in recovery. Examples of these skills include asking for help, setting limits, sharing emotions with others, or writing down feelings in a journal. Counselors can help clients explore feelings and create individual ways of management. For instance, counselors can help clients identify the feelings of sadness by asking where in their bodies they experience that feeling. Once the feeling is identified, they can share it with a sponsor, group member, or friend instead of repressing it (as would be the old behavior).

When clients relapse, typically they have their own brand of trouble they get into. One client, for example, would almost always obtain another drunk driving ticket when he relapsed. Another client would end up in the local detoxification clinic, only to be informed again that his job was on the line. Counselors need to have patience and a helping spirit when working with relapsing clients. Many times, clients will call and report to their counselors that they have used again and could they come back in for counseling. Following the relapse, clients can reengage in counseling, review their previous plan, add new strategies to the plan, and act on new behavior. In conjunction with treatment and counseling is the importance of outside support meetings and the role spirituality plays in the recovery process.

Summary

This chapter focused primarily on relapse and relapse prevention and how to address the thoughts, emotions, and behavior of a client who may be struggling with relapse issues.

Identification of other compulsive and addictive behaviors and options for referral were also outlined so as to provide the counselor with information on appropriate care.

Exploration Questions From Chapter 11

1. What are your views on relapse?
2. What are your thoughts on spirituality and the recovery process?
3. How are religion and spirituality similar? Different?
4. Explore how you would use group counseling in the relapse prevention process.
5. How might you implement ideas from this chapter into your internship or work site?

Suggested Activities

1. Attend 12-step meetings (e.g., AA, NA, Al-Anon, Adult Children of Alcoholics) as well as alternative support groups (e.g., Secular Organizations for Sobriety, Women for Sobriety). Compare and contrast your experiences.
2. Identify for yourself how you could use the relapse prevention information to help prevent counselor burnout.

Appendix 11.A
Example of Warning Sign Card

Isolation --"Reclining Chair"

Clients write one word on the left side of an index card. On the right side they write a word that personalizes the word on the left. In this case, the client picked a reclining chair in his home where he sits and drinks in isolation. Once the client visualizes the chair and can see the many nights of isolative drinking and drugging, he can begin to make changes in behavior that will be conducive for recovery. Change could include moving the reclining chair to another room or getting rid of it altogether. By identifying the reclining chair, the client realizes how much time is spent at home alone and therefore uses it as an indicator of isolation.

Clients then create 10–15 warning sign cards, which are placed in order with the help of the counselor. The client can use the cards daily like flash cards to identify which warning signs are present for that particular day or week. The client can read them each morning and share them with supportive people in the family or in 12-step meetings. The cards are a way in which the client stays aware of thoughts, feelings, and behaviors that, when ignored, contribute to the relapse cycle.

Whereas one side of the card is a warning sign, the opposite side is the recovery skills needed to manage the warning sign. Counselors and support people can help clients brainstorm management possibilities for each of the warning signs. The new management strategies are written on the backside of the card to provide options other than repeating the same behavior again.

Spirituality and Support Groups
in Recovery

In this chapter we outline the importance and relevance of spirituality in the recovery process and how support groups can play a significant factor in the success of clients wrestling with addiction issues. In our work, we have found a substantial overlap across the individual's sense of spirituality and their recovery efforts and process. Though an individual's spiritual center is not always apparent or made overt, there are powerful forces and reserves clients can call upon in their efforts to recover and move in a more meaningful and positive direction. Many addiction treatment centers in the United States introduce clients to spirituality-based recovery found in the 12-step program of Alcoholics Anonymous (AA). According to W. R. Miller (1998), religious or spiritual involvement reduces the risk of substance abuse while increasing the necessary involvement (which is a correlate with recovery). Miller found that addicted clients who practiced the 12-steps were more likely to remain abstinent than those treated with other nonspiritual-based therapies. Miller also found evidence that AA involvement was associated with increased positive outcomes in outpatient treatment. He also found that meditation-related interventions were associated with a reduction in substance abuse and found evidence that AA involvement was associated with positive outcomes following inpatient treatment. In a similar study, Johnsen (1993) discovered a trend toward the use of prayer and meditation by individuals abstaining from alcohol and drugs. Johnsen suggested the evidence indicated spirituality is more than intangible and could be identified as a significant strength used by the recovering person. A study by Piderman, Schneekloth, Pankratz, Maloney, and Altchuler (2007) found that after only 3 weeks of addiction treatment, subjects reported significantly greater spiritual well-being, more frequent participation in private religious practices, an increase in the use of positive religious beliefs to cope with their addiction, greater involvement in AA, and greater confidence about remaining sober. A similar study found a significant increase in patient spiritual well-being over the course of 2 weeks in an inpatient addiction treatment program (C. W. Brooks & Matthews, 2000). Gorski and Miller (1986) asserted AA as the single most effective treatment for alcoholism. Evidence exists that those who have participated in spiritually-based programs have made the most significant movement in their recovery from addiction (Green, Fulhlove, & Fulhlove, 1998).

An 8-year federally funded study, Project Match (Project Match Research Group, 1997), examined alcoholic patients in three types of outpatient care: 12-step facilitation, cognitive–behavioral therapy, and motivational enhancement therapy. All had comparable results; however, the individuals in each group who attended AA had more abstinent days with 12-step facilitation than with cognitive–behavioral therapy (Project Match Research Group, 1997). White (1998) and Peteet (1993) noted that most alcohol and drug treatment programs use AA's 12-step recovery philosophy. On the basis of these data, they believed spirituality plays a central role in the process of recovery.

Spirituality and Religion

W. R. Miller (1998) identified three differentiations between religion and spirituality. The first is that spirituality is understood typically at a personal and individual level, whereas religion is more of a social phenomenon, with an organized structure and numerous purposes, one being to develop spirituality in the entire congregation. The second differentiation is that spirituality defies boundaries, whereas religion is defined by boundaries, beliefs, practices, and rituals (Kurtz & Ketcham, 1992).

Finally, it is possible that various forms of religion may distort one's spirituality and that it may obscure personal experiences and beliefs. Spirituality is an aspect of alcoholism recovery involving more than a consideration of specified religious principles. It contains the belief that individuals are but a part of a larger and more vast reality and are charged with participation rather than a domination role in that existence (Chapman, 1996). George Valliant (1983), a significant figure in alcoholism research, in one of his most classic writings described the pain, suffering, and emptiness of alcoholics and suggested that these symptoms were connected with a spiritual void in need of spiritual healing.

According to Prezioso (1987), "Spirituality is key to treatment and recovery because addiction, I believe, is a spiritual as well as a physical disease" (p. 233). Chapman (1996) suggested that spirituality is an important aspect in the treatment of alcohol dependence. According to Grof (1987a), Western civilization has lost connection with the inner life and, as a result, has attempted to fill this void with chemicals. He further suggested that a person cut off from his or her spiritual sources will have challenges in finding real satisfaction through external pursuits. "It is well known among professionals that to be successful, the treatment and rehabilitation programs in this field have to include the spiritual aspect" (Grof, 1987b, p. 3). Jacquelyn Small (1987) stated, "If the recovering addict has been taught nothing about how to connect with his inner wisdom, and leaves the treatment program believing some expert 'fixed' him, he can do nothing but become, once again, dependent on something or someone to worship outside of himself"(p. 24). The counselor is encouraged to explore spiritual aspects of the client's existence in order to prevent relapse (Chapman, 1996).

Surrender and Compliance

Harry Tiebout, M.D., a psychiatrist who worked with alcoholic patients and wrote about surrender as a factor in getting sober, described the recovery process as a conversion that resulted in a positive experience after an act of surrender (Hanna, 1992; Speer & Reinert, 1998). Tiebout went on to say that surrender occurs when clients accept reality unconsciously. Members in AA might say this is when they realized that in order to get sober they needed to accept life on life's terms. That initial shift occurs in Step 1 of AA with the second word *admitted*, whereby the acceptance of loss of control is admitted and thus the act of surrender can occur (Dyslin, 2008).

Compliance, on the other hand, is accepting reality on a conscious level but not on an unconscious level. The result is typically compliant behavior that results in later use. For instance, a client comes to treatment because his wife says that unless he discontinues drinking, their marriage will be over. He complies and enters treatment; follows the rules; stops drinking; attends group therapy, AA, and individual counseling; and admits he is an alcoholic. However, deep inside he knows that once his wife's concerns have been addressed he can return to what he perceives as "controlled" drinking. Externally he is compliant; internally he has not shifted. This is because he does not believe his drinking is out of control. That is not to say, as he is complying with treatment, that he might not find his new life without alcohol enjoyable. However, when the conversion occurs, it is the foundation of the recovery process that is further supported by a higher power (Brown, 1985; Dyslin, 2008).

Support Groups

Pick up a local newspaper and look in the classifieds under the section for support groups. You will probably find many listed in your area of the country. This is not by accident. Support groups work. If you have attended one, you are probably privy to the sense of "something bigger" happening within the room (and as to be expected, beyond the walls). Of course, not all support groups are the same. But in many instances, this sense of something bigger reflects the combined spiritual presence of those in attendance. Additionally, in many support groups, the members are each arriving at *his or her* unique sense of a "higher power."

Building on the notion that the spiritual self cannot possibly be separated from the person (and in this case, person with an addiction), support groups typically offer a collective place to strengthen the individual's sense of personal and communal spirituality. The fellowship found in the meetings creates an environment of support and hope.

Alcoholics Anonymous

The most widely known support group is that of Alcoholics Anonymous (AA). To understand the basic tenets of AA, one must first be aware of the rich history leading to the cofounding and development of this support network for recovering people around the world. World Services, the service organization of AA, estimates that there are over 2,000,000 members of AA around the world in over 180 countries (AA, 2009a). AA was cofounded in 1935 by two men, Dr. Bob Smith, a surgeon from Akron, Ohio, and Bill Wilson, a stockbroker from New York. Along with the history of the development of AA, we also want to share a piece of Bill Wilson's personal spiritual journey through his process of addiction and recovery. Many clients we have worked with have had their own unique spiritual journey that was intertwined with the use of drugs and/or alcohol.

William Griffith Wilson was born on November 26, 1895, in Dorset, Vermont. The eldest of two children, his early life was filled with loneliness and heartbreak, making his first drinking experience an overwhelmingly powerful one. Robert Thomsen's (1975) book contains a description of Bill Wilson's first use of alcohol:

> Soon he had the feeling that he wasn't the one being introduced but that people were being introduced to him: he wasn't joining groups, groups were forming around him. It was unbelievable. And at the sudden realization of how quickly the world could change, he had to laugh and he couldn't stop laughing. . . . It was a miracle. There was no other word. A miracle that was affecting him mentally, physically, and as he would soon learn, spiritually too. Still smiling, he looked at the people around him. These were not superior beings. They were his friends. They liked him and he liked them. . . . He could hear the whine of a saxophone, little waves of voices rising, falling, but now they in no way ran against the overwhelming joy he was feeling. His world was all around him, young and fresh and loving, and as he made his way down the drive he moved easily, gracefully, as though—he knew exactly how he felt—all his life he had been living in chains. Now he was free. (pp. 97–98)

This was a profound, alcohol-induced spiritual experience that sent Bill into alcoholic oblivion for many years as he sought to replicate that feeling of freedom. It wasn't until he lay in his hospital bed many years later, in alcohol withdrawal, that he had a similar experience, except on this occasion he lost his compulsion to drink.

> My depression deepened unbearably and finally it seemed to me as though I were at the bottom of the pit. I still gagged badly on the notion of a Power greater than myself, but finally, just for the moment, the last vestige of my proud obstinacy was crushed. All at once I found myself crying out, "If there is a God, let Him show Himself! I am ready to do anything, anything!"
>
> Suddenly the room lit up with a great white light. I was caught up into an ecstasy which there are no words to describe. It seemed to me, in the mind's eye, that I was on a mountain and that a wind not of air but of spirit was blowing. And then it burst upon me that I was a free man. Slowly the ecstasy subsided. I lay on the bed, but now for a time I was in another world, a new world of consciousness. All about me and through me there was a wonderful feeling of Presence, and I thought to myself, "So this is the God of the preachers!" A great peace stole over me and I thought, "No matter how wrong things seem to be, they are all right, Things are all right with God and His world." (AA, 1957, p. 63)

This conversion experience, his reading from William James's (1929) *The Varieties of Religious Experience* as introduced by Ebby T. (a long-term friend who also was an alcoholic), Dr. William Silkworth (Bill's physician), exposure to the Oxford Group, and Dr. Carl Jung's belief that the "cure" for alcoholism was found in the Latin words *spiritus contra spiritum* (or "treating the spirits with spirit"), all contributed to Bill's getting sober and culminating in that first meeting with Dr. Bob Smith. The meeting of the two men resulted in the development of AA as we know it today (Kurtz, 1979).

The Oxford Group was evangelical in nature and encouraged members to live a daily life of spiritual values. It had four tenets, which were purity, honesty, unselfishness, and love. The Oxford Group influenced Bill and Bob in the creation of AA (Cheevers, 2004). The ideas of a conversion experience and humility were significant in their understanding of the Oxford Group (Kurtz, 1979).

In addition to the Oxford Group were the observations by Dr. Carl Jung in a letter to Bill regarding his work with Rowland H., a client. Carl Jung significantly contributed to the idea that recovery from alcoholism was most hopefully treated with spiritual means and that the alcoholic needed to place him- or herself in a religious atmosphere to undergo a conversion experience (Hanna, 1992). All of these combined factors helped Bill maintain sobriety long enough to meet Dr. Bob Smith.

Up until Bob met Bill, he had not been able to maintain sobriety. Not only did Bill tell Bob about his drinking story and subsequent sobriety but also Bob told Bill his story, for the first time sharing it with another human being. It was at this meeting where AA was born (AA, 2009b). Bob soon got sober, never to drink again, and the two set off to help other alcoholics. Within 4 years, over 100 sober alcoholics developed from this new phenomenon called AA. By 1939 they wrote and crafted the 12 steps of AA and included it in the main text of AA, commonly referred to as the *Big Book*. In 1941 the *Saturday Evening Post* printed an article on AA, and by the end of that year there were an estimated 6,000 members (AA, 2009b). These steps have been used by other support groups for many issues (e.g., eating, sexual behavior, gambling, relationships). These steps are not a mandate but rather a suggested path to sobriety and a spiritual awakening.

Twelve Steps of AA (AA, 2001)

Step 1: We admitted we were powerless over alcohol—that our lives had become unmanageable.

Step 2: Came to believe that a Power greater than ourselves could restore us to sanity.

Step 3: Made a decision to turn our will and our lives over to the care of God, *as we understood Him.*

Step 4: Made a searching and fearless moral inventory of ourselves.

Step 5: Admitted to God, to ourselves, and to another human being the exact nature of our wrongs.

Step 6: Were entirely ready to have God remove all these defects of character.

Step 7: Humbly asked Him to remove our shortcomings.

Step 8: Made a list of all persons we had harmed, and became willing to make amends to them all.

Step 9: Made direct amends to such people wherever possible, except when to do so would injure them or others.

Step 10: Continued to take personal inventory and when we were wrong promptly admitted it.

Step 11: Sought through prayer and meditation to improve our conscious contact with God, *as we understood Him,* praying only for knowledge of His will for us and the power to carry that out.

Step 12: Having had a spiritual awakening as a result of these steps, we tried to carry this message to alcoholics and to practice these principles in all our affairs.

Using and Understanding the 12 Steps

Step 1: We admitted we were powerless over alcohol—that our lives had become unmanageable.

This step is significantly placed first in the 12 steps. It sets the foundation from which clients can build a recovery program. The word *admitted* suggests that clients have admitted to themselves that when they use drugs and/or alcohol (a) they are powerless to control their consumption, and (b) the harder they try, the more out of control they get. The myth is that addicts and alcoholics are powerless to do anything about their addiction, which is false. On the contrary, once clients detoxify or stop using long enough to completely remove the chemicals from their system, they have the power and choice to make the necessary changes in their thoughts and behaviors. The second aspect of this step states life is unmanageable as a result of the addiction. Recovery is about not picking up the first drink or drug while addressing those aspects of life that are unmanageable from years of using and drinking. Counselors can help clients during this step by discussing the emotions related to unmanageability and powerlessness and helping focus the control they do have over their behavior.

Step 2: Came to believe that a power greater than ourselves could restore us to sanity.

This step indicates a process. "Came to believe" means it is not instantaneous and takes time. A "power greater than ourselves" suggests that individuals consider a power greater than oneself that could "restore sanity." This is asking a great deal from clients who may hear or interpret it immediately as being asked to believe in God. This step is actually only asking to consider that a greater power could restore one to sanity. For example, an AA or Narcotics Anonymous (NA) meeting is a power greater than one person, and for many early in recovery, that meeting is their higher power. At the end of each meeting clients may feel better and increasingly connected, allowing "sane" thoughts to emerge. "A higher power is specifically meant not to be the equivalent of any religious denomination or one's notion of God, but rather is an internal, individual conception of a Spirit that is broad, all inclusive, and accessible to all who sincerely seek it" (MacKinnon, 2004, p. 8).

Step 3: Made a decision to turn our will and lives over to the care of God, *as we understood Him.*

Making a decision does not necessarily mean clients are ready to act. It says, "made a decision to turn our will and lives," or our egos, over to the care of God, which is up to the clients' interpretation. God for some is *Good Orderly Direction*, whereas others view God as nature or the support group. For some it may be a Christian God, and for others it may be Buddha or the Universe. When Bill and Bob crafted the steps they were careful to allow one's own interpretation and "understanding" of God to be embraced.

Step 4: Made a searching and fearless moral inventory of ourselves.

Many times during the counseling process, clients are engaged in inventory work. This step suggests clients make a "moral inventory" of resentments, fears, and value-conflicting behaviors. The counselor can help clients list and discuss those feelings associated with the inventory. Feelings of shame, embarrassment, and guilt are usually a part of this step. Also important for the client is to identify and list positive attributes, strengths, and useful characteristics of self.

Step 5: Admitted to God, to ourselves, and to another human being the exact nature of our wrongs.

For clients to complete a thorough inventory, they need to have stopped drinking and developed a sense of support in recovery. Identifying immoral behavior in Step 4 is a powerful and painful process. Counselors can help clients with Step 5 by supporting and listening to their process. Generally, fifth steps are heard by sponsors, clergy members, and sometimes counselors.

Step 6: Were entirely ready to have God remove all these defects of character.

Once the character flaws in Steps 4 and 5 have been identified and shared with another human being, Step 6 asks clients to have their higher power, or the God of their understanding, remove the defects of character. Actually, Steps 4 and 5 outline areas for growth that can be addressed in counseling. For example, if an identified character flaw is manipulation, the counseling sessions could focus on how to become more honest in getting needs met rather than manipulating others.

Step 7: Humbly asked Him to remove our shortcomings.

This step is an act of letting go of old behaviors and allowing new behaviors and choices to surface. Essentially, as the client matures and grows in some ways, he or she may hold onto old behaviors because of familiarity and what the behaviors provided in the past.

Step 8: Made a list of all persons we had harmed and became willing to make amends to them all.

Another myth is that alcoholics and addicts don't take responsibility for their actions because of their "disease." Nothing could be furthest from the truth. In Step 8, the client identifies and lists "all persons we had harmed" and then "became willing" to make amends. It doesn't say that the client will at this point; it just says, "became willing." Counselors can help clients discuss the process of identifying names and for what reasons the individuals were selected.

Step 9: Made direct amends to such people wherever possible, except when to do so would injure them or others.

Counselors can discuss with clients the possible responses from potential individuals who have been harmed and help prepare clients for negative responses. Discussion in the sessions assesses whether making amends would "injure them or others" in the process.

Step 10: Continued to take personal inventory and when we were wrong promptly admitted it.

Helping clients continually take a daily and personal inventory maintains internal honesty. Clients may have a daily routine that structures a nightly reflection of the day or a time to write in a journal. This step is critical in keeping clients on top of their recovery program. If they do not continue with an inventory, old thoughts and resentments may surface. "Resentment is the number one offender. It destroys more alcoholics than anything else" (AA, 1976, p. 64).

Step 11: Sought through prayer and meditation to improve our conscious contact with God, *as we understood Him,* praying only for knowledge of His will for us and the power to carry that out.

The counselor can help clients maintain spiritual connection with a higher power or God by encouraging discussion of such entities in session. Counselors can also provide breathing exercises or guided imagery in sessions to help with relaxation and conscious contact of a higher power.

Step 12: Having had a spiritual awakening as a result of these steps, we tried to carry this message to alcoholics and to practice these principles in all our affairs.

Bill Wilson did not have the luxury of the first 11 steps. He had a spiritual awakening first and then started with Step 1. Bill's spiritual experience brought him to another alcoholic, Bob Smith, and they in turn have spread spirituality and fellowship throughout the world. The fellowship of AA, the connection with other people, a God of a personal understanding, and reaching out to others is the foundation of the AA philosophy. Counselors can best help clients by discussing values, beliefs, and areas needing spiritual attention. Father Martin consolidates the steps into these few words: "Trust God, Clean House, Help Others" (Maher, 1997, p. 79).

Information for Counselors as Clients Work a Program of Recovery

In addition to working the 12 steps of AA are other suggested areas that clients can become involved with to deepen their connection in recovery. The following are constructs counselors need to be familiar with when working with clients who attend AA or NA meetings:

- *Identifying a home group:* Helping clients find a 12-step meeting that they feel comfortable with and live near is important. This group is called a "home" group because clients attend this particular meeting on a regular basis and make sure it is part of their regular weekly meeting routine.
- *Sponsorship:* A sponsor is an individual in recovery who has been clean and sober for an extended period of time and who continually works a 12-step program. Sponsors help "sponsees" work the 12 steps of AA, give support, challenge thinking, and provide whatever is appropriate and necessary at the time. Some sponsors talk with their "pigeons," or sponsees, on a daily basis, whereas others may talk with them every few days. Sponsors are a connection to the program of AA or NA and provide a mentorlike relationship to newcomers. Sponsors generally have sponsors of their own and maintain regular contact with them as well.

- *Service work*: This is volunteer work to help the functioning of each meeting locally and regionally. Service can be setting up chairs for the meeting or making coffee. Service work can also include the opening and closing of the meeting facility, chairing a meeting, or being the treasurer and collecting donations. Service work helps newcomers stay involved and introduces them to others in recovery.
- *90 and 90*: This means an individual is attending 90 meetings in 90 days in order to develop support or reconnect (usually after time away from the program), to renew a recovery program, or after a relapse.
- *Use of slogans*: "Easy Does It," "Keep It Simple, Stupid" (or "Sweetheart"), "Let Go and Let God," and "One Day at a Time" are some of the primary slogans used by recovering members to help keep life simple, to take it easy, let go of ego, and to do it 24 hours a day.
- *Chip system*: Depending on the meeting and where in the country it is located, a poker chip system offers to its members a chip for their first 24 hours of sobriety; 3, 6, and 9 months of sobriety; plus a year and subsequent years of sobriety. Many times sponsors will buy a medallion for yearly celebrations, which are followed with a party or small gathering after the meeting.
- *The three meetings*: At each meeting there are three meetings: (a) the before meeting where individuals congregate and reconnect, (b) the actual meeting itself where there may be a speaker or a discussion, and (c) the after meeting where members go out for meals and socialize. The importance for clients to involve themselves in each of the three aspects of the meeting is important for developing support and fellowship.
- *Closed and open meetings*: Closed meetings are offered only to those individuals who are attending because they have a desire to stop drinking or using. Open meetings are open to those interested in finding out more about AA or NA, which includes family members, clergy, counselors, or students learning about addiction. Those reading this text and planning to work with this population in general would best serve their clients by going to open meetings to learn about the workings of AA or NA.
- *Clubhouses*: AA or NA clubhouses allow members, day or night, to have a place to talk with other recovering members. The clubhouses provide a place to be sober, to talk about recovery, play games, or just relax.
- *Intergroup*: This is a location where individuals volunteer to answer the AA or NA hotline, distribute AA or NA reading materials, and answer questions received either in person or on the phone. Intergroup provides the listing of meetings in a given locality and information to the newcomer or traveler from a new town in search of 12-step meetings.

Alternative Ideologies and Support in Recovery

Rational Recovery

Because some clients may stop treatment, resist certain approaches, or have a negative reaction to therapy (support groups) that offers strong connections to spirituality, we have included the following model. Although this approach is no longer as present in mainstream recovery, it is an important alternative for some clients.

Rational Recovery (RR) was started in the mid 1980s by Jack Trimpey, who developed an extensive cognitive–behavioral therapy group network. Professional counselors hosted RR groups within their practices and/or agencies. In 1994, the nonprofit board of RR attempted to seize control of the name Rational Recovery; however, their legal attempt failed, resulting in changes in RR. The nonprofit board is now known as SMART Recovery.

SMART Recovery provides information about self-recovery through addictive voice recognition technique (AVRT), which helps addicted clients recover "without the use of groups, shrinks, or rehabs" (RR, 2004, ¶2). Trimpey (RR, 2004, ¶5) suggested that AVRT is not compatible with group formats and that "you will not want to congregate with others who would reinforce that crippling dependent belief." The "addictive voice" is what is believed to be the cause of addiction and not a disease or medical process.

RR is critical of 12-step recovery groups. "We do not care about their spiritual visions and gratitude toward AA/NA, because in spite of all their piety and enthusiasm, they are still in the jaws of addiction, staying sober one-day at a time, engaged in occult spirituality, languishing in the social ghetto of recovery groups"(RR, 2004, ¶27). Instead, RR incorporates traditional values of individual responsibility, self-restraint, and moral judgment. In fact, "AVRT directs one back to his or her original family values, especially the concepts of choosing right over wrong, ideas that are usually understood by age five" (RR, 2004, ¶27). Clients and counselors interested in this approach can go to the Web site (www.rational. org) and access the AVRT comprehensive remedy for addiction.

This approach to sobriety has been found, according to the RR Web site, to be beneficial to individuals who do not want to engage in discussion with others in a support network fashion or who have negative reactions to words such as *higher power, God,* or *spirituality.* Further, this approach purports to be easy, simple, straightforward, and can be accessed through the Internet.

Women for Sobriety

Developed in 1975 by Dr. Jean Kirkpatrick, this approach addresses issues for women struggling from alcoholism through the use of a support network (Ardell, 1996). Women for Sobriety (WFS) is the first self-help program for women that takes into consideration the special issues women deal with in getting sober and in ongoing recovery. The program of WFS is based on positive thinking, metaphysics, meditation, group dynamics, and the pursuit of health through nutrition. "Kirkpatrick felt that female alcoholics experience chronic low-self-esteem partly because of societal stigmatization of alcoholic women. . . . Instead, WFS attributes sobriety to a woman's own power and state of mind"(Ardell, 1996, p. 6).

WFS groups exist all over the United States and Canada and are facilitated by WFS certified moderators who have good sobriety records and are thoroughly acquainted with the WFS program and philosophy. Meetings generally occur weekly for 90 minutes. This program has 13 affirmations that are suggested for members to say each morning and evening:

1. I have a life-threatening problem that once had me.
   I now take charge of my life. I accept the responsibility.
2. Negative thoughts destroy only myself.
   My first conscious act must be to remove negativity from my life.
3. Happiness is a habit I will develop.
   Happiness is created, not waited for.
4. Problems bother me only to the degree I permit them to.
   I now better understand my problems and do not permit problems to overwhelm me.
5. I am what I think.
   I am a capable, competent, caring, compassionate woman.
6. Life can be ordinary or it can be great.
   Greatness is mine by a conscious effort.
7. Love can change the course of my world.
   Caring becomes all important.

8. The fundamental object of life is emotional and spiritual growth.
   Daily I put my life into a proper order, knowing which are the priorities.
9. The past is gone forever.
   No longer will I be victimized by the past, I am a new person.
10. All love given returns.
    I will learn to know that others love me.
11. Enthusiasm is my daily exercise.
    I treasure all moments of my new life.
12. I am a competent woman and have much to give life.
    This is what I am and I shall know it always.
13. I am responsible for myself and for my actions.
    I am in charge of my mind, my thoughts, and my life. WFS (1999)

WFS's sole purpose is to help women recover from problem drinking through connecting with others who are or were in similar circumstances. WFS is not affiliated with AA, although members may attend both AA and WFS meetings. WFS believes that for many women, alcohol was used to combat stress, isolation, and loneliness. For some, such feelings resulted in dependency. WFS also believes the basis of addiction is physiological and recommends total and complete abstinence. They require a desire to discontinue drinking and for a new life.

This support group was created out of the specific needs of women in recovery. As such, this modality can be a viable option for female clients. It can also be used in conjunction with AA or NA, depending on clients' willingness or desire to try different meetings. The limitation with WFS may be in the limited number of meetings that are available in any given area.

Secular Organizations for Sobriety

Jim Christopher founded Secular Organizations for Sobriety (SOS, 2000) in the mid 1980s after 17 years of alcoholism. He felt there were others like himself who wanted sobriety through personal responsibility and reliance on self. He also felt that since addiction was supported as a biochemical/physical illness, a higher power was not compatible with current research, and therefore is not an aspect of SOS. This approach is an alternative for those uncomfortable with the spiritual aspects found so widely in 12-step meetings. SOS separates sobriety from religion and spirituality and does not rely on the sense of a higher power for sobriety. However, the support of other alcoholics and addicts is a very important aspect of recovery where abstinence is recommended. There is a commitment to abstaining and that a first step is to acknowledge being an alcoholic or addict (SOS, 2000).

SOS meetings are found in every state in the United States and in many countries throughout the world. In 1987, SOS was recognized by the California courts to be an approved alternative to AA as a support group for offenders and those mandated for participation in a group.

As was for Mr. Christopher, this type of support group may appeal to clients with a strong reaction to the words *God, higher power,* or *spirituality* and are looking for an alternative to AA or NA.

Moderation Management

Moderation Management (MM), for many drinkers, is a first step in exploring drinking patterns. It is a behavioral change program with a national support group, which promotes early self-awareness of risky drinking and moderate drinking as a realistic goal. The support groups encourage those concerned about their drinking to either cut back or discontinue altogether. MM believes alcohol abuse versus dependency is a learned behavior or habit, not a disease. MM recognizes that those who are dependent on alcohol may have difficulty moderating their drinking. According to MM, "approximately 30% of MM members go on to abstinence based programs" (MM, 2003, ¶5).

MM encourages members to take responsibility for their own recovery, help others in the MM program, and by so doing, help themselves. The MM program also suggests that self-esteem and management are keys to recovery and that members need to treat each other with respect and dignity (MM, 2003).

MM's Nine Steps Toward Moderation and Positive Lifestyle Changes

1. Attend meetings, online groups, and learn about the program of MM.
2. Abstain from alcoholic beverages for 30 days and complete Steps 3 through 6 during this time.
3. Examine how drinking has affected your life.
4. Write down your life priorities.
5. Take a look at how much, how often, and under what circumstances you had been drinking.
6. Learn the MM guidelines and limits for moderate drinking.
7. Set moderate drinking limits and start weekly "small steps" toward balance and moderation in other areas of your life.
8. Review your progress and update your goals.
9. Continue to make positive lifestyle changes and attend meetings whenever you need ongoing support or would like to help newcomers.

A moderate drinker, as outlined by MM (MM, 2003),

- considers an occasional drink to be a small, though enjoyable, part of life.
- has hobbies, interests, and other ways to relax and enjoy life that do not involve alcohol.
- usually has friends who are moderate drinkers or nondrinkers.
- generally has something to eat before, during, or soon after drinking.
- usually does not drink for longer than an hour or two on any particular occasion.
- usually does not drink faster than one drink per half hour.
- usually does not exceed the .055% blood alcohol content, which is the moderate drinking limit.

This support group may appeal to drinkers in the contemplation–action stages of change (Prochaska & DiClemente, 1986). Those dependent on alcohol, and who are honest with their appraisal, may find their ability to moderate drinking difficult for any significant length of time and may move on to an abstinent-based support network. This type of group could help individuals determine, on their own, whether they lack the ability to control drinking.

Preparing Clients for Referral to Support Groups

Riordan and Walsh (1994) suggested that there are significant benefits to making a referral earlier in the therapeutic process to a support group. Timing, however, is important when making the referral. Usually a prime time for support group referral occurs following a binge on alcohol or drugs. Such behavior and the resultant consequences usually make the client more receptive to recommendations.

Determining the type of group that might be best suited to the client's needs and personality can be of substantial benefit to the client (Riordan & Walsh, 1994). Providing information, location, and a general idea of what the meeting will be like can be very helpful in preparing clients for attendance. Counselors may have contact names of members who attend meetings on a regular basis. Such individuals who are open to being contacted by newcomers can potentially help facilitate the referral and reduce the anxiety of the client.

Based on the previously provided information on various support groups, counselors can present a menu of support groups in the area that can help empower clients to be able to have a choice in their recovery. Most treatment programs working with addicted clients are likely to refer to AA or NA. This is, in part, because AA and NA are cited as the most commonly effective and available treatments for addiction (Brown, 1985; Flores, 1997; Kurtz, 1979). However, counselors who work independently of a treatment program and are working with clients who are ambivalent about discontinuing their using have choices among a variety of support groups. A client may initially develop a therapeutic relationship with the counselor and attend an MM meeting, only to determine that he or she could not control his or her drinking. A referral to SOS or AA could be the next step, depending on the willingness of the client and his/her reaction to the words *God* or *higher power.*

Counselors need to be familiar with the unique support resources in their community. It is critical for counselors to know if meetings exist in their area or not. It would also be helpful for counselors to attend each type of meeting or read pertinent information about each support network. Keeping specific reading materials, Web sites, and pamphlets in the office can also provide clients with useful resources. Counselors may discover that although they would like to refer a female alcoholic client to WFS, there may not be a meeting in the area and AA may be the only support group available. Counselors would then need to know if there were specific women's AA groups and help discuss the 12 steps in the session.

Summary

As a result of reading this chapter, counselors should be able to identify the relapse cycle and how to intervene with clients in the cycle. The reader should also have a basic understanding of AA and its 12 steps, in addition to a variety of other support groups and approaches. Significant in the reading is the idea of spirituality playing a part in recovery. Finally, helping clients prepare for their first meeting and aspects of the referral process are important to clients.

Exploration Questions From Chapter 12

1. How do you believe or not believe spirituality to be a part of recovery?
2. Which support groups might you use in your counseling?
3. How do you see support groups helping your clients?
4. What are your conceptions and misconceptions about 12-step meetings?
5. How many support groups are there in your area for addiction?

Suggested Activities

1. Attend one of each type of support group to determine for yourself what the experience is like going to your first meeting. Record your emotions and discuss with a friend.
2. Talk to individuals who you know attend support meetings and find out how the meetings help them.

Addictions Training, Certification, and Ethics

This chapter begins with information on the training and education of counselors for substance abuse issues. It continues with a discussion of ethics in relation to addiction certification and codes of ethics for associations, certifications, and licenses. Finally, professional boundaries and the importance of supervision and ethical decision making (including impaired professionals) are explored.

Training and Education of Counselors for Substance Abuse Issues

A study by Morgan, Toloczko, and Comly (1997) surveyed 70 counseling programs accredited by the Council for Accreditation of Counseling and Related Educational Programs (CACREP). Of the programs surveyed, only 21 (30%) required courses in substance abuse or dependency. Eighty-seven percent of the respondents reported that they placed students for practicum or field in institutions providing primary alcohol and drug counseling and that 11% of the graduating students accepted positions in these programs. The results of this study suggested that a significant proportion of counseling students are being placed in internship sites serving substance-abusing clients with minimal or no course work in substance abuse counseling. Further, a proportion of those students are accepting positions as alcohol and drug counselors.

Standards for an addiction counseling specialty with CACREP have been approved by its board of directors and are included in Appendix 13.A at the end of this chapter (CACREP Standards, 2009). The approval of these standards by CACREP provides a clear and needed understanding of preparation for work with this population. Historically, the absence of course work specifically on addiction was that "addictions counseling is the only counseling specialty that developed outside of university settings" (Matthews, 1998, p. 3). Matthews stated that the original addiction counselors were recovering addicts and alcoholics. He believed that nonrecovering students should be required to increase self-awareness and recognize their personal issues. For those students already working an active recovery program, a self-awareness process by the nature of being sober and clean is already occurring. However, for the vast majority of counselors-in-training who are not in recovery, the question is posed, "How might students increase their self-awareness and begin to experientially understand their clients' recovery process?"

The following are experiential suggestions for counselors who want to better understand the process their clients may go through when initiating treatment and beginning a recovery program. It is suggested that counselors do the following:

1. *Discontinue a substance or behavior for 4–5 weeks:* Counselors are encouraged to select a substance (e.g., caffeine, sugar, alcohol, nicotine) or a behavior (e.g., video games, spending money) that will be challenging and bring about discomfort when abstaining from it. As the abstinence process is initiated, counselors can record their feelings and talk with others about the discomfort. The abstinence should be approximately 4 to 5 weeks, which is the length of various inpatient treatment programs. This abstinence project allows counselors to begin to understand cravings, preoccupation, relapse, and a host of other issues clients will discuss in treatment.

2. *Attend support meetings:* Because a vast majority of treatment programs follow the 12 steps of Alcoholics Anonymous (AA), attending at least five open AA or Narcotics Anonymous (NA) meetings and five open Al-Anon or Adult Children of Alcoholics meetings will help counselors begin to understand the philosophy of the 12 steps and to potentially negate myths they had before attendance. Through attendance, students experientially understand what it is like to attend their first meeting and what actually occurs in meetings. It is also encouraged for counselors to attend other support meetings (e.g., Women for Sobriety or Secular Organizations for Sobriety) with permission of the group members.

3. *Construct a family tree:* Counselors are encouraged to explore any alcohol, drug addiction, or abuse within their families (parents, brothers, sisters, uncles, aunts, grandparents). Having counselors recognize patterns within their own families will help with understanding how behaviors can be generational.

4. *Present the 12 steps:* Having small groups present the 12 steps experientially helps to bring a deeper personal recognition of the steps.

5. *Visit a drug and alcohol facility:* Counselors are encouraged to visit local resources for outpatient and inpatient services. This gives an opportunity for students to observe the facility, talk with personnel, and better understand the process of recovery.

6. *Evaluate personal drug and alcohol use:* This is important for counselors to explore, not only for personal reasons but also for clinical reasons. For example, if a counselor's daily consumption of alcohol is 10 drinks and a client comes in stating he "drinks only 8 drinks per night," the counselor is probably not going to view the client's drinking as problematic, and thus not address it as an issue in counseling. Therefore, this personal evaluation should also be a part of the experiential process.

The previous suggestions help counselors understand what their clients may go through experientially when entering a treatment and recovery process. If counselors remain abstinent from a substance or behavior, attend AA or NA meetings, visit a rehabilitation program, explore their family and personal history for addiction, and experientially present on the 12 steps, they will have a substantially more profound understanding of the changes that face clients as opposed to simply reading the information in a textbook.

Project Taproot, a holistic addiction education program at the College of William and Mary, categorized student training into three categories: academic, experiential, and self-work (Matthews, 1998). Students learned information on addiction, explored experientially by means of the suggestions above, and as a result acquired grist for personal counseling. The combination of the factors helped counselors demonstrate increased realness, genuineness, and the ability to be present with clients. One of the theoretical approaches used in that training program was transpersonal counseling.

Transpersonal Approach to Addiction Counseling

White (1998) suggested that there are those who work in addiction who are professionals by their education and then there are those who are professionals by their experience. He believes an effective treatment team combines both. He also recognizes that with the increasing professionalism of addiction counselors, those without the proper formal education are leaving the field. The transpersonal approach to counseling is a bridge for those academics, not in personal addiction recovery, to understand "from the heart" the internal transformation that occurs in recovery with many of their patients. Flores (1988) stated, "While I do not completely believe that a person has to be an addict or an alcoholic in order to help and treat one, I do believe a person has to leave the realm of objectivity and immerse themselves as much as possible in the subjective experience of the other who has sought help" (p. 382).

Transpersonal counseling is a combination of psychoanalytic, behavioral, and humanistic psychologies, with transpersonal experiences. The word *trans* indicates "beyond the personal" (Strohl, 1998). Knowing the mind and knowing the heart bring together the spiritual dimension (Boorstein, 1996). Abraham Maslow helped create the Association for Transpersonal Psychogy (Sutich, 1965). He believed there was a stage beyond self-actualization, which is the transcendence of self. The transpersonal counseling approach integrates the counselor's sense of a personal spiritual journey with the unique spiritual journey of the client.

C. G. Jung (1933) elaborated on the path of healers and the significance of healers meeting their own needs in order to help their clients:

> At all events the doctor must consistently try to meet his own therapeutic demands if he wishes to assure himself of a proper influence on his patient. All these guiding principles in therapy confront the doctor with important ethical duties which can be summed up in the single rule: be the man through whom you wish to influence others. Mere talk has always been considered hollow, and there is no trick, however cunning, by which one can evade this simple rule for long. The fact of being convinced, and not the subject-matter of conviction it is this which has always carried weight. . . . Who can enlighten his fellows while still in the dark about himself, and who can purify if he is himself unclean? (p. 51)

C. G. Jung described the client–therapist relationship as being dialectical. He believed it to be a conversation between two people where knowledge is used only as a tool. The goal of treatment is transformation or the disappearance of egohood. Jung made references to a process that is much greater than the therapeutic relationship where the doctor can smooth the path for the patient in order to attain an attitude that offers the least resistance to the overall experience (C. G. Jung, 1933).

As a result, healers must reach an understanding of the client predicament as well as the resolution and subsequent transcendence. Without this awareness, the healer may feel helpless, and the state of both healer and client may grow worse (Dossey, 1984; Guggenbuhl, 1982; Muktananda, 1982). An important assumption here is that the counselor is not doing the healing, but rather it is a process occurring within the client and between the client and counselor. The counselor, however, must be willing to participate in his or her own spiritual growth and healing for this to happen (May, 1977). According to Grof (1987b), those counselors who are closed to the deeper levels of unconsciousness will ultimately be less effective with those clients whose psychopathology has roots in these deeper levels.

Small (1982) related the importance of helpers helping themselves before they can help others on their journies. She believes that counselors and healers act as the primary catalyst for the process of self-creation:

> Awareness and a willingness to work on ourselves provide the springboard for this inward, upward journey that takes us first into ourselves and finally beyond ourselves in service of others . . . real helpers are fellow travelers, who invite others to discover the meaning of their suffering, relieve suffering wherever they can, but who resist interfering with another's free will. (Small, 1982, p. 247)

These past few quotes imply the importance of the counselor's personal growth and its relationship to client empathy and understanding. If counselors do not understand their own inner spirit, it most likely will be difficult for them to help access this inner spirit within clients (Dossey, 1984; Guggenbuhl, 1982; Muktananda, 1982). The more secure counselors are in their own philosophical base, the more they will emit the quality of potency, which is one of the traits that research has found in high-functioning counselors (Small, 1987). In this way, the client resonates to an authentic person (counselor) who as a willing guide uses his or her whole self in relation to the client's path of recovery and healing (Small, 1987).

Transpersonal counselors differ from other therapists by the orientation, scope, and spiritual perspective they take in working with clients. *All* of the information presented by the client is useful in therapy. Transpersonal counselors believe in the client's potential to self-heal and achieve health beyond what is normally considered (Strohl, 1998). Cortright (1997) believed that transpersonal psychotherapy is a natural match with addictions treatment, allowing an integration of the many varied psychotherapeutic approaches while promoting recovery in a spiritual context. Counselors must commit to the process of self-examination and acceptance while living in the moment (Strohl, 1998). As counselors take care of their needs, examine their unfinished business, and seek to grow as authentic and genuine human beings, the sacred space between therapist and client can be the beginning of a trusting and growing experience for the client.

National Associations and Certifications

In 1974 the National Association of Alcoholism and Drug Abuse Counselors (NAADAC) formed as a national organization representing counselors around the country in the alcohol and drug counseling field. NAADAC offers three certifications: the National Certified Addiction Counselor I (NCACI), the National Certified Addiction Counselor II (NCACII), and the Master Addiction Counselor (MAC), where each has specific requirements for eligibility. The MAC requires a master's degree, whereas the NCACI and the NCACII do not (NAADAC, 2008, ¶2).

The Comprehensive Alcohol Abuse and Alcohol Prevention, Treatment, and Rehabilitation Act passed in the early 1970s, providing money to states for treatment of alcoholic patients (Banken & McGovern, 1992). In addition to such monies was the creation of the National Institute of Drug Abuse and the National Institute for Alcohol Abuse and Alcoholism. In combination, this was the beginning of specific training for alcohol and drug counselors (Banken & McGovern, 1992). Many of the initial addictions counselors were primarily members of AA whose main credential was their own recovery from alcoholism (Moyer, 1994; Valle, 1979). In the early years of the addiction field, "nondegreed, recovering addicts or alcoholics were recognized as qualified counseling professionals for substance abuse counseling" (West, Mustaine, & Wyrick, 1999, p. 36).

The National Board for Certified Counselors (NBCC, 2008), the International Association of Addiction and Offender Counselors (IAAOC), and the American Counseling Association (ACA) recognized this specialty need and cocreated the Master Addictions Counselor (MAC, which is not the same as NAADAC's MAC). NBCC provides a National Certified Counselor (NCC) credential requiring counselors to obtain a master's degree in counseling or related field as well as completing supervision hours and passing the National Counselors Examination. Upon meeting each requirement, counselors may call themselves an NCC and are eligible, with further supervision in addiction, addiction courses, and passing a standardized exam, to become an MAC. This specialty certification attests to the knowledge, skills, and abilities of master's level addiction counselors.

On the other hand, the Certified Addiction Counselor (CAC) credential frequently "does not have the educational qualifications necessary to meeting existing licensure guidelines; therefore, CACs frequently do not qualify for reimbursement from the managed care organizations" (Mustaine, West, & Wyrick, 2003, p. 105).

The International Certification Reciprocity Consortium is an international certification board for addiction that allows for reciprocity should a counselor move to an approved participating state or country. Counselors are able to maintain their CAC certification without having to go through an entirely new process in another state.

A study by Mustaine et al. (2003) found among 31 states surveyed and the District of Columbia, 12.5% required an associate's degree as a minimum requirement for certification as a CAC, 9.4% required a bachelor's degree, and none required a master's degree. The remainder required only the minimum of a high school diploma or equivalent. All of the respondents required a minimum number of years as a counselor and the successful completion of a written examination. In no cases were the applicants required to have a master's degree.

Why Have a Certification or Licensure Specialty in Addiction?

Banken and McGovern (1992) surveyed alcohol and drug counselors regarding their opinion of whether substance abuse counseling was a specialty or a distinct profession. The results indicated that most substance abuse counselors identified the discipline as a specialty rather than a distinct profession. This indicates that in addition to training and course work in generalist counseling, counselors require specific information, training, and supervision on substance abuse clients. Managed care moved addictions treatment into the mainstream of mental health care where certification and licensure in addiction are now more critical than personal recovery or experiential knowledge of AA recovery (Hoffmann, Halikas, Mee-Lee, & Weedman, 1991).

Those counselors graduating from graduate programs interested in addictions treatment with no personal recovery experience may find themselves working in treatment programs that have a strong spiritual component. According to Sebenick (1997), these counselors may be skeptical of spirituality in the treatment and recovery process. Graduate programs need to better prepare counselors to not only be empathic but also to be spiritually sensitive of the counselor and the client (Matthews & Hollingsworth, 1999).

The literature suggests that a large proportion of counselors are drawn to the field of addictions counseling on the basis of their own recovery experience and have minimal training or education. The Association for Addiction Professionals outlines ethical standards for counselors who are members of NAADAC. NAADAC consists of alcoholism and drug abuse counselors who believe in the dignity and worth of human beings (NAADAC, 2004, ¶1). This national association provides addiction counselors with a sense of professional unity through a national conference, quarterly updates, an addiction resource magazine, and legislative updates. NAADAC members agree to abide by the ethical standards that underlie the following nine principles (NAADAC, 2004):

1. *Nondiscrimination:* Diversity among colleagues and clients is affirmed, regardless of age, gender, sexual orientation, ethnic/racial background, religious/spiritual beliefs, marital status, political beliefs, or mental/physical disability.
2. *Client welfare:* Essentially, this principle states that the member will do no harm and exercise respect, sensitivity, and insight. The primary professional responsibility of the counselor is loyalty to the welfare of clients and to work in counseling regardless of who actually pays his or her fees.
3. *Client relationship:* This principle states basically that the client is free to make his or her own decision regarding treatment. The counselor is also charged with providing informed consent regarding nature, extent, and fees involved in services.
4. *Trustworthiness:* Counselors have the responsibility to act consistently within the bounds of a known moral universe, to fulfill both personal and professional commitments, and to safeguard fiduciary relationships.

5. *Compliance with the law:* Counselors are aware of the law and the relevant regulations and the duty to observe them while reserving the right to commit civil disobedience.
6. *Rights and duties:* Essentially the counselor understands the personal and professional commitments and network of rights and duties and is willing to work to the best of his or her ability to fulfill those duties.
7. *Dual relationships:* Counselors approach the therapeutic relationship from an equal standpoint and will not take unfair advantage of those who are vulnerable and exploitable.
8. *Preventing harm:* It is understood that each action and decision has a potential implication to benefit or harm clients. Counselors will consider the impact of those decisions prior to carrying them out.
9. *Duty of care:* Counselors say they will maintain a safe, supportive environment with clients, colleagues, and other employees.

The *ACA Code of Ethics* (2005) and the NAADAC (2004) code of ethics are similar, which is helpful to those who are members of both organizations. Both ACA and NAADAC are in existence to help consumers of services. ACA is comprised of specialty divisions, one of which focuses on addiction (IAAOC). NAADAC promotes prevention, intervention, treatment, and education of substance-abusing and addicted individuals, as well as those suffering from other addictions such as gambling, sex, and food. NAADAC is focused on addiction, whereas ACA focuses on counseling with specialty divisions. Within each association's ethical code are the limitations and constraints for the release of confidential information (Toriello & Benshoff, 2003).

Working With Clients: Confidentiality and Informed Consent

Clients entering treatment or counseling have the right to confidentiality. Confidentiality protects clients from harm or injury resulting from information being shared outside the counseling session. Because confidentiality is such an important aspect of developing a therapeutic relationship, it requires attention and discussion during the first session. Although many licensing boards require counselors to create informed consent forms before initiating counseling services, it is also good clinical preparation and an ethical responsibility (ACA, 2005).

An informed consent identifies for clients the necessary information concerning counselors and the counseling process. Information recommended for inclusion on consent forms are specialty training, certificates, certifications, licenses, education held by the clinician, fees for service, crisis and cancellation policies, theoretical approaches, confidentiality and the limitations therein, referrals, and insurance usage (Corey, Corey, & Callanan, 2007). Clients are asked to sign the informed consent to officially document that they have been informed about counseling procedures. The informed consent, however, does not document that the client agrees with the information; rather, the form simply indicates that they have been informed, at which time clients receive a copy of the informed consent.

The informed consent typically contains a statement about confidentiality and the restrictions counselors have with regard to breaking confidential information. Depending on the license, certification, or association counselors hold or belong to, potential ethical dilemmas are created. If counselors are members of ACA, they abide by its code of ethics. If counselors are members of NAADAC, they abide by that code of ethics. However, if the counselors are members of ACA, NAADAC, and have licenses to practice as counselors and are also CACs, these individuals have four ethical codes from which they work.

Additionally, there are federal guidelines to follow for substance dependent clients in facilities receiving federal funding. Federal alcohol and drug guidelines for patients (where *patient* is defined as any individual who has applied for or been given a diagnosis or treatment for alcohol or drug abuse) at a federally assisted program (where the program receives federal monies to provide addiction treatment) that includes any individual who, after arrest on a criminal charge, is identified as an alcohol or drug abuser for determining eligibility to participate in a program (Code of Federal Regulations, 2000, p. 18), state that the program can only break confidentiality if

1. The patient *consents in writing* (release of information), which includes (Code of Federal Regulations, 2000)
    a. Specific name or designee of program or person permitted to make disclosure.
    b. Name of individual of organization to which the disclosure is to be made.
    c. The name of the client.
    d. The purpose of the disclosure.
    e. How much and what type of information to be disclosed.
    f. Signature of the client, and when the client is a minor or is adjudicated as mentally incompetent, the signature of the authorized person to provide consent.
    g. Date when the consent is signed.
    h. A statement on the consent that allows revocation at any time during treatment except to the extent the program or person who is to make the disclosure has already acted in reliance on it.
    i. The date, event, or condition in which the release expires if not revoked before. This date or event or condition must insure that the consent will last no longer than reasonably necessary to serve the purpose that it is given.
2. The disclosure is allowed by a *court order* (ordered by the judge). The court order may authorize confidential disclosure from a client in the course of diagnosis, treatment, or referral for treatment only if
    a. The information to be disclosed would protect against threat to life or injury, including suspected child abuse/neglect and verbal threats against a third party.
    b. The information is needed in connection with an investigation or prosecution of an extremely serious crime (e.g., threatens loss of life, serious bodily injury, homicide, rape, kidnapping, armed robbery, assault with a deadly weapon, child abuse).
    c. The information is connected with litigation in which the client offers testimony or evidence pertaining to the confidential communication (Code of Federal Regulations, 2000, p. 23).
3. The disclosure is made to medical personnel in a medical emergency or to qualified personnel for research, audit, or program evaluation.

A treatment program may disclose client information to those persons within the criminal justice system who have made participation in the program a condition of the disposition of any criminal proceedings against the patient or of the patient's parole. Disclosures are limited to client's involvement in the program, prognosis, progress, and relapse history.

Federal law and regulations do not protect any information about a crime committed by a patient either within the program or against any person who works for the program or about any threat to commit such a crime. Federal laws and regulations also do not protect information about suspected child abuse or neglect from being reported under state law to appropriate state or local authorities (Code of Federal Regulations, 2000).

In 1974 the California Supreme Court reversed the appellate court division and in 1976 made the final decision that a counselor who knows or should have known that a patient poses a serious danger of violence and who does not attempt any type of reasonable effort or care to protect the intended victim or notify police, can be held liable (Tarasoff v. Regents of the University of California). The court further stated the disclosure is made only if it is necessary to avert danger to others.

Counselors licensed and working in alcohol and drug treatment programs that receive federal funding may find counseling ethics and federal law in conflict. The crucial point for counselors working with addicted clients is to be knowledgeable of local/county, state, and federal law as well as the code of ethics for certifications and licenses that they hold. Licensure and certification boards as well as national organizations have made diligent efforts to develop ethical codes of conduct and practice that work together rather than are in opposition of each other. Therefore, holding multiple credentials and being a member of national organizations is generally not a problem. However, dilemmas do occur when the ethical codes and licensure ethics conflict with federal law. For example, the following is a portion of ACA's (2005) ethical code B.1. Respecting Client Rights:

B.1.b. Respect for Privacy. Counselors respect client rights to privacy. Counselors solicit private information from clients only when it is beneficial to the counseling process.

B.1.c. Respect for Confidentiality. Counselors do not share confidential information without client consent or without sound legal or ethical justification.

B.1.d. Explanation of Limitations. At initiation and throughout the counseling process, counselors inform clients of the limitations of confidentiality and seek to identify foreseeable situations in which confidentiality must be breached.

B.2. Exceptions

B.2.a. Danger and Legal Requirements. The general requirement that counselors keep information confidential does not apply when disclosure is required to protect clients or identified others from serious and foreseeable harm or when legal requirements demand that confidential information must be revealed. Counselors consult with other professionals when in doubt as to the validity of an exception. Additional considerations apply when addressing end of life issues. *(See A.9.c.)*

B.2.b. Contagious, Life-Threatening Diseases. When clients disclose that they have a disease commonly known to be both communicable and life threatening, counselors may be justified in disclosing information to identifiable third parties, if they are known to be at demonstrable and high risk of contracting the disease. Prior to making a disclosure, counselors confirm that there is such a diagnosis and assess the intent of the clients to inform the third parties about their disease or to engage in any behaviors that may be harmful to an identifiable third party.

B.2.c. Court-Ordered Disclosure. When subpoenaed to release confidential or privileged information without a client's permission, counselors obtain written, informed consent from the client or take steps to prohibit the disclosure or have it limited as narrowly as possible due to the potential harm to the client or the counseling relationship.

B.2.d. Minimal Disclosure. To the extent possible, clients are informed before confidential information is disclosed and are involved in the discloser decision-making process. When circumstances require the disclosure of confidential information, only essential information is revealed.

One of the most glaring conflicts is between ACA's (2005) *Code of Ethics* on confidentiality (i.e., duty to warn, protect client, and contagious diseases) and the federal regulations for confidentiality with a drug and alcohol client. Federal confidentiality law for alcohol and drug clients is very specific about the information that can be released and under what conditions (Ward, 2002). This creates a potentially challenging dilemma for counselors who are licensed as psychologists, social workers, or counselors and working in drug and alcohol facilities that receive federal funding.

With this potential ethical conflict, the importance of supervision cannot be overemphasized. Counselors do not need to and should not make these decisions alone (i.e., in a vacuum) and need to document case notes for each session (Mitchell, 2007). Professional counselors obtain support, feedback, instruction, and consultation on potential ethical dilemmas. Legal consultation is recommended to ensure support from the agencies or programs. Counselors need to be aware of their local and state regulations as well as the policies of the programs in which they work in order to be best informed and to help their clients.

The Process of Ethical Decision Making

Each day, counselors find themselves negotiating ethical dilemmas. Supervision, knowledge of ethical codes, agency policies, and state and /federal laws help guide clinicians to ethical decisions involving their clients. Additionally, Herlihy and Corey (2006) outlined five principles intended to facilitate ethical behaviors of counselors:

- *Autonomy* refers to independence and self-determination. Under this principle, counselors respect the freedom of clients to choose their own directions, make their own choices, and control their own lives. We have an ethical obligation to decrease client dependency and foster independent decision making. We refrain from imposing goals, avoid being judgmental, and are accepting of different values. Although many alcohol and drug clients are mandated to counseling and treatment, they still choose to what degree they will engage in treatment. Counselors respect the client's decision to discontinue treatment; however, they need to inform clients of the potential consequences from the referring sources should they discontinue.

- *Nonmaleficence* means to do no harm. As counselors, we must take care that our actions do not risk hurting clients, even inadvertently. We have a responsibility to avoid engaging in practices that cause harm or have the potential to result in harm. An example of doing no harm is for the counselor to avoid any potential dual relationships, such as meeting the client for coffee or going to a 12-step meeting together.

- *Beneficence* means to promote good, or mental health and wellness. This principle mandates that counselors actively promote the growth and welfare of those they serve. An example is a counselor who encourages clients to explore their creative side, facilitating increased enjoyment of the recovery process.

- *Justice* is the foundation of our commitment to fairness in our professional relationships. Justice includes consideration of such factors as quality of services, allocation of time and resources, establishment of fees, and access to counseling services. This principle also refers to the fair treatment of an individual when his or her interests need to be considered in the context of the rights and interests of others. An example of justice is a counselor who works with a client's financial situation and doesn't limit services because of the client's inability to pay the full rate.

- *Fidelity* means that counselors make honest promises and honor their commitments to clients, students, and supervisees. This principle involves creating a trusting and therapeutic climate in which people can search for their own solutions and taking care not to deceive or exploit clients (Herlihy & Corey, 2006, pp. 9–10).

In addition to following the Herlihy and Corey (2006) principles, counselors also need structure for ethical decision making. Veterans as well as novice counselors benefit from a pragmatic, methodical decision-making process. With practice and clinical experience, counselors develop a sense of what to look for and how to approach various ethical challenges. Initially though, it can be quite overwhelming. As such, the following guidelines from Corey et al. (2007) are outlined to help with the process.

The first aspect of making an ethical decision is to *clarify and outline the dilemma*. Is the dilemma related to federal, state, or local laws and the ethical code? Or is the dilemma related to ethics and the agency policy? Experienced counselors may describe the initial conflict as a feeling within their body that is uncomfortable and creates internal dissonance. Once the dilemma has been clarified, counselors need to *address all the issues surrounding this dilemma*. An example of an ethical issue may be administrators pushing for ever-higher patient census without increasing the number of professional staff providing appropriate care and discharge planning. Next is a *thorough review of all pertaining ethical codes* as prescribed by the counselor's certifications, licenses, and associations. Next is *gathering the information* for consultation and supervision, where the information and conflict can be discussed with an outside professional counselor. The objectivity provided offers counselors an increased opportunity to brainstorm many options and the potential ramifications of the dilemma. It also serves as action in terms of ethical behavior to consult with colleagues. Documentation of recommendations and suggestions by the consultation is important for clinical records. If the final decision ever comes to be questioned, either through the legal system, an insurance agency, or ethical/licensing board, documentation of proactive consultation in the client record helps justify the course of action. The next step in ethical decision making is to *consider and review all of the options* and possibilities for each decision. Reviewing the many possibilities is important in this stage of the process. Thinking about how the ethical decision will impact not only clients but also the lives of others, counselors, the agency, and surrounding staff is critical. Corey et al. (2007) suggested that once a tentative decision has been made, the counselor should reconsider each of the five principles cited above before making a final decision. Finally, *make the decision* on what seems to be the best course of action based on the information given. Following the decision, other aspects of the client's case may surface, which may require further ethical exploration (and possibly a change in course regarding the previous decision).

Below are three case examples that present ethical dilemmas. The first case focuses on dual relationships, the second case deals with confidentiality, and the third case addresses managed care.

Ethical Dilemmas With Ethical Dilemmas

Case of Kurt: Dual Relationship

Kurt works as a mental health counselor in a rural community. He is one of two counselors in the county providing mental health services. Although the agency where he works does not provide formal alcohol and drug treatment on an outpatient basis, he does see clients who are in the initial stages of considering treatment. He also works with clients following treatment on continuing mental health issues. Kurt has worked in this community for the past 10 years and enjoys the country life as well as his work with clients. Most of his clinical time is composed of assessments, individual and family counseling, and on occasion group therapy. The agency is small and the pay is minimal. His coworker, Anne, spends 50% of her time seeing clients in their homes or in far-reaching areas of the counties in their area. The remaining time she spends in the main office.

One of the clients referred to Kurt was from an outpatient alcohol and drug program in another county. The client, Sal, had completed 4 months of outpatient treatment and was referred to Kurt for ongoing care to address Sal's lifelong history of depression. During the initial session, Kurt realized that Sal worked at the car dealership where he took his car for inspection and mechanical problems. Because it was a small dealership, the chance Sal would work on his car at some point was high. Kurt also realized that Anne had limited training in addiction recovery issues and depression. Following the session with Sal, Kurt contemplated a number of issues. The first was his certainty that Sal would inevitably work on his car. The second issue was the lack of professional mental health resources (i.e., counselors) in the area, and third was Sal's need for ongoing counseling, which at times involved suicidal plans.

Given this information, review the five principles and the decision-making process with regards to the following questions:

1. If you were Kurt, would you work with Sal as a client? Why or why not?
2. Is there a potential ethical dilemma? Why or why not?
3. If Kurt took on Sal as a client, what would he need to be careful of (precautions) when working with Sal in counseling?
4. If Kurt did not take Sal on as a client, what would he need to do? How might he need to handle it?
5. How might Anne play a part in Kurt's decision process?
6. With whom might Kurt consult to make the final decision?

Case of Katherine: Confidentiality

Katherine works in a college counseling center composed of five other counselors. Many of the clients she works with in therapy are alcohol and drug abusers referred by the judicial program at the university. Many of her alcohol- and drug-abusing clients resist counseling, complying only because of the required five sessions they need to attend in order to satisfy the university's alcohol and drug policy. Most of the clients are willing to sign a release of information regarding their attendance in counseling to the dean of students, however, rarely to anyone else. One morning as Katherine was copying intake forms, a police officer from the community presented himself very authoritatively at the front desk, demanding to see the file on a client Katherine was seeing for counseling. The police officer became quite intimidating, stating that anyone resisting his request could be subject to legal action. Upon immediate reflection, Katherine realized the police officer had the same last name as the client whose file was being requested. The student had just been referred by the district justice for counseling because of his alcohol and drug arrest for underage drinking and being drunk in public. At that moment the officer was called on his radio for immediate response to an accident. The officer said he would return after his call to review the file.

Given this information, address the following questions:

1. Can a police officer demand to see a client file? Under what conditions, if any?
2. Under what conditions can Katherine breach confidentiality?
3. Who might she want to consult with?
4. Should she let him review the file?
5. Should Katherine tell the client that his father was in to see his chart?
6. If you were Katherine, how might you talk to the officer when he returned?

Case of Bruce: Managed Care

Bruce, an outpatient alcohol and drug counselor, handles 50 to 60 clients who are insured through managed care. His agency is an approved program with this managed care company and typically provides 20 visits per client per year. One of his clients is a relapser, having been to at least three inpatient programs and at least five outpatient programs over the past 10 years. However, this treatment experience appeared to be helping her address and take action on a number of issues. For years she had been unwilling to leave her abusive relationship; now she was living in a women's recovery house. She was also unwilling to leave her job as a waitress in an upscale restaurant downtown; now she was returning to school to finish her degree. And finally, she had begun discussing issues of trauma she had not been willing to talk about before in treatment. In addition, she was going to AA meetings on a regular basis, had obtained a sponsor, and was even making coffee at one of the meetings. She truly had made great strides. Unfortunately, her insurance company discontinued coverage for individual counseling, stating that her initial goals for treatment had been reached and she could continue with her outside support and halfway house but that they were unwilling to continue payment for individual therapy.

Bruce believes his client is working very hard in recovery and is beginning to address issues that have significantly contributed to her relapse process. Bruce feels she finally has the safety and support of her recovery house to help her deal with the issues she is slowly bringing out in individual therapy. She has been sober this time for 7 months, the most she has ever been clean and sober since she began using at age 12.

To make the situation more challenging, Bruce's agency is under new management and unless the client is willing to self-pay, she needs to be referred to a local community agency, where the waiting list is 6 months long. The new director will not allow counselors to continue to see clients unless they pay full price for therapy.

Given the issues and circumstances presented, address the following questions using the five principles and decision-making process:

1. Is there an ethical dilemma? Review your code of ethics to determine what that ethical dilemma might be.
2. How might Bruce work to obtain benefits from the insurance company? What might be his strategy, knowing his prior relationship with the company?
3. How might Bruce interact with the new director of the agency? What dilemma does his edict place upon Bruce and the rest of his clients with the same insurance?
4. Do you think Bruce should keep the client or should he refer her?
5. How might he justify either action?
6. How might Bruce include the client in this process?

Each of these scenarios presents a potential or current ethical dilemma to the counselor. In the first case there is the potential for a dual relationship in a rural community where there are limited resources. In the second case there is an authority figure demanding access to records, using his position as justification for breaking confidentiality. And in the third case, two businesses are either trying to save or make money at the expense of the client. Scenarios such as these could happen each day in the life of a counselor and at times can seem overwhelming.

Maintaining Professional Boundaries and Avoiding Dual Relationships

Ethically, it is important for counselors to be open to professional as well as personal growth. This includes being able to receive feedback and supervision and being willing to enter personal therapy if needed. When counselors ignore personal needs, neglect supervision or consultation, or are unwilling to seek help, professional boundaries become exponentially unclear while the potential for dual relationships increases. Ethical training should consist of role playing, knowledge of ethical codes, case studies and dilemmas for discussion, as well as decision-making practice (St. Germaine, 1997; Toriello & Benshoff, 2003).

In a survey of 40 addiction certification boards in the United States, 33 required ethics training for initial certification, and of those boards, 29 of them required 6 contact hours, 1 board required 9 contact hours, and 3 boards required 15 contact hours of ethics training. The total number of ethical complaints was 372, with the top 3 related to issues of professional boundaries and dual relationships: having a sexual relationship with a current client (61 complaints), unable to effectively perform duties because of alcohol, drugs, or other conditions (46 complaints), and practicing without a certificate (37 complaints; St. Germaine, 1997). A similar survey with licensed professional counselors revealed the top three complaints as practicing without a license (27%), sexual relationship with a client (both current and former, 20%), and other (15%; Neukrug, Healy, & Herlihy, 1992).

Self-care for counselors is not only sage advice but also an ethical mandate. Counselors not open to self-examination may find themselves on a slippery slope leading to boundary problems with clients. Figure 13.1 shows a continuum of boundary crossing that outlines a path to unethical behavior.

The continuum presupposes that counselors are not in regular supervision. This is why supervision is critically important. For counselors feeling depressed, overwhelmed, isolated, and disconnected, meeting needs through clients is a serious breach of the counselor role. Add to this a possible overidentification with clients because the counselor is a recovering addict or alcoholic and/or there is a lack of supervision, and client harm results. In a national survey, St. Germaine (1997) found that 52% of CACs were recovering alcoholics or addicts and that 47.5% of those counselors encountered their clients outside of therapy

---

PHASE I-Isolation/Minimization of Feelings

Increase in counselor self-disclosure to the client, but not for clinical reasons
Professional isolation from colleagues; reduced supervision or missing supervision
Loss of interest in activities outside of work; sole interest is work and longer hours
Feelings of isolation; disconnection from others; avoiding feelings

Inappropriate boundary crossing can start with a counselor who is feeling isolated, disconnected from family and friends as well as colleagues. The initial signs may be minimized feelings and minor depression where feelings are suppressed and energy levels are low. A counselor, if in supervision, might be asked about his/her appearance and depressed affect. However, those not involved in regular supervision or working as solo practitioners are at risk for isolation and depression.

PHASE II-Avoidance

Finds affirmation from clients as very important; meeting own needs through client
Tends to avoid client's difficult issues; not wanting to offend in order to keep clients in counseling
Counseling sessions take on the feeling of a social meeting rather than therapy
Sharing more and more personal information with client

Counselors begin to avoid client issues that are emotionally laden. Sessions may take on the feeling of two friends getting together to drink coffee, at which time the counselor shares more about his or her life. Through this avoidance the client is not being attended to and the counselor is developing a social relationship rather than therapeutic one and is meeting his or her own needs.

PHASE III-Social and Sexual Attraction and Acting Out Behaviors

Agree to meet outside of the therapy time for social activity
Meets for longer than counseling hour with clients of attraction
Sexual attraction to clients; not sharing in supervision
Calling clients at home under the guise of counseling concerns
Fostering client dependency
Complimenting client in a flirtatious manner
Fantasizing about client; preoccupation
Making inappropriate gestures in counseling session
Sexual contact with client

This counselor has avoided the client's feelings surrounding his or her presenting issue while meeting his or her needs as the counselor, starting initially by minimizing feelings.

Figure 13.1. Continuum of Inappropriate Boundary Crossing

sometimes and 21.4% encountered them frequently or daily. The NAADAC conducted a study in 1994 and found 58% of its membership in recovery. Because an increasing number of counselors is in recovery, exploration into dual relationships and the need for clarification is ethically important (Doyle, 1997; Hecksher, 2007). Dual relationships, as defined by Herlihy and Corey (2006), occur "when professionals assume two roles simultaneously or sequentially with a person seeking help" (p. 1). Doyle explored the various ethical dilemmas as they related to dual relationships and recovering counselors by outlining five areas.

The first of these areas is *confidentiality and anonymity*. In this area Doyle described the challenges counselors face when attending AA or support meetings and clients see him or her at the meeting. The counselor's anonymity has been jeopardized as well as the comfort level in that person sharing in the meeting. If or when the counselor discloses to the client that he or she is in recovery, it places a new light on the therapeutic relationship. "The sharing of private information about one's recovery, its challenges, and its successes, while conceivably therapeutic, also may lead to the relationship becoming more personal than professional if caution is not used" (Doyle, 1997, p. 430).

Another area is *self-help meetings*. Clients and counselors who attend the same support meetings create opportunities for counselors to discover things that may not be beneficial to their client's clinical success. For instance, what if the counselor disclosed how he or she almost relapsed? Or if the client admitted in the group that he or she had used alcohol or drugs again, would the counselor use that information in the next therapy session? Would the counselor report that to the probation officer, who needs to know if the client is using? These questions and certainly more, according to Doyle (1997), place the counselor in a challenging position. He indicated that some communities offer self-help meetings for professionals, such as Caduceus (support meetings for helping professionals, such as physicians, nurses, counselors, etc.), where this duality would be avoided.

The third area is *social relationships*. Doyle (1997) described the social aspect of AA when members get together after the meetings for coffee and conversation. In rural communities this can be particularly challenging. It can place the counselor and the client in an interesting position. Should the counselor continue with the same meeting? Should the counselor go for coffee knowing one of the participants will be his or her client? He also brings up the question, "At what point and after how much time does attendance with former clients become acceptable?" (p. 432).

Sponsorship is another area. Members of AA or other 12-step support groups are advised to obtain a sponsor early in recovery for support. Doyle (1997) questioned whether or not counselors should sponsor their clients, whether current or past. He found in AA literature, *AA Guidelines: For Members Employed in the Alcoholism Field* (AA, n.d.) that collective responses (totaling over 600 years of sobriety) from members working in the field of addiction (totaling 400 years of professional experience) recommended not to sponsor current or past clients and to keep the two roles distinct.

The last area is *employment*. It is fairly common for treatment centers to hire former patients who have successfully remained sober and clean and who possess the credentials to be an addiction counselor. The dual relationship occurs when a previous client is hired and potentially is supervised by his or her counselor when he or she went through treatment. Our experience in the field suggests that this occurrence happens and can present interesting dynamics. One of the programs where I (Ford) worked had a counselor who had been hired after having been sober for 8 years, became certified, and obtained his master's degree in counseling. He was then hired and directly supervised by the counselor who provided treatment to him 8 years before.

Doyle (1997) suggested that counselors in recovery review and examine all ethical codes that would apply (i.e., certifications, licenses, associations, standards of practice) before working in the counseling field. He also suggested that recovering counselors consult with experienced and seasoned colleagues. Third, he suggested that counselors consider the wide range and variety of meetings offered and to minimize dual relationships in their recovery program. Finally, he suggested that self-disclosure of the counselor's recovery should be used judiciously.

Impaired Professionals

Addiction to alcohol and drugs is not discriminatory but rather it is an equal opportunity illness. When professionals become impaired, other lives many times are at stake. Therefore, monitoring boards, detoxification protocols, and extensive treatment regimes intervene and follow the progress of these professionals with great intensity and concern. Professionals such as surgeons, commercial airline pilots, nurses, pharmacists, lawyers, mental health counselors, addictions counselors, and FBI/CIA operatives are a few of the categories of impaired professionals who require special attention.

State licensing boards typically have monitoring protocols for individuals impaired from alcohol or drug use. Their main interest is in protecting the consumer from harm while obtaining help for the addicted professional. Involvement with monitoring programs can be initiated in a number of ways. Consumers may register a complaint with licensing boards for reasons ranging from intoxication on the job to unprofessional behavior and incompetent work. Professional boards receive the complaint and make the decision whether or not to investigate the complaint and the professional in question. Generally, once a professional has been identified as having a drug or alcohol problem, he or she is referred for treatment and continuous monitoring. Depending on the state, a separate entity will supervise and monitor the professional's treatment involvement, abstinence from drugs and alcohol, attendance in self-help meetings, meetings with monitoring staff, and help him or her comply with treatment recommendations. This monitoring process can last up to 5 or 6 years, depending on the profession and the monitoring organization. Licensing boards work collaboratively with the monitoring organization by placing the individual's license in a probationary status, pending continuous compliance with treatment recommendations. Licensing boards may decide to suspend licenses until a time when the individual has provided documentation of compliance with the monitoring organization. The professional can petition the licensing board to restore or provisionally restore the license, again, pending continuous monitoring. Because the loss of a license is the professional's livelihood, compliance with monitoring organizations is usually quite high. Because of the potential for lethality with consumers, monitoring organizations use hair follicle drug screening as well as standard random urine screens. In cases where relapse occurs, the professional may lose his or her license to practice immediately and may be referred to longer term treatment.

I (Ford) facilitated a weekly group consisting of impaired professionals for over 3 years. It was, without a doubt, one of the highlights of my professional career. Doctors, lawyers, surgeons, teachers, police officers, and nurses each shared the common bonds of addiction as well as being professionals in their chosen fields. Each group member was a witness to each other's recovery over the years. In addition to the group, many were monitored weekly through urine screens, contacts with sponsors and monitors, as well as attendance at AA and NA meetings. For some, the shame and fear of jeopardizing others' lives because of their addiction were very powerful, which helped propel them early in recovery.

Summary

This chapter reviewed the importance of counselors knowing the codes of ethics for each association, license, and certification. A counselor may hold a license and an addiction certification, resulting in conflicting practices. This chapter has helped to clarify and address those areas.

Because many counselors who treat addiction are also in recovery, special attention was given to dual relationships and how to negotiate potential ethical dilemmas that present themselves in treatment. Finally, the area of impaired professionals was addressed to help counselors realize that they are not immune to becoming impaired from addictive use.

Exploration Questions From Chapter 13

1. What ethical situations are you most concerned about?
2. Identify resources, support, and supervision and how you would use them for ethical dilemma discussions.
3. Have you ever known a practitioner to be unethical? If so, what responsibilities do you have?
4. Why are ethical codes and standards of practice important for counselors as well as clients?
5. Identify potential dual relationships with clients in the work setting you are currently in.

Suggested Activities

1. Review your code(s) of ethics for each association, organization, certification, or licensure you hold or are a member of and compare and contrast them. Identify how they may conflict and ask other clinicians how they handle this.
2. Discuss with other drug and alcohol counselors in the field how they handle ethical issues and identify the most common ethical dilemma they encounter on a regular basis.

Appendix 13.A
CACREP Standards for Addiction Counseling

Students who are preparing to work as addiction counselors will demonstrate the professional knowledge, skills, and practices necessary to work in a wide range of addiction counseling, treatment, and prevention programs, as well as in a mental health counseling context. Counselor education programs preparing counselors to work with addictions must provide evidence that student learning has occurred in the following domains listed below. However, the following program area standards listed below are in addition to the requirements found in Sections I–III of the CACREP 2009 *Standards*. In other words, the addiction counseling standards do not stand alone but in addition to the core Sections I–III. (Note: The chapter numbers within parentheses indicate chapters from this book.)

Foundations

A. *Knowledge*
   1. Understands the history, philosophy, and trends in addiction counseling. (ch. 4, 5)
   2. Understands ethical and legal considerations specifically related to the practice of addiction counseling. (ch. 13)
   3. Knows the roles, functions, and settings of addiction counselors, as well as the relationship between addiction counselors and other mental health professionals. (ch. 4–6)
   4. Knows the professional organizations, competencies, preparation standards, and state credentials relevant to the practice of addiction counseling. (ch. 13)
   5. Understands a variety of models and theories of addiction related to substance use and other addictions. (ch. 5)
   6. Knows the behavioral, psychological, physical health, and social effects of psychoactive substances and addictive disorders on the user and significant others. (ch. 3, 4, 8)
   7. Recognizes the potential for addictive disorders to mimic a variety of medical and psychological disorders and the potential for medical and psychological disorders to coexist with addiction and substance abuse. (ch. 4, 7)
   8. Understands factors that increase the likelihood for a person, community, or group to be at risk for or resilient to psychoactive substance use disorders. (ch. 5)
   9. Understands the impact of crises, disasters, and other trauma-causing events on persons with addictions. (ch. 9)
   10. Understands the operation of an emergency management system within addiction agencies and in the community. (ch. 4)
B. *Skills and Practice*
   1. Demonstrates the ability to apply and adhere to ethical and legal standards in addiction counseling. (ch. 13)
   2. Applies knowledge of substance abuse policy, financing, and regulatory processes to improve service delivery opportunities in addictions counseling. (ch. 6)

Counseling, Prevention, and Intervention

C. *Knowledge*
1. Knows the principles of addiction education, prevention, intervention, and consultation. (ch. 3–8)
2. Knows the models of treatment, prevention, recovery, relapse prevention, and continuing care for addictive disorders and related problems. (ch. 11)
3. Recognizes the importance of family, social networks, and community systems in the treatment and recovery process. (ch. 8)
4. Understands the role of spirituality in the addiction recovery process. (ch. 12)
5. Knows a variety of helping strategies for reducing the negative effects of substance use, abuse, dependence, and addictive disorders. (ch. 4–6)
6. Understands the principles and philosophies of addiction-related self-help programs. (ch. 12)
7. Understands professional issues relevant to the practice of addiction counseling, including recognition, reimbursement, and right to practice. (ch. 13)
8. Understands the principles of intervention for persons with addictions during times of crises, disasters, and other trauma-causing events. (ch. 8, 9)

D. *Skills and Practices*
1. Uses principles and practices of diagnosis, treatment, and referral of addiction and other mental and emotional disorders to initiate, maintain, and terminate counseling. (ch. 1, 4, 5)
2. Individualizes helping strategies and treatment modalities to each client's stage of dependence, change, or recovery. (ch. 4, 5, 12)
3. Provides appropriate counseling strategies when working with clients with addiction and co-occurring disorders. (ch. 4)
4. Demonstrates the ability to use procedures for assessing and managing suicide risk. (ch. 4, 5)
5. Demonstrates the ability to provide counseling and education about addictive disorders to families and others who are affected by clients with addictions. (ch. 8)
6. Demonstrates the ability to provide referral to self-help and other support groups when appropriate. (ch. 12)
7. Demonstrates the ability to provide culturally relevant education programs that raise awareness and support addiction and substance abuse prevention and the recovery process. (ch. 2, 4, 5, 11)
8. Applies current record-keeping standards related to addiction counseling. (ch. 13)
9. Demonstrates the ability to recognize his or her own limitations as an addiction counselor and to seek supervision or refer clients when appropriate. (ch. 13, 14)

Diversity and Advocacy

E. *Knowledge*
1. Understands how living in a multicultural society affects clients with addictions. (ch. 2)
2. Understands current literature that outlines theories, approaches, strategies, and techniques shown to be effective when working with specific populations of clients with addictions. (ch. 2)
3. Knows public policies on local, state, and national levels that affect the quality and accessibility of addiction services. (ch. 6, 11, 13)
4. Understands effective strategies that support client advocacy and influence public policy and government relations on local, state, and national levels to enhance equity, increase funding, and promote programs that affect the practice of addiction counseling. (ch. 13)

F. *Skills and Practices*
1. Maintains information regarding community resources to make appropriate referrals for clients with addictions. (ch. 4, 5)
2. Advocates for policies, programs, and/or services that are equitable and responsive to the unique needs of clients with addictions. (ch. 4, 5)
3. Demonstrates the ability to modify counseling systems, theories, techniques, and interventions to make them culturally appropriate for diverse populations of addiction clients. (ch. 1, 2, 4, 10)

Assessment

G. *Knowledge*
1. Understands various models and approaches to clinical evaluation for addictive disorders and their appropriate uses, including screening and assessment for addiction, diagnostic interviews, mental status examination, symptom inventories, and psychoeducational and personality assessments. (ch. 4)
2. Knows specific assessment approaches for determining the appropriate level of care for addictive disorders and related problems. (ch. 6, 7)
3. Understands the assessment of biopsychosocial and spiritual history. (ch. 5, 12)
4. Understands basic classifications, indications, and contraindications of commonly prescribed psychopharmacological medications so that appropriate referrals can be made for medication evaluations and so that the side effects of such medications can be identified. (ch. 3, 4)

H. *Skills and Practices*
1. Selects appropriate comprehensive assessment interventions to assist in diagnosis and treatment planning, with an awareness of cultural bias in the implementation and interpretation of assessment protocols. (ch. 2–7)
2. Demonstrates skill in conducting an intake interview, a mental status evaluation, a biopsychosocial history, a mental health history, and a psychological assessment for treatment planning and case management. (ch. 4)
3. Screens for psychoactive substance toxicity, intoxication, and withdrawal symptoms; aggression or danger to others; potential for self-inflicted harm or suicide; and co-occurring mental and/or addictive disorders. (ch. 4)
4. Helps clients identify the effects of addiction on life problems and the effects of continued harmful use or abuse. (ch. 4, 13)
5. Applies assessment of clients' addictive disorders to the stages of dependence, change, or recovery to determine the appropriate treatment modality and placement criteria in the continuum of care. (ch. 4, 5)

Research and Evaluation

I. *Knowledge* (entire text)
1. Understands how to critically evaluate research relevant to the practice of addiction counseling.
2. Knows models of program evaluation for addiction counseling treatment and prevention programs.
3. Knows evidence-based treatments and basic strategies for evaluating counseling outcomes in addiction counseling.

J. *Skills and Practice*
1. Applies relevant research findings to inform the practice of addiction counseling.
2. Develops measurable outcomes for addiction counseling programs, interventions, and treatments.
3. Analyzes and uses data to increase the effectiveness of addiction counseling programs.

Diagnosis

K. *Knowledge*
  1. Knows the principles of the diagnostic process, including differential diagnosis, and the use of current diagnostic tools, such as the current edition of the *Diagnostic and Statistical Manual of Mental Disorders* (*DSM*). (ch. 4, 5)
  2. Knows the impact of co-occurring addictive disorders on medical and psychological disorders. (ch. 4, 5)
  3. Understands the established diagnostic and clinical criteria for addictive disorders and describes treatment modalities and placement criteria within the continuum of care. (ch. 4–6)
  4. Understands the relevance and potential cultural biases of commonly used diagnostic tools as related to clients with addictive disorders in multicultural populations. (ch. 2, 4–6)

L. *Skills and Practices*
  1. Demonstrates appropriate use of diagnostic tools, including the current edition of the *DSM*, to describe the symptoms and clinical presentation of clients with addictive disorders and mental and emotional impairments. (ch. 4)
  2. Is able to conceptualize an accurate multi-axial diagnosis of disorders presented by clients and communicate the differential diagnosis with collaborating professionals. (ch. 4)

These standards are from CACREP, 2009, *Addiction Counseling*, p. 17. Copyright 2009 by CACREP. Reprinted with permission.

Chapter

14

The Importance of Counselor Self-Care

Not all counseling is the same. I (Bill) have worked with clients on many different types of issues and concerns, ranging from suicidal clients needing inpatient care after going through the detoxification process to sixth-grade students fighting over who is who's best friend (that day). Not all clients present with the same issues, and not all counselors have the same stressors each day. But just as no client's "experienced pain" is greater than or less than another's, we have found that every counselor (including us) faces powerful stressors in working with their particular population(s). Our best advice is that all of us must continue to develop effective, proactive coping mechanisms to help us handle the plethora of stressors that inevitably emerge in our work.

For counselors working directly with addicted populations, there seems to be an increased level of stress related to clients presenting with life and death issues (e.g., homicidal ideation, suicidal ideation, medical emergencies), career issues (e.g., loss of job, poor work performance), and family (e.g., divorce, abuse or neglect, family disowning).

In this final chapter we address the well-being of counselors and their self-care. In our collective experience, we have found that those who choose to work with addicted clients and their families will be significantly challenged and in need of resources for balance. Striving for balance is important for counselors because it helps to maintain healthy therapeutic boundaries with clients while promoting effective and ethical clinical care. With this in mind, we present the following, which is an unfortunate and all too familiar scenario that can lead to burnout.

It's been a long day and you have just finished a counseling session with your seventh client of the day. You have at least an hour of progress notes to record and a group to facilitate before venturing home. Your agency expects you to maintain a caseload of 60 outpatient clients and schedule at least 35 individual clients per week. This means scheduling at least 40 clients per week, knowing that you will only see 25 to 30 clients for counseling that week. On this particular day you forgot to eat lunch and realize you needed to go to the bathroom 2 hours ago. You never touched the coffee you made at 10:00 a.m., and you left your lunch in the car. When you go out to the receptionist you receive 15 messages to return and have at least three letters to write for court dispositions at the end of the week.

You get the picture. Unfortunately, many counselors live day-to-day, week-to-week repeating this scenario, thinking little about personal time for basic needs. Self-care is an incredibly important aspect to counselor well-being and an area where many struggle. High stress, minimal pay, lack of support and supervision, and very challenging clients are ingredients for burnout in this profession. This scenario exists in many agencies and treatment programs around the country; however, little has been provided to counselors on the topic of self-care. We ask our clients to take risks, share painful emotions, and to stay active on a regular basis. But do we heed the same suggestions? The following are ideas that most of us have already come up with for our clients, except now they are for you, the reader, to consider: personal counseling, supervision, self-help meetings, continuing education and training, nutrition, meditation, exercise, leisure activities, and detachment.

Personal Counseling

Yalom (2005) suggested that students should become clients during their training to best experience what it is like to be a client. This experience can also initiate healing in areas that may interfere with effective therapy. Corey et al. (2007) strongly urged counselors to be aware of their own defenses, conflicts, and unfinished business and how they impact the counseling relationship. Self-knowledge, according to Matthews (1998), is the key to empathy.

Personal issues of the counselor may be revealed in counseling relationships as a need to fix clients, to remove clients' emotional pain, to be perfect, to assume too much responsibility for client change, or as a fear of doing harm to clients (Corey et al., 2007). They further suggested that counselors enter therapy during the course of instruction and as needed throughout their counseling career. "It is ethically imperative for counselors to take care of themselves and to heal themselves" (Corey et al., 2007, p. 39). "One's own personal therapy is a very important asset to providing quality therapy" (Flores, 1997, p. 533). Flores believes the group leader who understands what it feels like to be a client will be more sensitive to issues presented in group therapy.

Supervision

"Clinical supervision, especially in the field of alcohol and drug abuse, is essential if therapists are to successfully manage all of their countertransferential considerations that are likely to be evoked by these patients" (Flores, 1997, p. 534). Clinical supervision may involve administrative discussion; however, the main focus in supervision allows the supervisee a forum for discussion about cases, personal and professional introspection, and internal reactions to clients with intention on treatment goals. Bernard and Goodyear (2004) defined supervision as

> an intervention that is provided by a senior member of a profession to a junior member or members of that same profession. This relationship is evaluative, extends over time, and has the simultaneous purposes of enhancing the professional functioning of the junior member(s), monitoring the quality of professional services offered to the clients she, he, or they see(s), and serving as a gatekeeper for those who are to enter the particular profession. (p. 4)

Supervision allows counselors an environment to explore clinical issues. These discussions can result in constructive and supportive feedback. This process provides counselors a forum to enhance clinical as well as case management skills. There are counselors who write exceptional clinical notes and treatment plans, yet have difficulty working with resistance in counseling sessions. Supervisors play a significant role in helping counselors understand where these difficulties originate while discussing options for counselors. Supervisors need to maintain the role of supervisor and not the role of the supervisee's counselor. Although personal issues may surface in supervision sessions, supervision is not counseling. "Therapeutic interventions with supervisees should be made only in the service of helping them become more effective with clients: To provide therapy that has broader goals is an ethical misconduct" (Bernard & Goodyear, 2004, p. 9). Supervisors need to continually be aware of boundaries in the supervisory role, otherwise trainees may become confused and treat supervision as therapy.

The benefits to supervision allow counselors a time to clinically debrief and to receive feedback, validation, and a sense of confidence for future sessions. Supervision also helps identify countertransference issues with their supervisees. Video- or audiotapes or live supervision are three methods for effective supervision. That being said, counselor self-reports continue to be used as a common method of clinical supervision (Bernard & Good-year, 2004). The use of regular supervision prevents counselor burnout and provides an environment for clinical discussion, typically increasing counselor job satisfaction and ethical conduct.

Wellness Model in Supervision

Because balance, personal counseling, and supervision are so important to counselor well-being, a model of counselor wellness was developed (Myers & Sweeney, 2005; Myers, Sweeney, & White, 2002). Myers et al. (2002) discussed five aspects of wellness that can be applied to counselor well-being during the supervision process. The first of these aspects is spirituality, which is differentiated from religion. Spirituality is seen as transcendence from the material and is connected with ideas of the cosmos and universe, thus providing connection. The second aspect examines self-direction and includes self-worth, sense of control, realistic beliefs, emotionally aware, creativity, problem solving, sense of humor, nutrition, exercise, self-care, stress management, and cultural and gender awareness. The ability to address each of these aspects contributes to the wellness of the counselors. The third aspect addresses work and leisure, where both of these factors are fulfilling in a meaningful and productive manner. The fourth aspect is friendship at both individual and community levels, where support is critical to the development and maintenance of well-being. The concept of love is the final aspect of the wellness model, where intimate, romantic, and loving relationships factor into a healthy and vibrant support network.

Supervisors can use this model to help promote balance and well-being in the lives of their supervisees. Because counseling requires a great deal from counselors, wellness is paramount. Using the wellness model developed by Myers et al. (2002) during the supervisory process can help keep focus not only on client care but also on counselor care.

Self-Help Support Meetings

As referenced in the above model, community support is important for counselors and their well-being. Many counselors working in the field of addictions are recovering addicts and alcoholics, come from addicted families, or are in both categories. Self-help meeting attendance for counselors in the mental health field who have family or friends who are alcoholics or addicts is strongly encouraged. Support meetings such as Families Anonymous, Al-Anon, Adult Children of Alcoholics, or Co-Dependency Anonymous can help those needing support and provides counselors with an understanding of detachment and the emotional impact of addiction.

For counselors in addiction recovery, it is important that they focus on attending to their own recovery program outside of the workplace. Setting limits and boundaries is very important, particularly if clients attend the same Alcoholics Anonymous or Narcotics Anonymous meetings.

Continuing Education and Training

In addition to support, credentialing and training help counselors keep on the cutting edge of counseling techniques. Most licensing and certification boards require practitioners to obtain continuing education hours in order to maintain their credentials. For those not licensed or certified, continuing education and training is essential for ongoing professional growth. Training in a specific area not only enhances the current base of knowledge but also provides new ideas and approaches for client care. This helps counselors increase their clinical skills and fosters a sense of responsibility to the profession and to the clients in their care. It also helps counselors stay up-to-date on information and technology.

Nutrition and Hydration

As described in the initial scenario, counselors generally are not good at eating regularly or drinking the needed amounts of liquids or water per day. Instead, meals tend to be rushed and sugared drinks are consumed. Counselors who eat on the run and consume caffeine and sugared drinks, may find themselves having low energy later in the day or on their shift. By eating small, healthy snacks throughout the day or shift, making time for meals, drinking at least eight glasses of water a day, and avoiding sugar and caffeine, counselors can maintain their energy.

Breathing Exercises and Imagery

In between the meetings, sessions, and paperwork, counselors should make time to close their eyes, even if for only 5 minutes, and practice breathing deeply and imagining a peaceful and serene location. Breathing mindfully centers the mind and slows the body down. Imagery takes the mind to peaceful places and brings about brief and needed pleasure to a potentially very hectic schedule. Counselors who practice this even a few times per week may find good results and an increase in energy, which can be taken into counseling sessions.

Exercise, Stretching, and Therapeutic Environment

Counseling is typically a sedentary activity. Over time, counselors are prone to developing back problems or neck strains from extensive sitting. It is important for counselors to take regular breaks throughout the day and, if possible, to stretch their leg and shoulder muscles. In addition to stretching, exercises such as walking, running, or hiking can help maintain physical well-being and release tension from sitting. Exercise is good for the body and helps focus the mind and redirect mental preoccupation away from work. Obtaining a back cushion can be helpful in maintaining counselor posture.

Counselors should consider creating a counseling space that fosters harmony, peace, and serenity. If possible, the room should have pleasing colors, comfortable chairs, and appropriate lighting. However, both of our first offices had plastic sheets stapled on the windows, smelled of mildew, and didn't have pictures on the walls. The first thing we did was to take the plastic off the windows, rearrange the furniture, and hang colorful artwork to make the rooms comfortable and more therapeutic. Although not ideal, with some effort they became quite comfortable rooms for counseling.

Hobbies and Leisure Activities

Once counselors leave their offices, it is important to find other activities that bring them enjoyment. Those who constantly work without leisure activities increase their risk for burnout. Developing hobbies or interests provides relief to an already stressful vocation. Making time to play is of utmost importance, particularly for those working in the drug and alcohol field.

Detaching

Leaving work at work is sometimes a challenge for counselors (especially those new to the field) because the nature of what we do involves the lives of others. That being said, we advise that detaching from work will help prevent burnout. Here are a few suggestions for detaching. First, make time after each counseling session to write clinical notes instead of waiting until the end of the day. Not only is it a good habit to get into but it will also prevent mistakes and confusion of client information. It will also bring closure each day with those clients.

Second, when leaving work, whether by car or some other form of transportation, pick a location on the route home to be your detaching point, which transitions you home. For example, I (Ford) had a 45-minute commute for one of my jobs, and I picked a spot along the highway that was my detaching point. Once I passed it, the evening was mine, and my work was complete until the next day.

Burnout Prevention

These suggestions are methods in which to avoid or minimize burnout. Burnout at some level is inevitable during the course of a counselor's career. Counselors will, hopefully, identify their burnout warning signs and make shifts in behavior so as to not continue on the burnout path. Usually when counselors become burned out they exhibit the behaviors or feelings of being cynical, tired, lacking energy, angry, depressed, or blaming clients for not improving. In addition, counselors in burnout find the more they work, the less they feel they have accomplished anything. As a result they try harder, only to become more burned out, depressed, and less productive.

So how does a counselor become burned out? Simple, by not taking care of one's needs: emotionally, physically, intellectually, and spiritually. Ironically, it is a parallel process that counselors work on with their clients in treatment. Counselors need to take time and eat healthy foods, avoid excessive sugar and caffeine consumption, stretch, exercise, and be stimulated spiritually as well as intellectually through training and educational opportunities.

Counselor self-care can be initiated in counselor education programs during field or internship experiences. Educational programs need to work with students on developing self-care plans that can be used throughout their careers. "With the current reality of higher caseloads, the infusion of managed care, and the reduction of personnel resources, enhancing the spiritual well-being of counselors may also help prevent occupational stress and burnout" (C. W. Brooks & Matthews, 2000, p. 31).

The intent here is to help counselors see the continued importance of self-care and how it relates to counselor well-being, and ultimately how it affects ethical decision making and setting healthy boundaries. Counselors who find themselves tired and losing empathy for clients will also begin to lose objectivity and increase their chances of inappropriate boundary decisions in therapy.

Counselor Support System

The work of counselors is done largely in isolation from other professionals. Unless there is regular supervision or an attempt by counselors to maintain connection, counselors are many times on their own to work with clients. The following five areas are important for counselors in the development of a support system.

Professional Support Network (Counselors, Peers, Supervisors)

Counselors want to develop trusting clinical relationships with other counselors, peers, and supervisors. This is the first line of support for counselors. The beginning counselor needs as much support and clinical supervision as possible. The seasoned counselor also needs support and supervision and is just as susceptible to counselor burnout.

Family and Friend Support Network (Partner, Children, Parents)

At the end of a long day, a phone call from a friend, partner, or child can be the best medicine. Counselors need to fill up their energy tanks with resources and support from others.

Mentors (Professional, School, Other)

This aspect of the counselors' support system is crucial to professional development. Counselors who have professors and other professionals who are willing to listen and provide guidance are invaluable.

Faith/Fellowship/Social Supports (Religious, Spiritual, Social Supports)

This area of counselor support is personal. It may range from attendance at church to involvement with Alcoholics Anonymous. This aspect of the support system generally enriches the soul and spirit of the counselor.

Leisure Activities and Private Time (Reading, Gardening, Meditation)

As discussed previously, activities that bring about enjoyment are encouraged. In addition, quiet, reflective time can allow counselors to meditate on their personal as well as professional intentions.

Summary

The application of the wellness model and the counselor support system as well as the other suggestions for counselors will provide options for enhancing counselor well-being. Ultimately, how counselors take care of themselves affects the work they do with clients. If counselors are too tired, resentful, hungry, and isolated, it generally leads to burnout, which impacts clients. It is our hope that this chapter motivates counselors to initiate or enhance a program of wellness in order to develop a balanced well-being.

Exploration Questions From Chapter 14

1. What do you do to maintain balance in your life?
2. Who are the people you most admire and why?
3. Think about counseling professionals who you look up to. How do they maintain creativity in their lives?
4. How do self-care and ethical behavior relate?
5. How do you know when you are burning out?

Suggested Activities

1. Plan one day per week to have fun.
2. Take time each day to laugh and enjoy the moments between sessions, groups, meetings, or classes.

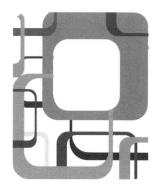

References

Ackerman, R. J. (1983). *Children of alcoholics: A guidebook for educators, therapists, and parents* (2nd ed.). Holmes Beach, FL: Learning Publications.

Adinof, B. (2004, November/December). Neurobiologic processes in drug reward and addiction. *Harvard Review in Psychiatry, 12*(6), 305–320.

Ahia, C. E., & Martin, D. (1993). The danger-to-self-or-others exception to confidentiality. In T. P. Remley, Jr. (Series Ed.), *The ACA legal series* (pp. 1–65). Alexandria, VA: American Counseling Association.

Alcoholics Anonymous. (1957). *Alcoholics Anonymous comes of age.* New York: AA World Services.

Alcoholics Anonymous. (1976). (3rd ed.). New York: AA World Services.

Alcoholics Anonymous. (2001). (4th ed.). New York: AA World Services.

Alcoholics Anonymous. (2005). Retrieved January 16, 2009, from http://www.alcoholics-anonymous.org/

Alcoholics Anonymous. (2009a). *A. A. at a glance.* Retrieved January 16, 2009, from http://www.aa.org/lang/en/catalog.cfm?origpage=10&product=83

Alcoholics Anonymous. (2009b). *A. A. timeline–origins: 1935–1944.* Retrieved January 16, 2009, from http://www.aa.org/aatimeline/

Amaro, H., Whittaker, R., Coffman, G., & Heeren, T. (1990). Acculturation and marijuana and cocaine use: Findings from HHANES 1982-1984. *American Journal of Public Health, 80,* 54–60.

American Counseling Association. (2005). *ACA code of ethics.* Alexandria, VA: Author.

American Psychiatric Association. (2000). *Diagnostic and statistical manual of mental disorders* (4th ed., text rev.). Washington, DC: Author.

American Society of Addiction Medicine. (1996). *Patient placement criteria for the treatment of substance-related disorders* (2nd ed.). Chevy Chase, MD: Author.

Amico, J. M., & Niesen, J. (1997, May/June). Sharing the secret: The need for gay-specific treatment. *The Counselor,* 12–15.

Ansbacher, H. L., & Ansbacher, R. R. (1956). *The individual psychology of Alfred Adler: A systematic presentation in selections from his writings.* New York: Harper & Row.

Ardell, D. (1996, Spring). Another alternative to AA. *Ardell Wellness Report, 42,* 6.

Ashworth, M., Gerada, C., & Dallmeyer, R. (2002, November). Benzodiazepines: Addiction and abuse. *Drugs: Education, Prevention & Policy, 9*(4), 389–397.

Association for Specialists in Group Work. (2009). *Standards of practice.* Retrieved January 16, 2009, from http://www.asgw.org/PDF/Group_Stds_Brochure.pdf

Atkinson, D. R., Morten, G., & Sue, D. W. (Eds.). (1993). *Counseling American minorities* (4th ed.). Madison, WI: Brown & Benchmark.

Babor, T. F., De La Fuente, J. R., Saunders, J., & Grant, M. (1992). AUDIT: *The Alcohol Use Disorders Identification Test: Guidelines for use in primary health care.* Geneva, Switzerland: World Health Organization.

Bandura, A. (1969). *Principles of behavior modification.* New York: Holt, Rinehart & Winston.

Bandura, A. (1977). *Social learning theory.* Englewood Cliffs, NJ: Prentice Hall.

Banken, J. A., & McGovern, T. F. (1992). Alcoholism and drug abuse counseling: State of the art consideration. *Alcoholism Treatment Quarterly, 9,* 29–53.

Bateson, G. (1971). The cybernetics of self: A theory of alcoholism. *Psychiatry, 34*(1), 1–18.

Beattie, M. (1987). *Codependent no more: How to stop controlling others and start caring for yourself.* San Francisco: HarperCollins.

Beatty, R. L., Geckle, M. O., Huggins, J., Kapner, C., Lewis, K., & Sandstrom, D. J. (1999). Gay men, lesbians, and bisexuals. In B. S. McCrady & E. E. Epstein (Eds.), *Addictions: A comprehensive guidebook* (pp. 542–551). New York: Oxford Press.

Beck, A. T., Steer, R. A., & Brown, G. K. (1996). *Manual for the Beck Depression Inventory-II.* San Antonio, TX: Psychological Corporation.

Benshoff, J. J., Harrawood, L. K., & Koch, D. S. (2003). Substance abuse and the elderly: Unique issues and concerns. *Journal of Rehabilitation, 69,* 43–49.

Bensley, L. S., & Wu, R. (1991). The role of psychological reactance in drinking following alcohol prevention messages. *Journal of Applied Social Psychology, 21,* 1111–1124.

Bepko, C., & Krestan, J. (1985). *The responsibility trap: A blueprint for treating the alcoholic family.* New York: The Free Press.

Bernard, J. M., & Goodyear, R. K. (2004). *Fundamentals of clinical supervision* (3rd ed). Boston: Allyn & Bacon.

Bertalanffy, L. V. von. (1968). *General system theory.* New York: Braziller.

Bijttebier, P., Goethals, E., & Ansoms, S. (2006). Parental drinking as a risk factor for children's maladjustment: The mediating role of family environment. *Psychology of Addictive Behaviors, 20*(2), 126–130.

Black, C. (1981). *It will never happen to me.* New York: Ballantine Books.

Blum, K., Noble, E. P., Sheridan, P. J., Montgomery, A., Ritchie, T., Jagadeeswaran, P., et al. (1990). Allelic association of human dopamine D2 receptor gene in alcoholism. *Journal of the American Medical Association, 263,* 2055–2060.

Blumenthal, S., Bell, V., Neumann, N. U., Schuttler, R., & Vogel, R. (1989). Mortality and rate of suicide among first admission psychiatric patients. In S. D. Platt & N. Kreitman (Eds.), *Current research on suicide and parasuicide: Selected proceedings of the Second European Symposium on Suicidal Behavior* (pp. 58–66). Edinburgh, Scotland: Edinburgh University Press.

Boorstein, S. (1996, Winter). Transpersonal context and interpretation. *ATP Newsletter,* 5–8.

Bradshaw, J. (1988). *Healing the shame that binds you.* Deerfield Beach, FL: Health Communications.

Brock, G. W., & Barnard, C. P. (2009). *Procedures in marriage and family therapy* (4th ed.). Boston, MA: Pearson Education.

Bronfenbrenner, U. (1976). *Reality and research in the ecology of human development: Masters lectures on developmental psychology.* Washington, DC: American Psychological Association.

Bronfenbrenner, U. (1988). Interacting systems in human development. In N. Bolger, A. Caspi, G. Downey, & M. Moorehouse (Eds.), *Persons in context: Developmental processes* (pp. 25–49). New York: Cambridge University Press.

Bronson, M., Swift, R., & Peers, E. (2005). Withdrawal charts: A clinical tool for the management of drug withdrawal symptoms. *Clinical Update, 12,* 1–2.

Brooks, A. J., Malfait, A. J., Brooke, D., Gallagher, S. M., & Penn, P. E. (2007). Consumer perspectives on co-occurring disorders treatment. *Journal of Drug Issues, 37*(2), 299–320.

Brooks, C. W., & Matthews, C. O. (2000). The relationship among substance abuse counselors' spiritual well being, values, and self-actualizing characteristics and the impact on clients' spiritual well being. *Journal of Addictions & Offender Counseling, 21*, 23–33.

Brown, S. (1985). *Treating the alcoholic: A developmental model of recovery.* New York: Wiley.

Bryan, C. J., & Rudd, M. D. (2006). Advances in the assessment of suicide risk. *Journal of Clinical Psychology, 62*(2), 185–200.

Bureau of Labor Statistics. (2008). *Occupational outlook handbook.* Retrieved October 2, 2008, from http://www.bls.gov/oco/ocos067.htm

Cabaj, R. P. (2000). Substance abuse, internalized homophobia, and gay men and lesbians: Psychodynamic issues and clinical implications. *Journal of Gay & Lesbian Psychotherapy, 3*, 5–24.

Caldiero, R. M., Parran, T.V., Adelman, C. L., & Piche, B. (2006). Inpatient initiation of buprenorphine maintenance vs. detoxification: Can retention of opioid-dependent patients in outpatient counseling be improved? *American Journal on Addictions, 15*(1), 1–7.

Campbell, P. R. (1996*). Population projections for states by age, sex, race and Hispanic origin: 1995-2025.* Washington, DC: Bureau of the Census.

Carnes, P., Delmonico, D. L., & Griffin, E. (2001). *In the shadows of the net: Breaking free of compulsive online sexual behavior.* Center City, MN: Hazelden Foundation.

Carter, B., & McGoldrick, M. (1999). *The expanded family lifecycle: Individual, family and social perspectives* (3rd ed.). Boston: Allyn & Bacon.

Castro, F. G., Proescholdbell, R. J., Abeita, L., & Rodriguez, D. (1999). Ethnic and cultural minority groups. In B. S. McCrady & E. E. Epstein (Eds.), *Addictions: A comprehensive guidebook.* New York: Oxford Press.

Celentano, D. D., & McQueen, D. V. (1984). Multiple substance use among women with alcohol-related problems. In S. C. Wilsnack & L. J. Beckman (Eds.), *Alcohol problems in women* (pp. 91–116). New York: Guilford Press.

Centers for Disease Control and Prevention. (2004). Web-based Injury Statistics Query and Reporting System (WISQARS). Available from National Center for Injury Prevention and Control Web site, www.cdc.gov/ncipc/wisqars

Chang, C. Y. (2003). Counseling Asian Americans. In N. A. Vacc, S. B. DeVaney, & J. M. Brendel (Eds.), *Counseling multicultural and diverse populations* (4th ed., pp. 73–92). New York: Brunner-Routledge.

Chao, J., & Nestler, E. J. (2004). Molecular neurobiology of drug addiction. *Annual Review of Medicine, 55*(1), 113–132.

Chapman, R. J. (1996). Spirituality in the treatment of alcoholism: A worldview approach. *Counseling and Values, 41*(1), 39–51.

Cheevers, S. (2004). *My name is Bill W.* New York: Simon and Schuster.

Christensen, C. P. (1989). Cross-cultural awareness development: A conceptual model. *Counselor Education and Supervision, 28*, 270–289.

Clark, L. W. (Ed.). (1993). *Faculty and student challenges in facing cultural and linguistic diversity.* Springfield, IL: Charles C Thomas.

Clinicians add cultural element to relapse prevention model. (1998). *Alcoholism and Drug Abuse Weekly, 10*, 1–4.

Cloninger, C. R., Bohman, M., & Sigvardsson, S. (1981). Inheritance of alcohol abuse: Cross fostering analysis of adopted men. *Archives of General Psychiatry, 38*, 861–868.

Cloninger, C. R., Sigvardsson, S., & Bohman, M. (1996). Type I and Type II alcoholism: An update. *Alcohol Health & Research World, 20*(1), 18–23.

Cochran, B. N., & Cauce, A. M. (2006). Characteristics of lesbian, gay, bisexual, and transgender individuals entering substance abuse treatment. *Journal of Substance Abuse Treatment, 30*, 135–146.

Code of federal regulations. (2000, October). Washington, DC: U.S. Government Printing Office.

Coleman, E. (1985). Developmental stages of the coming-out process. In J. C. Gosiorek (Ed.), *A guide to psychotherapy with gay and lesbian clients* (pp. 31–44). New York: Harrington Park Press.

Collins, R., Parks, G., & Marlatt, G. A. (1985). Social determinants of alcohol consumption: The effects of social interaction and model status on the self-administration of alcohol. *Journal of Consulting and Clinical Psychology, 53*, 189–200.

Cooper, M. L., Russell, M., Skinner, J. B., Frone, M. R., & Mudar, P. (1992). Stress and alcohol use: Moderating effects of gender, coping, and alcohol expectancies. *Journal of Abnormal Psychology, 101*, 139–152.

Copersino, M. L., Boyd, S. J., Tashkin, D. P., Huestis, M. A., Heishman, S. J., Dermand, J. C., et al. (2006). Cannabis withdrawal among non-treatment-seeking adult cannabis users. *American Journal on Addictions, 15*, 8–14.

Corey, G. (2005). *Theory and practice of counseling and psychotherapy* (7th ed.). Belmont, CA: Thomson Higher Education.

Corey, G., Corey, M. S., & Callanan, P. (2007). *Issues and ethics in the helping professions* (7th ed.). Pacific Grove, CA: Brooks/Cole.

Cortright, B. (1997). *Psychotherapy and spirit: Theory and practice in transpersonal psychotherapy*. Albany: State University of New York Press.

Couch, R. D. (1995). Four steps for conducting a pregroup screening interview. *Journal for Specialists in Group Work, 20*, 18–25.

Council for Accreditation of Counseling and Related Educational Programs. (2009). CACREP Standards. *Addiction Counseling*, p. 17. Retrieved January 16, 2009, from http://www.cacrep.org/2009standards.html

Craig, R. J. (2004). *Counseling the alcohol and drug dependent client: A practical approach*. Boston: Allyn & Bacon.

Crnkovic, A. E., & DelCampo, R. L. (1998). A systems approach to the treatment of chemical addiction. *Contemporary Family Therapy: An International Journal, 20*(1), 25–36.

Csiernik, R. (2002). Counseling for the family: The neglected aspect of addiction treatment in Canada. *Journal of Social Work Practice in the Addictions, 2*(1), 79–92.

Cuellar, I., Arnold, B., & Gonzales, G. (1995). Cognitive referents of acculturation: Assessment of cultural constructs in Mexican Americans. *Journal of Community Psychology, 23*, 339–356.

Cunningham, W. (2004). The myths of manhood: Addressing men's addiction and recovery through relational therapy. *Addiction Professional*, 26–31.

Cutler, M. (2004, October). *Ways to teach multicultural counseling*. Paper presented at the North Central Association for Counselor Education and Supervision Conference, St. Louis, MO.

Dar, K. (2006). Alcohol use disorders in elderly people: Fact or fiction? *Advanced Psychiatric Treatment, 12*, 173–181.

Darrow, S. L., Russell, M., Cooper, M. L., Mudar, P., & Frone, M. R. (1992). Sociodemographic correlates of alcohol consumption among African-American and White women. *Women and Health, 18*(4), 35–51.

Davis, S. R., & Meier, S. T. (2001). *The elements of managed care: A guide for helping professionals*. Belmont, CA: Brooks/Cole.

Dawson, D. A., Grant, B. F., Chous, S. P., & Pickering, R. P. (1995). Subgroup variation in U.S. drinking patterns: Results of the 1992 National Longitudinal Alcohol Epidemiologic Study. *Journal of Substance Abuse, 7*, 331–334.

DeJong, P., & Kim Berg, I. (2008). *Interviewing for solutions* (3rd ed.). Belmont, CA: Thomson Higher Education.

Delmonico, D. L., & Griffin, E. (2002). The challenge of treating compulsive sex. *Counselor: The Magazine for Addiction Professionals, 3*, 14–20.

Dempsey, C. L. (1994). Health and social issues of gay, lesbian, and bisexual adolescents. *Families in Society: Journal of Contemporary Human Services, 75*(3), 160–167.

Deutsch, C. J. (1984). Self-reported sources of stress among psychotherapists. *Professional Psychology: Research and Practice, 15*, 833–845.

Devine, C., & Braithwaite, V. (1993). The survival roles of children of alcoholics: Their measurement and validity. *Addiction, 88*, 69–78.

Devore, W., & Schlesinger, E. G. (1996). *Ethnic-sensitive social work practice* (4th ed.). Boston: Allyn & Bacon.

Dickoff, H., & Lakin, M. (1963). Patients' views of group psychotherapy: Retrospections and interpretations. *International Journal of Group Psychotherapy, 13*, 61–73.

Diller, J. V. (2004). *Cultural diversity: A primer for the human services* (2nd ed.). Belmont, CA: Brooks/Cole.

Donovan, D. M., Kivlahan, D. R., Doyle, S. R., Longabaugh, R., & Greenfield, S. F. (2006). Concurrent validity of the *Alcohol Use Disorders Identification Test (AUDIT)* and *AUDIT* zones in defining levels of severity among out-patients with alcohol dependence in the COMBINE study. *Addiction, 101*, 1696–1704.

Dossey, L. (1984). *Beyond illness*. Boulder, CO: Shambala Publishing.

Doyle, K. (1997). Substance abuse counselors in recovery: Implications for the ethical issues of dual relationships. *Journal of Counseling & Development, 75*, 428–432.

Drake, R. E., Bartels, S. J., Teague, G. B., Noordsy, D. L., & Clark, R. E. (1993). Treatment of substance abuse in severely mentally ill patients. *Journal of Nervous and Mental Disease, 181*, 606–611.

Dyslin, C. (2008). The power of powerlessness: The role of spiritual surrender and interpersonal confession in the treatment of addictions. *Journal of Psychology & Christianity, 27*(1), 41–55.

Elkashef, A., Holmes, T., Bloch, D., Shoptaw, S., Kampman, K., Reid, M., et al. (2005, March). Retrospective analyses of pooled data from CREST I and CREST II trials for treatment of cocaine dependence. *Addiction, 100*, 91–101.

Erikson, E. H. (1963). *Childhood and society*. New York: Norton.

Evans, K., & Sullivan, J. M. (1990). *Dual diagnosis: Counseling the mentally ill substance abuser*. New York: Guilford Press.

Ewing, J. A., & Rouse, B. A. (1970, February). *Identifying the hidden alcoholic*. Paper presented at the 29th International Congress on Alcoholism and Drug Dependence, Sydney, Australia.

Farber, B. A. (1983). Psychotherapists' perceptions of stressful patient behavior. *Professional Psychology: Research and Practice, 14*, 697–705.

Fawcett, J., & Busch, K. A. (1995). Stimulants in psychiatry. In A. F. Schatzberg & C. B. Nemeroff (Eds.), *Textbook of psychopharmacology* (pp. 417–435). Washington, DC: American Psychiatric Association Press.

Federal Drug Administration. (n.d.). *Controlled Substances Act, 1970*. Retrieved January 13, 2009, from http://www.fda.gov/opacom/laws/cntrlsub/cntlsba.htm

Fifield, L. H., Latham, J. D., & Phillips, C. (1977). *Alcoholism in the gay community: The price of alienation, isolation, and oppression*. Los Angeles, CA: Gay Community Services Center.

Fiorentine, R. (2001). Counseling frequency and the effectiveness of outpatient drug treatment: Revisiting the conclusion that "more is better." *American Journal of Drug and Alcohol Abuse, 27*(4), 617–631.

Fisher, G. L., & Harrison, T. C. (2005). *Substance abuse: Information for school counselors, social workers, therapists, and counselors* (3rd ed.). Boston: Allyn & Bacon.

Flores, P. (1988). *Group psychotherapy with addicted populations*. New York: Haworth Press.

Flores, P. J. (1997). *Group psychotherapy with addicted populations: An integration of twelve-step and psychodynamic theory* (2nd ed.). New York: Haworth Press.

Flynn, P. M., & Brown, B. S. (2008). Co-occurring disorders in substance abuse treatment: Issues and prospects. *Journal of Substance Abuse Treatment, 34*(1), 36–47.

Fowler, T., Shelton, K., Lifford, K., Rice, F., McBride, A., Nikolov, I., et al. (2007). Genetic and environmental influences on the relationship between peer alcohol use and own alcohol use in adolescents. *Addiction, 102*, 894–903.

Friedmann, P. D., Lemon, S. C., Stein, M. D., & D'Aunno, T. A. (2003). Community referral sources and entry of treatment-naive clients into outpatient addiction treatment. *American Journal of Drug and Alcohol Abuse, 29*(1), 105–115.

Fukuyama, M. A. (1990). Taking a universal approach to multicultural counseling. *Counselor Education and Supervision, 30,* 6–18.

Gallagher, R. P. (Ed.). (2005). *National Survey of Counseling Center Directors.* International Association of Counseling Services, Inc. (Monograph Series 80). Pittsburgh, PA: University of Pittsburgh.

Garrett, J. T., & Garrett, M. W. (1994). The path of good medicine: Understanding and counseling Native Americans. *Journal of Multicultural Counseling and Development, 22,* 134–144.

Garrett, M. T. (2003). Counseling Native Americans. In N. A. Vacc, S. DeVaney, & J. M. Brendel (Eds.), *Counseling multicultural and diverse populations: Strategies for practitioners* (4th ed., pp. 27–54). New York: Brunner-Routledge.

Geary, B. B. (2001). Assessment in Ericksonian hypnosis and psychotherapy. In B. B. Geary & J. K. Zeig (Eds.), *The handbook of Ericksonian psychotherapy* (pp. 1–17). Phoenix, AZ: The Milton H. Erickson Foundation Press.

Gibson, P. (1989). Gay male and lesbian youth suicide. In G. Remafedi (Ed.), *Death by denial: Studies of suicide in gay and lesbian teenagers* (pp. 15–68). Boston: Alyson.

Gideon, W. (1975). *Individual and group involvement: A recovery process for the alcoholic.* Houston, TX: University of Houston.

Gladding, S. (2003). *Group work: A counseling specialty* (4th ed.). Upper Saddle River, NJ: Merrill Prentice Hall.

Gloria, A. M., Ruiz, E. L., & Castillo, E. M. (2004). Counseling and psychotherapy with Latino and Latina clients. In T. B. Smith (Ed.), *Practicing multiculturalism: Affirming diversity in counseling and psychology* (pp. 167–189). Boston: Pearson Education.

Gold, M. S., & McKewen, M. (1995). Trends in hallucinogenic drug use: LSD, 'ecstasy,' and the rave phenomenon. *Directions in Substance Abuse Counseling, 3*(3), 3–11.

Goldberg, R. (1997). *Drugs across the spectrum.* Englewood, CO: Morton.

Goldenberg, H., & Goldenberg, I. (2008). *Family therapy: An overview* (7th ed.). Belmont, CA: Thomson Higher Education.

Gomberg, E. S. L. (1991). Comparing alcoholic women with positive vs. negative family history [Abstract]. *Alcoholism: Clinical and Experimental Research, 15*(2), 363.

Gomberg, E. S. L. (1993). Women and alcohol: Use and abuse. *Journal of Nervous and Mental Disease, 181,* 211–219.

Gomberg, E. S. L. (1994). Risk factors for drinking over a woman's life span. *Alcohol Health and Research World, 18*(3), 220–227.

Gomberg, E. S. L. (1999). Women. In B. S. McCrady & E. E. Epstein (Eds.), *Addictions: A comprehensive guidebook* (pp. 527–541). New York: Oxford Press.

Good Tracks, J. G. (1973). Native American non-interference. *Social Work, 17,* 30–34.

Goodwin, D. W. (1989). Alcoholism. In H. I. Kaplan & B. J. Sadock (Eds.), *Comprehensive textbook of psychiatry* (Vol. V). Baltimore: Williams & Wilkins.

Gorski, T. (1989). *Passages through recovery: An action plan for preventing relapse.* Center City, MN: Hazelden Press.

Gorski, T. T., & Miller, M. (1986). *Staying sober: A guide for relapse prevention.* Independency, MO: Independence Press.

Grant, B. F. (1997). Prevalence and correlates of alcohol use and *DSM-IV* alcohol dependence in the United States: Results of the National Longitudinal Alcohol Epidemiologic Survey. *Journal of Studies on Alcohol, 58,* 464–473.

Grant, B. F. (2000). Estimates of U.S. children exposed to alcohol use and dependence in the family. *American Journal of Public Health, 90,* 112–115.

Gravitz, H. L., & Bowden, J. D. (1985). *Guide to recovery: A book for adult children of alcoholics.* Holmes Beach, FL: Learning Publications.

Green, L., Fulhlove, M., & Fulhlove, R. (1998). Stories of spiritual awakening: The nature of spirituality in recovery. *Journal of Substance Abuse Treatment, 15*(4), 325–331.

Grilo, C. M., Becker, D. F., Anez, L. M., & McGlashan, T. H. (2004). Diagnostic efficiency of *DSM-IV* criteria for borderline personality disorder: An evaluation in Hispanic men and women with substance use disorders. *Journal of Consulting and Clinical Psychology, 72,* 126–131.

Grof, S. (1987a). Spirituality, addiction and western science. *ReVision, 10*(2), 5–18.

Grof, S. (1987b). Spirituality, alcoholism, and drug abuse: Transpersonal aspects of addiction. *ReVision, 10*(2), 3–4.

Gross, J. (1998, April 22). Youths tie tobacco use to marijuana. *The New York Times.* Retrieved January 23, 2009, from http://www.nytimes.com

Group therapy works well for addiction. (1997). *Behavioral Health Treatment, 2,* 1–3.

Guggenbuhl, C. N. (1982). *Power in the helping professions.* Dallas, TX: Spring Publications.

Haaken, J. (1993). From Al-Anon to ACOA: Codependence and the reconstruction of caregiving. *Signs, 18*(2), 321–345.

Hall, C. S., & Lindsey, G. (1978). *Theories of personality* (3rd ed.). New York: Wiley.

Hall, C. W., & Webster, R. E. (2002). Traumatic symptomatology characteristics of adult children of alcoholics. *Journal of Drug Education, 32*(3), 195–211.

Hall, C. W., Webster, R. E., & Powell, E. J. (2003). Personal alcohol use in adult children of alcoholics. *Alcohol Research, 8*(4), 157–162.

Haly, J. (1986). *Uncommon therapy.* New York: W. W. Norton.

Hanna, F. J. (1992). Reframing spirituality: AA, the 12-steps and the mental health counselor. *Journal of Mental Health Counseling, 14*(2), 166–179.

Hanson, G., & Venturelli, P. J. (1998). *Drugs and society* (5th ed.). Boston: Jones & Bartlett.

Hartman, S., Staub, M., & Styer, J. (2002). *Women and addiction: Gender issues in abuse and treatment.* Wernersville, PA: Caron Foundation.

Hecksher, D. (2007). Former substance users working as counselors: A dual relationship. *Substance Use & Misuse, 42,* 1253–1268.

Helzer, J. E., Burnam, A., & McEvoy, L. T. (1991). Alcohol abuse and dependence. In L. Robins & D. A. Regier (Eds.), *Psychiatric disorders in America: The epidemiologic catchment area study* (pp. 81–115). New York: Free Press.

Herd, D. (1994). Predicting drinking problems among Black and White men: Results from a national survey. *Journal of Studies on Alcohol, 55,* 61–71.

Herlihy, B., & Corey, G. (2006). *ACA ethical standards casebook* (6th ed.). Alexandria, VA: American Counseling Association.

Hermos, J., Young, M., Lawler, E., Rosenbloom, D., & Fiore, L. (2007, October). Long-term, high-dose benzodiazepine prescriptions in veteran patients with PTSD: Influence of preexisting alcoholism and drug-abuse diagnoses. *Journal of Traumatic Stress, 20*(5), 909–914.

Herring, R. D. (1990). The clown or contrary figure as a counseling intervention strategy with Native American clients. *Journal of Multicultural Counseling and Development, 22,* 153–164.

Hicks, D. (2000). The importance of specialized treatment programs for lesbian and gay patients. *Journal of Gay & Lesbian Psychotherapy, 3,* 81–94.

Hingson, R. W., Heeren, T., Zakocs, R. C., Kopstein, A., & Wechsler, H. (2002). Magnitude of alcohol-related mortality and morbidity among U.S. college students ages 18–24. *Journal of Studies on Alcohol, 63,* 136–144.

Hiroi, N., & Agatsuma, S. (2005). Genetic susceptibility to substance dependence. *Molecular Psychiatry, 10,* 336–344.

Hoffmann, N. G., Halikas, J. A., Mee-Lee, D., & Weedman, R. D. (1991*). ASAM patient placement criteria for the treatment of psychoactive substance use disorders.* Washington, DC: The American Society of Addiction Medicine.

Hogan, J. A., Gabrielsen, K. R., Luna, N., & Grothaus, D. (2003). *Substance abuse prevention: The intersection of science and practice*. Boston: Allyn & Bacon.

Holmes, A., Hodge, M., Lenten, S., Fielding, J., Castle, D., Velakoulis, D., & Bradley, G. (2006). Chronic mental illness and community treatment resistance. *Australas Psychiatry, 14*(3), 272–276.

Hughes, T., & Eliason, M. (2002). Substance use and abuse in lesbian, gay, bisexual and transgender population. *Journal of Primary Prevention, 22*, 261–295.

Hulnick, H. R. (1977). Counselor: Know thyself. *Counselor Education and Supervision, 17*, 69–72.

Humfleet, G. L., & Amos, A., (2004). Is marijuana use becoming a "gateway" to nicotine dependence? *Addiction, 99*, 5–6.

Hutcheson, D. M., Everitt, B. J., Robbins, T. W., & Dickinson, A. (2001). The role of withdrawal in heroin addiction: Enhances reward or promotes avoidance? *Nature Neuroscience, 4*, 943–947.

Illicit drug use grows among the elderly. (2002, March 27). *Christian Science Monitor*, p. 3.

Institute of Medicine. (2003). *Unequal treatment: Confronting racial and ethnic disparities in health*. Portland, OR: National Academy Press.

Ivey, A. E., & Ivey, M. B. (2008). *Essentials of interviewing: Counseling in a multicultural world*. Belmont, CA: Thomson Higher Education.

James, W. (1929). *The varieties of religious experience*. New York: Random House.

Jayakody, R., Danziger, S., & Pollack, H. (2000). Welfare reform, substance use, and mental health. *Journal of Health Politics, Policy and Law, 25*, 623–651.

Jellinek, E. M. (1952). Phases of alcohol addiction. *Quarterly Journal of Studies on Alcohol, 13*, 673–674.

Jellinek, E. M. (1960). *The disease concept of alcoholism*. New Haven, CT: College and University Press.

Jenkins, R. (2007). Substance use and suicidal behavior. *Psychiatry, 6*(1), 16–18.

Johnsen, E. (1993). The role of spirituality in recovery from chemical dependency. *Journal of Addictions & Offender Counseling, 13*(2), 58–62.

Johnson, V. E. (1980). *I'll quit tomorrow*. San Francisco: Harper & Row.

Johnston, L. D., O'Malley, P. M., & Bachman, J. G. (2001). *Monitoring the future: National survey results on drug use, 1975–2000. Vol. I: Secondary school students* (NIH Publication No. 01–4924). Bethesda, MD: National Institute on Drug Abuse.

Johnston, L. D., O'Malley, P. M., Bachman, J. G., & Schulenberg, J. E. (2008). *Monitoring the Future national survey results on adolescent drug use: Overview of key findings, 2007* (NIH Publication No. 08-6418). Bethesda, MD: National Institute on Drug Abuse.

Jones, J. P., & Kinnick, B. C. (1995). Adult children of alcoholics: Characteristics of students in a university setting. *Journal of Alcohol and Drug Education, 40*(2), 58–70.

Jones-Webb, R. (1998). Drinking patterns and problems among African Americans: Recent findings. *Alcohol Health & Research World, 22*(4), 260–265.

Jongsma, A. E., & Peterson, L. M. (1999). *The complete adult psychotherapy treatment planner*. New York: Wiley.

Jung, C. G. (1933). *Modern man in search of a soul*. New York: Harcourt.

Jung, C. G. (1974). *The Bill W. Carl Jung letters*. New York: AA Grapevine.

Jung, J. (1994). *Under the influence: Alcohol and human behavior*. Pacific Grove, CA: Brooks-Cole.

Kerr, B. (1994). Review of the Substance Abuse Screening Inventory. In J. C. Conoley & J. C. Impara (Eds.), *The supplement to the eleventh mental measurements yearbook* (pp. 249–251). Lincoln: University of Nebraska Press.

Kessler, R. C., Berglund, P., Demler, O., Jin, R., Merikangas, K. R., & Walters, E. E. (2005). Lifetime prevalence and age-of-onset distributions of *DSM-IV* disorders in the National Comorbidity Survey Replication. *Archives of General Psychiatry, 62*, 593–602.

King, A. C., & Canada, S. A. (2004). Client-related predictors of early treatment drop-out in a substance abuse clinic exclusively employing individual therapy. *Journal of Substance Abuse Treatment, 26*, 189–195.

Kinney, J., & Leaton, G. (1995*). Loosening the grip: A handbook of alcohol information*. St Louis, MO: Times Mirror/Mosby.

Kirisci, L., Mezzich, A., & Tarter, R. (1995). Norms and sensitivity of the adolescent version of the drug use screening inventory. *Addictive Behaviors, 20*, 149–157.

Klinger, R. L., & Stein, T. S. (1996). Impact of violence, childhood sexual abuse, domestic violence and abuse on lesbian, bisexual, and gay men. In R. P. Cabaj & T. S. Stein (Eds.), *Textbook homosexuality and mental health* (pp. 801–818). Washington, DC: American Psychiatric Press.

Kohlberg, L. (1968). Moral development. In *International encyclopedia of social science*. New York: The Free Press.

Kohut, H. (1977). *The restoration of the self*. New York: International Universities Press.

Kouri, E. M., Pope, H. G., & Lukas, S. E. (1999). Changes in aggressive behavior during withdrawal from long-term marijuana use. *Psychopharmacology, 143*, 302–308.

Krahn, G., Farrell, N., Gabriel, R., & Deck, D. (2006). Access barriers to substance abuse treatment for persons with disabilities: An exploratory study. *Journal of Substance Abuse Treatment, 31*(4), 375–384.

Kübler-Ross, E. (1969). *On death and dying*. New York: Macmillan.

Kuhn, C., Swartzwelder, S., & Wilson, W. (2003). *Buzzed: The straight facts about the most used and abused drugs from alcohol to ecstasy* (2nd ed.). New York: Norton.

Kurtz, E. (1979). *Not God: A history of Alcoholics Anonymous*. Center City, MN: Hazelden Educational Services.

Kurtz, E., & Ketcham, K. (1992). *The spirituality of imperfection: Modern wisdom from classic stories*. New York: Bantam Books.

Laux, J. M., Newman, I., & Brown, R. (2004). Michigan Alcoholism Screening Test (MAST): A statistical validation analysis. *Measurement and Evaluation in Counseling and Development, 36*, 209–225.

Laux, J. M., Salyers, K. M., & Kotova, E. (2005). A psychometric evaluation of the SASSI-3 in a college sample. *Journal of College Counseling, 8*, 41–51.

Lawton, M. J. (1981). *The role of the rehabilitation counselor as a facilitative gatekeeper for the alcoholic and elicit drug abuser* (Rehabilitation Monograph Series No. V). Richmond: Virginia Commonwealth University.

Levin, S. M., & Kruger, J. (Eds.). (2000). *Substance abuse among older adults: A guide for social service providers*. Rockville, MD: Substance Abuse and Mental Health Services Administration.

Lewis, J. A., Dana, R. Q., & Blevins, G. A. (1994). *Substance abuse counseling: An individualized approach* (2nd ed.). Pacific Grove, CA: Brooks/Cole.

Lewis, R. G., & Gingerich, W. (1980). Leadership characteristics: Views of Indian and non-Indian students. *Social Casework, 61*, 494–497.

Lewis, V., & Allen-Byrd, L. (2007). Coping strategies for the stages of family recovery. *Alcoholism Treatment Quarterly, 25*(1/2), 105–124.

Li, L., & Ford, J. A. (1998). Illicit drug use by women with disabilities. *American Journal of Drug and Alcohol Abuse, 24*(3), 405–418.

Locke, D. C. (1998). *Increasing multicultural understanding: A comprehensive model* (2nd ed.). Thousand Oaks, CA: Sage.

Loue, S., & Ioan, B. (2007). Legal and ethical issues in heroin diagnosis, treatment, and research. *Journal of Legal Medicine, 28*, 193–221.

Maccio, E. M., & Doueck, H. J. (2002). Meeting the needs of the gay and lesbian community: Outcomes in the human services. *Journal of Gay & Lesbian Social Services, 14*, 55–73.

MacGowan, M. J. (2006). Measuring and increasing engagement in substance abuse treatment groups: Advancing evidence-based group work. *Journal of Groups in Addiction & Recovery, 1*(2), 53–67.

Mackay, P. W., & Marlatt, G. A. (1994, April). Relapse: A slip doesn't mean that treatment has failed. *Addiction Letter*, *10*(4), 4–5.

MacKinnon, S. V. (2004). Spirituality: Its role in substance abuse, treatment and recovery. *DATA: The Brown University Digest of Addiction Theory & Application*, *23*(7), 8–9.

Magura, S., Staines, G., Kosanke, N., Rosenblum, A., Foote, J., Deluca, M. D., et al. (2003). Predictive validity of the ASAM patient placement criteria for naturalistically matched vs. mismatched alcoholism patients. *American Journal on Addictions, 12*, 386–397.

Maher, J. (1997). *One step more: The life and work of Father Joseph C. Martin*. Havre de Grace, MD: Ashley.

Manhal-Baugus, M. (1998). The self-in-relation theory and women for sobriety: Female-specific theory and mutual help group for chemically dependent women. *Journal of Addictions and Offender Counseling, 18*(2), 78–85.

Manisses Communication Group. (1994). Relapse: A slip doesn't mean that treatment has failed. *Addiction Letter, 10*(4), 4–5.

Marlatt, A. (1996). Harm reduction: Come as you are. *Addictive Behaviors, 21*(6), 779–788.

Martin, D. G., & Moore, A. D. (1995). *Basics of clinical practice: A guidebook for trainees in the helping professions*. Prospect Heights, IL: Waveland Press.

Matano, R. A., & Yalom, I. D. (1991). Approaches to chemical dependency: Chemical dependency and interactive group therapy—A synthesis. *International Journal of Group Psychotherapy, 41*(3), 269–293.

Matta, J. (2004, April). *Motivational interviewing*. Paper presented at the American Counseling Association conference, Kansas City, MO.

Matthews, C. O. (1998). Integrating the spiritual dimension into traditional counselor education programs. *Counseling and Values, 43*, 3–18.

Matthews, C. O., & Hollingsworth, G. A. (1999). Transpersonal psychology: The bridge between heart and mind in addictions counselor education. *Journal of the Pennsylvania Counseling Association, 1*, 16–27.

Matto, H. C. (2004). Applying an ecological framework to understanding drug addiction and recovery. *Journal of Social Work Practice in the Addictions, 4*(3), 5–22.

May, G. (1977). The psychodynamics of spirituality: A follow-up. *Journal of Pastoral Care, 31*(2), 84–90.

McCombs, K., & Moore, D. (2002). *Substance abuse prevention and intervention for students with disabilities: A call to educators*. East Lansing, MI: National Center for Research on Teacher Learning. (ERIC Document Reproduction Service No. ED469441)

McDermut, W., Mattia, J., & Zimmerman, M. (2001). Comorbidity burden and its impact on psychosocial morbidity in depressed outpatients. *Journal of Affective Disorders, 65*, 289–295.

McGoldrick, M., Giordano, J., & Pearce, J. K. (Eds.). (1996). *Ethnicity and family therapy* (2nd ed.). New York: Guilford Press.

McGregor, C., Srisurapanont, M., Jittiwutikarn, J., Laobhripatr, S., Wongtan, T., & White, J. M. (2005). The nature, time course and severity of methamphetamine withdrawal. *Addiction, 100*, 1320–1329.

McHenry, B., & Korcuska, J. (2002). Identity development and resiliency in gay adolescents: Multicultural perspectives. *The South Dakota Counselor, 8*, 20–25.

Menninger, J. A. (2002). Assessment and treatment of alcoholism and substance-related disorders in the elderly. *Bulletin of the Menninger Clinic, 66*, 166–184.

Meyer, C. (2005, July 18). Prescription drug abuse in the elderly: How the elderly become addicted to their medications. *Associated Content*. Retrieved October 3, 2008, from http://www.associatedcontent.com/article/5731/prescription_drug_abuse_in_the_elderly.html

Miller, G. A. (1983). *Substance Abuse Subtle Screening Inventory*. Bloomington, IN: SASSI Institute.

Miller, N. S., & Gold, M. S. (1998). Management of withdrawal syndromes and relapse prevention in drug and alcohol dependence. *American Family Physician, 58*, 139–147.

Miller, W. R. (1998). Researching the spiritual dimensions of alcohol and other drug problems. *Addiction, 93*(7), 979–991.

Miller, W. R., & Rollnick, S. (1991). *Motivational interviewing: Preparing people for change.* New York: Guilford Press.

Miller, W. R., & Rollnick, S. (2002). *Motivational interviewing: Preparing people to change addictive behavior* (2nd ed.). New York: Guilford Press.

Minuchin, S. (1974). *Families and family therapy.* Cambridge, MA: Harvard University Press.

Minuchin, S., & Fishman, H. C. (1981). *Family therapy techniques.* Cambridge, MA: Harvard University Press.

Mitchell, R. (2007). *Documentation in counseling records* (3rd ed.). Alexandria, VA: American Counseling Association.

Moderation Management. (2003). *What is moderation management?* Retrieved January 16, 2009, from http://www.moderation.org/whatisMM/shtml

Moe, J., Johnson, J., & Wade, W. (2007). Resilience in children of substance users: In their own words. *Substance Use & Misuse, 42*, 381–398.

Moore, D., & Li, L. (2001). Disability and illicit drug use: An application of labeling theory. *Deviant Behavior, 22*(1), 1–21.

Morgan, O. J., Toloczko, A. M., & Comly, E. (1997). Graduate training of counselors in addictions: A study of CACREP-approved programs. *Journal of Addictions & Offender Counseling, 17*, 66–76.

Moyer, M. (1994, November). Addiction treatment then and now. *The Addiction Letter*, p. 4.

Muktananda, S. (1982). *Understanding your own mind, in ancient wisdom and modern science.* Albany: State University of New York Press.

Murphy, B.C., & Dillon, C. (2008). *Interviewing in action in a multicultural world* (3rd ed.). Belmont, CA: Thomson Higher Education.

Mustaine, B. L., West, P. L., & Wyrick, B. (2003). Substance abuse counselor certification requirements: Is it time for a change? *Journal of Addictions & Offender Counseling, 23*, 99–107.

Myers, J. E., & Sweeney, T. J. (Eds.). (2005). *Counseling for wellness: Theory, research, and practice.* Alexandria, VA: American Counseling Association.

Myers, J. E., Sweeney, T. J., & White, V. E. (2002). Advocacy for counseling and counselors: A professional imperative. *Journal of Counseling & Development, 80*, 394–403.

National Association of Alcoholism and Drug Abuse Counselors. (2004). *Ethics.* Retrieved January 16, 2009, from http://naadac.org/index.php?option=com_content&view=article&id=405&ltemid=73

National Association of Alcoholism and Drug Abuse Counselors. (2008). *Certification.* Retrieved January 16, 2009, from http://naadac.org/index.php?option=com_content&view=article&id=424&ltemid=77

National Association of Alcoholism and Drug Abuse Counselors Education and Research Foundation. (1995). *Income and compensation study of alcohol and drug counseling professionals.* Arlington, VA: Author.

National Board for Certified Counselors. (2008). *Master's addiction counselor.* Retrieved January 23, 2009, from http://www.nbcc.org/certifications/mac/Default.aspx

National Institute on Alcohol Abuse and Alcoholism. (1998, October). Alcohol and the liver: Research update. *Alcohol Alert, 42.* Retrieved January 23, 2009, from http://alcoholism.tqn.com/health/alcoholism/library/blnaa42.htm

National Institute on Alcohol Abuse and Alcoholism. (2003, April). Underage drinking: A major public health challenge. *Alcohol Alert, 59.* Retrieved January 23, 2009, from http://pubs.niaaa.nih.gov/publications/aa59.htm

National Institute on Alcohol Abuse and Alcoholism. (2006). NIAAA 2001–2002 NESARC [Data file]. Retrieved January 23, 2009, from http://niaaa.census.gov/index.html

National Institute on Disability and Rehabilitation Research. (1996). *NIDRR's core areas of research.* Retrieved January 23, 2009, from http://www.ed.gov/rschstat/research/pubs/core-area.html

National Institute on Drug Abuse. (1999, May). *Cocaine abuse and addiction* (NIH Publication No. 99-4342). Washington, DC: U.S. Government Printing Office.

National Institute on Drug Abuse. (2000, September). *Heroin: Abuse and addiction* (NIH Publication No.00-4165). Washington, DC: U.S. Government Printing Office.

National Institute on Drug Abuse. (2001, March). *Hallucinogens and dissociative drugs* (NIH Publication No. 01-4209). Washington, DC: U.S. Government Printing Office.

National Institute on Drug Abuse. (2002, January). *Methamphetamine abuse and addiction* (NIH Publication No. 02-4210). Washington, DC: U.S. Government Printing Office.

National Institute on Drug Abuse. (2004, March). *Inhalant abuse* (NIH Publication No. 00-3818). Washington, DC: U.S. Government Printing Office.

National Institute on Drug Abuse. (2005a, May). *Research report series: Heroin abuse and addiction* (NIH Publication No. 05-4165). Washington, DC: U.S. Government Printing Office.

National Institute on Drug Abuse. (2005b, July). *Prescription drugs: Abuse and addiction* (NIH Publication No. 01-4881). Washington, DC: U.S. Government Printing Office.

National Institute on Drug Abuse. (2005c, July). *Marijuana abuse and addiction* (NIH Publication No. 05-3859). Washington, DC: U.S. Government Printing Office.

National Institute on Drug Abuse. (2006a, July). *Cigarettes and other products.* Washington, DC: U.S. Government Printing Office. Retrieved January 13, 2008, from http://www.drugabuse.gov/pdf/infofacts/Tobacco06.pdf

National Institute on Drug Abuse. (2006b, August). *A research report: Steroid abuse and addiction* (NIH Publication No. 00-3721). Washington, DC: U.S. Government Printing Office.

Neff, J. A., Prihoda, T. J., & Hoppe, S. K. (1991). "Machismo," self-esteem, education and high maximum drinking among Anglo, Black, and Mexican-American male drinkers. *Journal of Studies on Alcohol, 52,* 458–463.

Neukrug, E. S., Healy, M., & Herlihy, B. (1992). Ethical practices of licensed professional counselors: An updated survey of state licensing boards. *Counselor Education and Supervision, 32*(2), 130–141.

Nidecker, M., DiClemente, C. C., Bennett, M. E., & Bellack, A. S. (2008). Application of the transtheoretical model of change: Psychometric properties of leading measures in patients with co-occurring drug abuse and severe mental illness. *Addictive Behaviors, 33*(8), 1021–1030.

Okun, B. F., Fried, J., & Okun, M. L. (1999). *Understanding diversity: A learning-as-practice primer.* Pacific Grove, CA: Brooks/Cole.

Ondus, K. A., Hujer, M. E., Mann, A. E., & Mion, L. C. (1999). Substance abuse and the hospitalized elderly. *Orthopedic Nursing, 18*(4), 27–36.

Parks, G. A. (Ed.). (2002). *Engaging college students: Motivational enhancement strategies for use in brief alcohol interventions and prevention programming.* Seattle: University of Washington, Addictive Behaviors Research Center.

Pavkov, T. W., McGovern, M. P., Lyons, J. S., & Geffner, E. S. (1992). Psychiatric symptomatology among alcoholics: Comparisons between African Americans and caucasians. *Psychology of Addictive Behaviors, 6*(4), 219–224.

Pedersen, P. (2003). Multicultural training in schools. In P. Pedersen & J. Carey (Eds.), *Multicultural counseling in schools* (2nd ed., pp. 190–210). Needham, MA: Allyn & Bacon.

Peele, S. (1989). *Diseasing of America: Addiction treatment out of control.* Lexington, MA: Lexington Books.

Pennington, H., Butler, R., & Eagger, S. (2000). The assessment of patients with alcohol disorders by an old age psychiatric service. *Aging & Mental Health, 4,* 182–185.

Pennsylvania Department of Health. (1999). *Pennsylvania's client placement criteria for adults.* Harrisburg, PA: Commonwealth of Pennsylvania.

Peteet, J. (1993). A closer look at the role of a spiritual approach in addictions treatment. *Journal of Substance Abuse Treatment, 10,* 263–267.

Piaget, J. (1954). *The construction of reality in the child.* New York: Basic Books.

Piderman, K., Schneekloth, T., Pankratz, V., Maloney, S., & Altchuler, S. (2007, May). Spirituality in alcoholics during treatment. *American Journal on Addictions, 16*(3), 232–237.

Pipes, R. B., & Davenport, D. S. (1999). *Introduction to psychotherapy: Common clinical wisdom* (2nd ed.). Boston: Allyn & Bacon.

Pope, H. G., & Katz, D. L. (1988). Affective and psychotic symptoms associated anabolic steroid use. *American Journal of Psychiatry, 145,* 487–490.

Presley, C. A., Meilman, P. W., & Lyeria, R. (1994). Development of the CORE Alcohol and Drug Survey: Initial findings and future directions. *Journal of American College Health, 42,* 248–258.

Prezioso, F. A. (1987). Spirituality in the recovery process. *Journal of Substance Abuse Treatment, 4,* 233–238.

Prochaska, J. O., & DiClemente, C. C. (1982). Transtheoretical therapy: Toward a more integrative model of change. *Psychotherapy: Theory, Research, and Practice, 19,* 276–288.

Prochaska, J. O., & DiClemente, C. C. (1984). *The transtheoretical approach: Crossing traditional boundaries of therapy.* Homewood, IL: Dow Jones/Irwin.

Prochaska, J. O., & DiClemente, C. C. (1986). Toward a comprehensive model of change. In W. R. Miller & N. Healther (Eds.), *Treating addictive behaviors: Processes of change* (pp. 3–27). New York: Plenum Press.

Prochaska, J. O., DiClemente, C. C., & Norcross, J. C. (1992). In search of how people change: Applications to the addictive behaviors. *American Psychologist, 47,* 1102–1114.

Project Match Research Group. (1997). Matching alcoholism treatments to client heterogeneity: Project Match posttreatment drinking outcomes. *Journal of Studies on Alcohol, 58*(1), 7–29.

Rando, T. A. (1995). Grief and mourning: Accommodating to loss. In H. Wass & R. Neimeyer (Eds.), *From dying: Facing the facts* (pp. 211–240). Washington, DC: Taylor & Francis.

Rational Recovery. (2004). *Frequently asked questions.* Retrieved January 2009, from http://www.rational.org/faq/html

Red Horse, J. G. (1980). Family structure and value orientation in American Indians. *Social Casework, 61,* 462–467.

Relapse prevention therapy and how it grew: An interview with Terence T. Gorski. (1999). *Behavioral Health Management, 19*(3), 33–35.

Remley, T. (2001, March). *Recognizing clients who are at risk of harming others.* Workshop presentation at the American Counseling Association conference, San Antonio, TX.

Rice, C. E., Dandreaux, D., Handley, E. D., & Chassin, L. (2006). Children of alcoholics: Risks and resilience. *The Prevention Researcher, 13*(4), 1–6.

Rigler, S. K. (2000). Alcoholism in the elderly. *American Family Physician, 61,* 1710–1716.

Riordan, R. J., & Walsh, L. (1994). Guidelines for professional referral to Alcoholics Anonymous and other twelve step groups. *Journal of Counseling & Development, 72,* 351–355.

Robins, L. N. (1966). *Deviant children grown-up.* Baltimore: Williams & Wilkins.

Robinson, R., Perry, V., & Carey, B. (1995). African Americans. In U.S. DHHS, PHS, SAMHSA, & CSAT, *Implementing cultural competence in the treatment of racial/ethnic substance abusers* (pp. 1–21). Rockville, MD: U. S. Department of Health and Human Services.

Rogers, C. R. (1957). The necessary and sufficient conditions of therapeutic personality change. *Journal of Consulting Psychology, 21,* 95–103.

Ross, H. E. (1989). Alcohol and drug abuse in treated alcoholics: A comparison of men and women. *Alcoholism: Clinical and Experimental Research, 13,* 810–816.

Rotheram-Borus, M. J., Hunter, J., & Rosario, M. (1994). Suicidal behavior and gay-related stress among gay and bisexual male adolescents. *Journal of Adolescent Research, 9,* 498–508.

Royce, J. E. (1989). *Alcohol problems and alcoholism: A comprehensive survey* (Rev. ed.). New York: Free Press.

Ruben, D. H. (2001). *Treating adult children of alcoholics: A behavioral approach (Practical resources for the mental health professional).* San Diego, CA: Academic Press.

Sanders, D. (1987). Cultural conflicts: An important factor in the academic failures of American Indian students. *Journal of Multicultural Counseling and Development, 15,* 81–90.

Sandmaier, M. (1992). *The invisible alcoholics: Women and alcohol* (2nd ed.). Blue Ridge Summit, PA: TAB Books.

Saunders, J. B., Aasland, O. G., Babor, T. F., De La Fuente, J. R., & Grant, M. (1993). Development of the Alcohol Use Disorders Identification Test (AUDIT): WHO collaborative project on early detection of persons with harmful alcohol consumption. *Addiction, 88,* 791–804.

Schmidt, A., Barry, K. L., & Fleming, M. F. (1995). Detection of problem drinkers: The Alcohol Use Disorders Identification Test. *Southern Medical Journal, 88*(1), 52–59.

Schmidt, E. (1996). Rational recovery: Finding an alternative for addiction treatment. *Alcoholism Treatment Quarterly, 14*(4), 47–57.

Schmidt, L. (1996). Addressing cultural issues in treatment. *The Addiction Letter, 12,* 3–5.

Schuckit, M. A. (1994). Low level of response to alcohol as a predictor of future alcoholism. *American Journal of Psychiatry, 151,* 184–189.

Schuckit, M. A., Anthenelli, R. M., Bucholz, K. K., Hesselbrock, V. M., & Tipp, J. (1995). The time course of development of alcohol-related problems in men and women. *Journal of Studies on Alcohol, 56,* 218–225.

Sears, J. T. (1997). Thinking critically/intervening effectively about heterosexism and homophobia: A twenty-five-year research retrospective. In J. T. Sears & W. L. Williams (Eds.), *Overcoming heterosexism and homophobia: Strategies that work* (pp. 13–48). New York: Columbia University Press.

Sebenick, C. W. (1997, January/February). Spirituality and AA recovery. *The Counselor, 1,* 14–17.

Secular Organizations for Sobriety. (2000). *Overview.* Retrieved January 16, 2009, from http://www.secularsobriety.org/overview.html

Shem, S., & Surrey, J. (1998). *We have to talk: Healing dialogues between men and women.* New York: Basic Books.

Shibuya, A., Yasunami, M., & Yoshida, A. (1989). Genotypes of alcohol dehydrogenase and aidehyde dehydrogenase loci in Japanese alcohol flushers and nonflushers. *Human Genetics, 82,* 14–16.

Siegel, B. (1986). *Love, medicine & miracles: Lessons learned about self-healing from a surgeon's experience with exceptional patients.* New York: Harper & Row.

Sinha, R., Robinson, J., Merikangas, K., Wilson, G. T., Rodin, J., & O'Malley, S. (1996). Eating pathology among women with alcoholism and/or anxiety disorders. *Alcoholism: Clinical and Experimental Research, 20,* 1184–1191.

Small, J. (1982). *Transformers: The artist of self-creation.* New York: Bantam Books.

Small, J. (1987). Spiritual emergence and addiction: A transpersonal approach to alcoholism and drug abuse counseling. *ReVision, 10*(2), 23–36.

Smith, T. B. (2004). *Practicing multiculturalism: Affirming diversity in counseling and psychology.* Boston, MA: Pearson Education.

Speer, R. P., & Reinert, D. F. (1998). Surrender and recovery. *Alcoholism Treatment Quarterly, 16*(4), 21–29.

St. Germaine, J. (1997). Ethical practices of certified addiction counselors: A national survey of state certification boards. *Alcoholism Treatment Quarterly, 15*(2), 63–72.

Star, J. E., Bober, D., & Gold, M. S. (2005). Double trouble: Depression and alcohol abuse in the adolescent patient. *Psychiatric Annals Special Issue: Alcohol Abuse, 35*(6), 496–502.

Staub, M. (2004, September). For women only: Making the case for gender-specific treatment. *Addiction Professional, 2*(5), 18–25.

Stephens, R. S. (1999). Cannabis and hallucinogens. In B. S. McCrady & E. E. Epstein (Eds.), *Addiction: A comprehensive guidebook* (pp. 121–140). New York: Oxford Press.

Stevens, P., & Smith, R. L. (Eds.). (2005). *Substance abuse counseling: Theory and practice* (3rd ed.). Upper Saddle River, NJ: Pearson Education.

Stolberg, V. B. (2006). A review of perspectives on alcohol and alcoholism in the history of American health and medicine. *Journal of Ethnicity in Substance Abuse, 5*(4), 39–106.

Stone, J. (1991). Light elements. *Discover, 12*(1), 12–16.

Straussner, S. L. (2002). Ethnic cultures and substance abuse. *Counselor: The magazine for addiction professionals, 3*, 34–37.

Streifel, C., & Servanty-Seib, H. (2006). Alcoholics Anonymous: Novel applications of two theories. *Alcoholism Treatment Quarterly, 24*(3), 71–91.

Stroebe, M., & Schut, H. (1999). The dual process model of coping with bereavement: Rationale and description. *Death Studies, 23*, 197–224.

Strohl, J. E. (1998). Transpersonalism: Ego meets soul. *Journal of Counseling & Development, 76*, 397–403.

Substance Abuse and Mental Health Services Administration. (1999). *National Household Survey on Drug Abuse: Population estimates 1998* (Office of Applied Studies Series H-9, DHHS Publication No. SMA 99-3327). Rockville, MD: Substance Abuse and Mental Health Services Administration. Retrieved January 23, 2009, from http://www.oas.samhsa.gov/NHSDA/Pe1998/TOC.htm

Substance Abuse and Mental Health Services Administration. (2003). *Overview of findings from the 2002 National Survey on Drug Use and Health* (Office of Applied Studies, NHSDA Series H-21, DHHS Publication No. SMA 03-3774). Rockville, MD: U.S. Department of Health and Human Services.

Substance Abuse and Mental Health Services Administration. (2005). *Results from the 2004 National Survey on Drug Use and Health: National findings* (Office of Applied Studies, NSDUH Series H-28, DHHS Publication No. SMA 05-4062). Rockville, MD: U.S. Department of Health and Human Services.

Sue, D.W., & Sue, D. (2008). *Counseling the culturally different: Theory and practice* (5th ed.). Hoboken, NJ: Wiley.

Sutich, A. (1965). Introduction. *Journal of Humanistic Psychology, 5*, 115–116.

Suzuki, S. (2006). *Zen mind, beginner's mind*. Boston: Shambhala Press.

Szapocznik, J., & Kurtines, W. M. (1989). *Break throughs in family therapy with drug-abusing and problem youth*. New York: Springer.

Tait, W. D. (2005). Psychopathology of alcoholism. *Journal of Abnormal and Social Psychology, 24* (4), 482–485.

Thomason, T. C. (1991). Counseling Native Americans: An introduction for non-Native American counselors. *Journal of Counseling & Development, 69*, 321–327.

Thomsen, R. (1975). *Bill W.: The absorbing and deeply moving life story of Bill Wilson co-founder of Alcoholics Anonymous*. Center City, MN: Hazelden.

Toriello, P. J., & Benshoff, J. J. (2003). Substance abuse counselors and ethical dilemmas: The influence of recovery and education level. *Journal of Addictions and Offender Counseling, 23*, 83–98.

Tuckman, B. W., & Jensen, M. A. C. (1977). Stages of small-group development revisited. *Group and Organizational Studies, 2*, 419–427.

United Nations Office on Drugs and Crime. (2004). *World drug report 2004* (Vol. 1, 1–22). New York: Author.

U.S. Bureau of the Census. (1996). *U.S. Census Bureau: The official statistics.* Retrieved January 23, 2009, from www.census.gov.gov/population/socdemo/race/black

U.S. Bureau of the Census. (2000). *Introductory data on American Indians: American Indian community profile and data center.* St. Paul, MN: American Indian Policy Center.

U.S. Department of Health and Human Services. (n.d.) *You can help: A guide for caring adults working with young people experiencing addiction in the family* (SAMHSA's Center for Substance Abuse Treatment, DHHS Publication No. PHD878, SMA 01-3544). Washington, DC: U.S. Government Printing Office. Retrieved October 3, 2002, from http://www.samhsa.gov/centers/csat/content/intermediaries

U.S. Department of Health and Human Services. (2007). *Results from the 2006 National Survey on Drug Use and Health: National findings* (Office of Applied Studies, NSDUH Series H-32, DHHS Publication No. SMA 07-4293). Rockville, MD: Substance Abuse and Mental Health Services Administration. Retrieved October 3, 2008, from http://www.oas.samhsa.gov/NSDUH/2K6NSDUH/2K6results.cfm#8.1.3

U.S. Department of Health and Human Services. (2008). *Results from the 2007 National Survey on Drug Use and Health: National findings* (NSDUH Series H-34, DHHS Publication No. SMA 08-4343). Rockville, MD: Substance Abuse and Mental Health Services Administration.

Vacc, N. A., DeVaney, S. B., & Brendel, J. M. (2003). *Counseling multicultural and diverse populations: Strategies for practitioners* (4th ed.). New York: Brunner-Routledge.

Valliant, G. E. (1983). *The natural history of alcoholism: Causes, patterns, and paths to recovery.* Cambridge, MA: Harvard University Press.

Valle, R. (1979). *Alcoholism counseling: Issues for an emerging profession.* Springfield, IL: Thomas.

Vanderlip, S. (2007, November/December). Addiction, the family secret. *Grand Magazine, 3*(6), 52–55.

Velasquez, M. M., Maurer, G. G., Crouch, C., & DiClemente, C. C. (2001). *Group treatment for substance abuse: A stages-of-change therapy manual.* New York: Guilford Press.

Wall, T. L., Shea, S. H., Chan, K. K., & Carr, L. G. (2001). A genetic association with the development of alcohol and other substance use behavior in Asian Americans. *Journal of Abnormal Psychology, 110,* 173–178.

Wallen, J. (1993). *Addiction in human development: Developmental perspectives on addiction and recovery.* New York: Haworth Press.

Walters, S. T., Vader, A. M., & Harris, T. R. (2007). A controlled trial of Web-based feedback for heaving drinking college students. *Prevention Science, 8*(2), 83–88.

Ward, K. (2002). Confidentiality in substance abuse counseling. *Journal of Social Work Practice in the Addictions, 2*(2), 39–52.

Washton, A. M., & Stone-Washton, N. (1990). Abstinence and relapse in outpatient cocaine addicts. *Journal of Psychoactive Drugs, 22,* 233–242.

Weber, G. (2008, January). Using to numb the pain: Substance use and abuse among lesbian, gay and bisexual individuals. *Journal of Mental Health Counseling, 30*(1), 31–48.

Wegscheider-Cruise, S. (1981). *Another chance: Hope and health for the alcoholic family.* Palo Alto, CA: Science and Behavior Books.

Wells, K. (1998). Treatment research at the crossroads: The scientific interface of clinical trials and effectiveness research. *American Journal of Psychiatry, 156*(1), 5–10.

Werth, J. L. (2002). Reinterpreting the Controlled Substances Act: Predictions for the effect on pain relief. *Behavioral Sciences and the Law, 20,* 287–305.

West, P. L., Mustaine, B. L., & Wyrick, B. (1999). State regulations and the ACA Code of Ethics and Standards of Practice: Oil and water for the substance abuse counselor. *Journal of Addictions and Offender Counseling, 20,* 35–46.

White, W. L. (1998). *Slaying the dragon: The history of addiction treatment and recovery in America.* Bloomington, IL: Chestnut Health Systems.

Wilsnack, S. C., Klassen, A. D., Schur, B. E., & Wilsnack, R. W. (1991). Predicting onset and chronicity of women's problem drinking: A five-year longitudinal analysis. *American Journal of Public Health, 81,* 305–318.

Wilsnack, S., & Wilsnack, R. (1991). Prevalence and magnitude of perinatal substance abuse exposures in California. *New England Journal of Medicine, 329*, 850–854.

Wilson, R. W., & Williams, G. D. (1989). Alcohol use and abuse among U.S. minority groups: Results from the 1983 National Health Interview Survey. In D. Spiegler et al. (Eds.), *Alcohol use among U.S. ethnic minorities* (pp. 399–410; NIAAA Research Monograph, 18, DHHS Publication No. ADM 89-1435). Washington, DC: U.S. Government Printing Office.

Witkiewitz, K., & Marlatt, G. A. (2004). Relapse prevention for alcohol and drug problems: That was Zen, this is Tao. *American Psychologist, 59*, 224–235.

Woititz, J. G. (1983). *Adult children of alcoholics.* Deerfield Beach, FL: Health Communications.

Women and alcohol: Keeping control. (2003, December). *Harvard Women's Health Watch, 11*, 1–3.

Women for Sobriety. (1999). *"New life" acceptance program.* Retrieved January 16, 2009, from www.womenforsobriety.org

Worden, J. W. (2002). *Grief counseling and grief therapy: A handbook for the mental health practitioner* (3rd ed.). New York: Springer.

Yalom, I. (2005). *The theory and practice of group psychotherapy* (5th ed.). New York: Basic Books.

Zucker, R. A., & Gomberg, E. (1986). Etiology of alcoholism reconsidered: The case for a biopsychosocial process. *American Psychologist, 41*, 783–793.

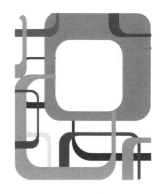

Index

Figures and tables are indicated by "f" and "t."

A

AA. *See* Alcoholics Anonymous
AA Guidelines: For Members Employed in the Alcoholism Field, 234
Abstinence
    counselor training and, 222
    defined, 40
    Moderation Management commitment to, 219
    Native American rates of, 21
    outpatient treatment and, 166
    Secular Organizations for Sobriety commitment
        to, 218
    spirituality and, 209
    treatment planning and, 36, 86
    withdrawal and, 52
ACA. *See* American Counseling Association
ACA Code of Ethics, 85, 115, 165, 226, 228
Acceptance of grief and loss, 158, 159
ACOA. *See* Adult Children of Alcoholics
Addictive voice recognition technique, 217
Adinof, B., 35
Adjourning of group counseling, 180
Adjusting to loss, 160–161
Adolescent substance abuse assessment, 71–72
Adult Children of Alcoholics (ACOA), 123, 149, 243
African American clients, 11–12, 17–19
Agonist therapy, defined, 71
AIDS. *See* HIV/AIDS
Al-Anon, 149, 243
Al-a-Teen, 149
Al-a-Tot, 149
Alcohol Use Disorders Identification Test (AUDIT), 74
Alcoholics Anonymous (AA)
    See also The Big Book
    abstinence and, 98, 115
    altruism and, 183
    counselor training and, 222, 234
    fellowship in recovery and, 163–164
    First Step, 163, 204

GLBT community and, 30
history of, 211–215
inpatient treatment, 119
instillation of hope and, 181
referrals to, 219–220
secular alternatives to, 218–219
spiritual orientation of, 4, 100, 209
treatment planning and, 117, 215–216
Twelve Steps, 34, 212–213
warning signs detected through, 201
Women for Sobriety as alternative to, 24–25, 217–218
Alcoholism
    adolescent abuse assessment, 71–72
    African American clients and, 17
    assessment instruments, 72–74. *See also*
        Assessment and diagnosis
    blood alcohol impairment, 42–44, 43t
    defined, 40
    drunk driving. *See* Driving under the influence (DUI)
    DSM-IV-TR criteria and, 69–71
    evaluation methods, 69–71
    genetic components and biological aspects, 95
    in post treatment referrals, 85
    screening methods, 44. *See also* Blood alcohol
        level; Breathalyzers
    suicide risk assessment and, 77–78
Alcoholism/abstention dichotomy in Native
    American clients, 21
ALDH2 (aldehyde, dehydrogenase gene), 21
Allen-Byrd, L., 136
Altchuler, S., 209
Alternative activities, 104
Altruism and group counseling, 183
American Counseling Association (ACA)
    code of ethics, 85, 115, 165, 226, 228
        Master Addictions Counselor credential, 224
        multicultural competencies for counselors, 13
American Society for the Promotion of Temperance, 98
American Society of Addiction Medicine (ASAM),
    levels of care, 116

(continued)